# INTEGRATED APPROACHES TO INFERTILITY, IVF AND RECURRENT MISCARRIAGE

*of related interest*

Biochemical Imbalances in Disease
A Practitioner's Handbook
*Edited by Lorraine Nicolle and Ann Woodriff Beirne*
*Foreword by David S. Jones*
ISBN 978 1 84819 033 7
eISBN 978 0 85701 028 5


Increasing IVF Success with Acupuncture
An Integrated Approach
*Nick Dalton-Brewer*
ISBN 978 1 84819 218 8
eISBN 978 0 85701 165 7

# INTEGRATED APPROACHES TO INFERTILITY, IVF AND RECURRENT MISCARRIAGE

## A HANDBOOK

EDITED BY JUSTINE BOLD AND
SUSAN BEDFORD

FOREWORD BY
PROFESSOR GAB KOVACS

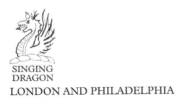

SINGING
DRAGON
LONDON AND PHILADELPHIA

Figure 6.1 (The stages of spermatogenesis) on page 135 is from
Shutterstock.com. Figure 14.1 (Zonal foot map) on page 333 is reproduced
with kind permission from the Association of Reflexologists.

First published in 2016
by Singing Dragon
an imprint of Jessica Kingsley Publishers
73 Collier Street
London N1 9BE, UK
and
400 Market Street, Suite 400
Philadelphia, PA 19106, USA

*www.singingdragon.com*

**Library of Congress Cataloging in Publication Data**
A CIP catalog record for this book is available from the Library of Congress

**British Library Cataloguing in Publication Data**
A CIP catalogue record for this book is available from the British Library

ISBN 978 1 84819 155 6
eISBN 978 0 85701 231 9

Printed and bound in Great Britain

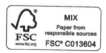

*Justine Bold dedicates this book to her family: Otto, Orin, John, David, Penny, David, Jason, Sarah, Lola and Jake.*

*Susan Bedford dedicates this book to her husband Richard and to their three gorgeous babies Sophie, William and Lucy.*

# Contents

# List of Tables, Figures and Boxes

## List of Tables

## List of Figures

# List of Boxes

# Foreword

Subfertility affects about one in six couples in the western world. While almost all causes of subfertility can now be treated, the available options can be very bewildering. Add in all the complementary treatments that may be used in conjunction with mainstream therapy, and patients become really confused.

Lots of information is available on the Internet, but most is not verified, and it is difficult to separate reliable evidence-based information from 'snake oil', pushed by a group or individual for personal commercial gain.

This publication, edited by two health professionals, has recruited a group of chapter authors, many with a 'nutrition and wellness' background, to update patients and their health professionals about the available treatments, including complementary therapies such as acupuncture, yoga and reflexology. Consumers can have the confidence that this information is provided by reputable experts.

The first chapter provides an overview of what to expect during infertility treatment, from a psychosocial point of view. There is a particularly useful table, outlining the consequences for community, economic, legal, religious and family affairs.

Chapter 2, written by a journalist with first-hand experience, describes various technical aspects of assisted conception, as well as providing a summary of the UK funding system – the 'postcode lottery'.

Chapter 3 concentrates on body weight and the effect on fertility of being under- or over-weight. It explains that excess fatty tissue promotes an over-secretion of oestrogens, and provides dietary advice on how to counter this.

There are separate chapters on female factors (Chapter 4), and male factors (Chapter 6).

Chapter 5, on endometriosis, puts forward suggestions on the effects of various foodstuffs and nutrients.

The effect of coeliac disease on fertility is discussed in Chapter 7, which benefits from being written by a gastroenterologist.

This is followed by Chapter 8, on immunological factors in reproduction, a controversial and poorly understood area.

Chapter 9 is a 'case-based' discussion of antiphospholipid syndrome and the theory of Natural Killer Cells (NKCells), and its possible treatment.

There is a very comprehensive chapter, Chapter 10, on diet, which includes all the possible micronutrients that have been implicated as factors in subfertility, or as possible therapeutic factors.

Chapter 11 concentrates on life-style factors, while Chapter 12 is directed at the woman of advanced maternal age.

The final three chapters, 13 to 15, are devoted to complementary medicine, discussing acupuncture, reflexology and yoga, respectively. The acupuncture chapter explains clearly the theory as to how acupuncture may change blood flow and improve implantation. It also gives a fair review of published studies and meta-analyses that have not shown any benefit from acupuncture as a therapeutic tool. The chapter discusses how this may be due to methodological problems of the studies, rather than to a lack of effect. The reflexology chapter explains the theory of the technique, highlighting that it is an 'overall wellness' effect, rather than a specific treatment for individual problems. In the chapter on yoga, the theory behind its effect on fertility is clearly outlined. It is also highlighted that, apart from any effect it may have on fertility, yoga has beneficial effects on mind and body.

This book will therefore be a helpful read for both professionals and consumers, especially those who have an interest in nutrition and complementary therapies.

*Gab Kovacs*
*Professor of O&G,*
*Monash University*
*August 2015*

# Acknowledgements

Justine Bold would like to thank her parents for their love and support, so she could develop this book at the same time as becoming a mother. She would also like to thank all the chapter authors for their contributions. She would like to thank John de Holland for proofreading, Dr Diane Haigney for checking Chapter 1 and Jo for being her cycle buddy and for proofreading. She would also like to thank her friend Sasha and immediate colleagues at the University of Worcester, Alison, Jane and Katie, and all the staff at Lydbrook Health Centre in Gloucestershire and Dr Sarah Matharu for their support through her own infertility journey. She would also like to acknowledge the help for her own treatment from information posted by Agate on the UK-based web forum Fertility Friends. She would finally like to thank Penny Abatzi and all staff at Serum in Athens for the successful cycle that resulted in the birth of her twin sons.

Susan Bedford would like to thank her husband Richard for all of his love and support (and cups of hot chocolate!) whilst working on this book. In addition, she would like to thank all of the chapter contributors for their hard work and commitment, as well as the fantastic team at Woking Nuffield and Frimley Park Hospital for the joy they have brought to so many people. In particular, she would like to thank Mr Andrew Riddle for his expertise and guidance throughout her own experience of assisted reproductive techniques (ART) and ultimately delivering all three beautiful babies. Finally, her close friends and colleagues, who have provided much-appreciated love, understanding and support throughout.

# Introduction

*Justine Bold BA (Hons), PgCHE, Dip BCNH, NTCC, CNHC Senior Lecturer Institute of Health & Society, University of Worcester, UK and Susan Bedford BSc (Hons), PGCE, MSc (Nut. Th), mBANT, CNHC*

## 1. Overview

This handbook is designed for professionals working with infertile couples considering or undergoing assisted reproduction (AR) or those going through fertility treatment themselves who want to know more about the evidence.

Estimates on the prevalence of infertility vary, but the Human Fertilisation and Embryology Authority (HFEA) in the UK estimated in 2013 that as many as one in seven heterosexual couples has problems conceiving, while Cahill and Wardle reported in 2002 that as many as one in six couples now turns to assisted reproductive techniques (ART) such as in vitro fertilisation (IVF) in their quest to have a child. The chapters that follow consider the factors underlying infertility, recurrent pregnancy loss and subfertility, as well as providing guidance on how patients can best be supported by evidence-based integrated approaches as they seek and undergo treatment.

The book includes material on lifestyle and nutritional factors, including coeliac disease, that can impact upon fertility. Key issues in reproductive immunology (RI), case histories and patients' stories are also presented. There are chapters on male and female factors and health conditions affecting fertility as well as a brief guide to different types of ART and supportive therapies such as counselling, acupuncture, reflexology and yoga. It is hoped that this information will inform the many health professionals and practitioners working with infertile couples, including doctors, nurses, counsellors and nutrition and complementary and alternative medicine (CAM) practitioners, along with those embarking on treatment, and so help to optimise treatment options and improve chances of success.

## 2. Why is this book needed?

Integrated approaches can offer patients both an improved experience and a greater chance of success, so this book aims to review the evidence and raise the awareness of the benefits of integrated solutions whilst offering opportunities for interdisciplinary learning. Health-related quality of life is severely reduced in patients experiencing infertility (Rashidi *et al.* 2008). It is hoped that greater understanding of the experience of infertility, recurrent pregnancy loss and fertility treatment might help foster a more supportive environment for patients/clients. Patient-centred care is associated with individual patient wellbeing (Gameiro, Canavarro and Boivin 2013).

### ··· BOX 1.1 ART FACTS AND FIGURES ·······

▶ A cross-sectional survey on access, effectiveness and safety of ART procedures performed in 53 countries during 2005 reports that 1,052,363 ART procedures resulted in an estimated 237,315 babies born.

▶ The availability of ART varied by country from 15 to 3982 cycles per million of population.

▶ Of all initiated fresh cycles, 62.9 per cent were intracytoplasmic sperm injection (ICSI).

(Zegers-Hochschild *et al.* 2014)

For many patients timely, appropriate intervention is key. Women in their late thirties or early forties especially need the right help quickly. Professionals of all kinds therefore need to be aware of issues that, if unaddressed, may reduce chances of success. Assisted reproduction is at present very costly and individuals or couples may only have one chance, and so optimising the many factors that could potentially reduce success is in the patients' best interest.

## 3. A brief overview of assisted reproduction

Infertility is the failure to conceive a child after one year of unprotected sex (Buckett and Bentick 1997; Johnson and Everitt 2000; Mosher and Pratt 1990; Templeton, Morris and Parslow 1996; Wallace and Kelsey 2010). Generally, within the developed world there is an increasing tendency to have children later in life, and this represents something of a challenge as the ability to conceive declines with age (Dunson and Baird 2004; Rowe 2006; Taylor 2003). Consequently, many couples trying to have a baby later in life find that they are unable to conceive naturally due to subfertility or infertility (Leridon 2004).

In the UK, data from the Office of National Statistics (ONS 1997, 2004) show an increase in the number of women who delay having children until their thirties. Cahill and Wardle (2002) reported that the percentage of births to women over the age of 30 had doubled in the previous 25 years. Recent data show that this trend is also prevalent in many other areas of the developed world. In the USA, for example, whilst general pregnancy rates are falling, including those to younger women, there are increases in pregnancy rates for the over-30 age group (Curtin *et al.* 2013). Women are generally at their most fertile between the ages of 22 and 26, and this often decreases dramatically after the age of 30, with a marked decline in fertility rates in women greater than 35 years of age (Magarelli, Pearlstone and Buyalos 1996). A typical 30-year-old woman has 12 per cent of the ovarian reserve she was born with, and has only 3 per cent at age 40 (Wallace and Kelsey 2010).

IVF is one of the main types of ART, and is a process by which egg and sperm cells are mixed outside the uterus in the lab, in vitro (Collins 1990). For IVF to be successful, the sperm must be viable, and able to fertilise healthy eggs. The woman's body also needs to be able to maintain a pregnancy (NICE 2004). Currently, experts in the area of fertility are using a variety of markers, tests and advice to assist in determining success via ART (Broekmans *et al.* 2006). Age in women is an important predictor of treatment outcome, as increasing age has been found to decrease IVF success rates (Piette *et al.* 1990). However, this doesn't mean that ART are inappropriate for couples when the woman is over a certain age, as individual factors need to be taken into account. Ovarian age does not always parallel chronological age, so a woman in her early forties may have a good fertility potential whilst a woman in her twenties may have premature ovarian failure (POF). As a result, many fertility clinics test a woman's fertility potential (ovarian reserve) in the initial stage of investigation before any treatment is considered (Lim and Tsakok 1997): medical assessment of ovarian reserve is thought to indicate the number of fertile years or predict the potential success that a woman may have (De Vet *et al.* 2002; Van Rooij *et al.* 2005; Visser *et al.* 2006). In reduced ovarian reserve there may be only limited potential for the ovaries to respond to stimulation. Fewer follicles may mature, so in IVF fewer oocytes may then be available for collection, possible fertilisation and thus embryo transfer. Poor response to ovarian stimulation is often a reason for cancellation of ART. These scenarios are investigated more thoroughly in Chapter 12 on assisted reproduction in women over 40. In the UK, at the time of writing this Introduction, the ovarian reserve test is available in the private sector but is not routinely used at a primary care level within the National Health Service. The editors both believe that more widespread assessment of ovarian reserve in younger women may be an important factor in helping women and couples to decide and plan when best to have children.

Infertility and lack of success of ART are often linked to medical factors affecting both sexes, but many research studies also suggest that dietary and lifestyle influences can affect fertility in both men and women and thus success of IVF (Crha *et al.* 2003; Derbyshire 2007; Westphal *et al.* 2004). Chapters are included in this book that investigate the evidence around these issues.

It is important to remember that ART success rates may also be influenced by medical history of the individuals undergoing treatment, their age, the expertise and experience of the consultant treating them, stress levels and diet (Templeton *et al.* 1996). Evidence also indicates that lifestyle is a factor that may affect IVF success, with obesity, high alcohol intake (which is commonly described as more than two drinks containing 10g of alcohol a day) (Grodstein, Goldman and Cramer 1994; Mello 1988), along with low intakes of anti-oxidants and minerals (Agarwal, Prabakaran and Said 2005), all being associated with reduced fertility in both sexes. Adverse lifestyles may induce changes in DNA sequences affecting the gametes and embryo development if conception occurs (Nafee *et al.* 2008).

There is some evidence that if optimum nutritional status is achieved and immunological/hormonal imbalances addressed, those individuals desiring to become pregnant will have a better chance of achieving successful conception, even with low ovarian reserve, and ultimately a healthy pregnancy will be achieved (Kennedy and Griffin 1998). This book aims to help healthcare practitioners consider the possible reasons and the evidence underpinning subfertility, recurrent pregnancy loss and infertility and address the many underlying factors that can reduce success rates of ART.

## 4. The editors

### Justine Bold

Justine is a senior lecturer at the University of Worcester in the UK in the Health and Applied Social Sciences Academic Unit. She has worked for over seven years on nutrition postgraduate programmes (MSc Nutrition & Health and MSc Nutritional Therapy). She is researching a PhD at the University of South Wales related to the experience of infertility. She has also worked as a nutritional therapy practitioner since 2003 with many clients with fertility and autoimmune issues. She has contributed to TV and radio programmes in the UK on the subject of infertility and ART. She has appeared on BBC news, BBC Radio 4 Woman's Hour, BBC Radio 4 Today programme, BBC The One Show, Radio 5 Live, Sky News, BBC Hereford & Worcester and Channel 5 News. She has written articles for both academic and consumer publications and presented at many conferences. She also contributed chapters on digestive health for a textbook, *Biochemical Imbalances in Disease* (Nicolle and Woodriff-Beirne 2010). She has personal experience of infertility and is now a mother to twins born in 2013.

### Susan Bedford

Susan is a highly experienced science teacher, specialising in biology and chemistry, with over sixteen years' experience in a variety of roles including senior management. She has an MSc in Nutritional Therapy from the University of Worcester and conducted her research in the area of fertility and nutrition. She is a fully qualified freelance nutritional therapist whose specialist area is fertility. She holds membership of the British Association for Applied Nutrition and Nutritional Therapy (BANT) and the Complementary and Natural Healthcare Council (CNHC). She has successfully worked with a variety of patients experiencing infertility issues and undergoing ART and has authored articles in relation to fertility for a leading nutritional company and a pre-conception charity.

## 5. Editorial approach to the book's development

The editors of this book both have children conceived through ART. Justine Bold has twins as a result of her sixth fertility treatment. Justine developed the concept for the book to make use of all she learnt through her infertility journey after feeling she had to piece together key information through the course of failed treatments. For example, reproductive immunological factors were not mentioned as possible contributing factors in her case but Justine only managed to carry a pregnancy to term with immune treatment and believes she wouldn't have her family without these issues being investigated and treated. She had to seek private treatment, some of this abroad.

Justine discussed the idea for the book with the other editor, Susan Bedford, who had been thinking similarly and they agreed to work on it in partnership. Susan says, 'I was lucky in that I was treated by a fantastic team and now have three gorgeous children as a result, although the journey to achieve them was not plain sailing by any stretch of the imagination. Throughout this time I became very interested in the role of nutrition in fertility and the effect that any underlying nutritional imbalances may exert on fertility. As a consequence I decided to study this area further. After completing my MSc in Nutritional Therapy, with my advanced study investigating the effect of nutrition and lifestyle and their impact on fertility, Justine and

I decided to develop this book together in the hope of helping others.'
Both Justine and Susan have contributed several chapters to this book
in addition to acting as editors.

## 6. Chapter contributors

The chapter contributors have a broad range of expertise and
experience. Some have medical backgrounds and work as doctors or
nurses, others currently work in the field of IVF or academia, and
some are leading professionals within a CAM discipline or therapy.
They are all passionate about the potential of integrated care and
believe it can improve patient experience and outcomes.

### Lisa Attfield

Lisa spent three years training to be a British Wheel yoga teacher in
her early thirties to help with her own infertility. She left a stressful
job in London to set up a small farm in rural Devon. Lisa was having
trouble conceiving in her late twenties, and after eight years of trying
the National Health Service (NHS) finally agreed to investigate and
she discovered that both she and her husband had fertility issues.
They were told that their only option was to pay privately for IVF
with ISCI. Lisa is now mother to three children, including twins
born in 2011, and she has recently produced her own Fertility Yoga
DVD. The DVD features a series of Hatha Yoga postures to benefit
reproductive health, breathing techniques and deep relaxations.
During Lisa's fertility journey she used many types of complementary
therapies to enhance her potential to conceive and to get into shape
for a healthy pregnancy.

### Louise Carder

Louise is a UK-based nutritional therapist holding memberships of
BANT, the Institute of Functional Medicine and the Royal Society of
Medicine. She is also a CNHC registrant. Louise has previously held
posts as Director and inaugural Head of Communications at BANT.
She works in a multidisciplinary clinic as a nutritional therapist, as an
independent practitioner consultant for the healthcare industry and

as a writer. Louise is currently undertaking research on autoimmunity, focusing on dietary lectins and immune-related infertility, ahead of further postgraduate study, and has spoken internationally on the subject of lectins.

## Clare Casson

Clare is a CNHC registered nutritional therapist with a special interest in natural and assisted fertility. She has her own private practice and also works alongside the medical team at the Zita West fertility clinic in London. The clinic combines evidence-based holistic therapies with leading-edge ART to achieve impressive results, including with clients who have been trying to conceive for several years. The clinic specialises in RI and also male infertility, with a programme pioneering DNA fragmentation testing in combination with targeted nutritional and lifestyle approaches to address the modifiable contributing factors to male infertility and subfertility.

## Deborah Cook

Deborah is a registered general nurse and nurse teacher, with over twenty years of clinical experience, mostly in Emergency Departments. Since October 2004 she has been a senior lecturer at the University of Worcester, teaching health assessment and emergency care. Since qualifying as a reflexologist in 2002, Deborah has used her existing knowledge of health and wellbeing to enhance her practice of this complementary therapy. She has also extended her basic training with Vertical Reflex Therapy and Hand Reflexology. Using these skills and experience she treats a wide range of clients with varying conditions, both in a private practice and for the local hospice.

## Natasha Claire Dunn

Natasha is a senior embryologist working in a Central London clinic. She received her BSc from La Trobe University, her Graduate Diploma in Reproductive Sciences from Monash University in Melbourne, Australia, and her Advanced Diploma of Medical Nutrition from the Australasian College of Natural Therapies (ACNT). Having trained at Genea, Natasha worked for several years at Monash IVF before moving to Barbados for a change of scenery (and more sunshine). She subsequently worked at a clinic in Rome for a short time, where she helped create a new laboratory. After returning to Australia, Natasha concentrated on studying Nutritional Medicine for two years while working at City Fertility Centre, Melbourne. While working at the London Fertility Centre, Natasha met Susan Bedford and Justine Bold, with whom she collaborated on this book. Outside of work, Natasha enjoys travelling in Europe with her close friend Kym, participating in triathlon events, and supporting charities.

## Karen MacGillivray-Fallis

Karen runs a successful nutritional therapy business in the UK in Harrogate, North Yorkshire, where she works with both private and corporate clients. After a long career in management, Karen undertook an MSc in Nutritional Therapy at the University of Worcester. She completed this in 2012. Her research investigated the dietary and lifestyle knowledge and behaviours of those wishing to conceive. Her particular fields of interest are reproductive health, mental wellbeing and behaviour change. She is a member of BANT, CNHC and the Nutrition Society. Karen is married with a young son and loves getting into the great outdoors at every opportunity.

## Kamran Rostami

Kamran is a Consultant Gastroenterologist and research scientist currently working at the Department of Gastroenterology in Alexandra Hospital, Redditchs in the United Kingdom. Kamran graduated from Carol Davila University of Medicine and Pharmacy, Bucharest, Romania in 1993 with a degree in Medicine. He earned a PhD degree in coeliac disease at the University of Amsterdam in 1998. He started his high training in Netherlands and completed his specialist training in the UK in January 2011. Over the last 12 years, he has focused his scientific interests on gluten-related disorders, and has established a series of platforms for their diagnosis and treatment.

## Mohammad Rostami-Nejad

Mohammad has worked as a research fellow at the Research Institute for Gastroenterology and Liver Diseases (RIGLD), Shahid Behehsti University of Medical Sciences, Tehran-Iran, since April 2005. He started research on coeliac disease on 2007 under the support and supervision of his brother Dr Kamran Rostami. He has scientific collaborations with different national and international centres and universities and has published two books on basic nutrition and diagnosis of coeliac disease in Persian in 2009 and 2010 as well as a book chapter in English. Mohammad was awarded a PhD in Clinical Immunology from VU University, Amsterdam, in 2012. He initiated the first coeliac diseases website in Persian: www.celiac.ir. Currently he is head of coeliac disease department at RIGLD and the Internal Editor of *Gastroenterology and Hepatology From Bed to Bench* (GHFBB), a journal published by the RIGLD at Shahid Beheshti University of Medical Sciences.

## Dian Shepperson Mills

Dian's research interests are in endometriosis, male and female infertility and the microbiome. She has published papers, abstracts and book chapters and lectured at scientific meetings worldwide. Dian organised Postgraduate Courses at the American Society for Reproductive Medicine (ASRM) (she was also Founder-Chair of the Nutrition SIG Special Interest Group in 1997). She is Director of the Endometriosis and Fertility Clinic within the Hale Clinic in London. She has published *Endometriosis: A Key to Healing and Fertility Through Nutrition* (Shepperson Mills and Vernon 2002). She is a trustee of the Endometriosis SHE Trust (UK) and the Institute for Optimum Nutrition (ION). She is also a member of the World Endometriosis Society and holds CNHC registration. She is also a member of the Royal Society of Medicine and BANT.

## Irina Szmelskyj

Irina is co-author of the book *Acupuncture for IVF and Assisted Reproduction: An Integrated Approach to Treatment and Management* (Szmelskyj and Aquilina 2014). She is a co-director and lead clinician of True Health

Clinics and is the founder of The Fertility Foundation. Over the last decade Irina has specialised in combining the use of evidence-based acupuncture alongside traditional acupuncture and integrating these approaches with conventional contemporary reproductive medicine. As a result she has acquired a wealth of experience and expertise in the management of patients with infertility issues and patients undergoing IVF. Irina has been invited to present at national and international conferences on this acupuncture subspecialty. She holds several academic posts, including Master of Science Degree lecturer, module leader and examiner. In 2006 she was the recipient of the British Acupuncture Council's nationally recognised Annual Research Excellence Award.

### Karen Veness

Karen is an award-winning journalist, copywriter and media professional who lives in Nottingham, England. Now a mother of two teenage daughters, her world changed in the mid-nineties when she and her husband James found themselves struggling to conceive. Privately funding their IVF treatment, they welcomed baby Holly in 1998, followed by Georgia a year later. Wanting time with her new, precious family, Karen decided to step back from the corporate world. She took up a position working for the UK patient charity, Infertility Network UK, to help educate people about infertility and encourage sufferers to speak out. She has written extensively about fertility issues and IVF and spoken at events throughout the UK and overseas. By telling her story, Karen hopes to provide a sense of camaraderie for individuals dealing with infertility and show how important it is never to give up hope.

## References

Agarwal, A., Prabakaran, S., and Said, T. (2005) 'Prevention of oxidative stress injury to sperm.' *Journal of Andrology 26*, 6, 654–660.

Broekmans, F., Knauff, E., Laven, J., Eijkemans, M., and Fauser, B. (2006) 'PCOS according to the Rotterdam consensus criteria.' *BJOG: An International Journal of Obstetrics and Gynaecology 13*, 1210.

Buckett, W., and Bentick, B. (1997) 'The epidemiology of infertility in a rural population.' *Association of Scandinavian Obstetricians and Gynaecologists 76*, 233–237.

Cahill, D., and Wardle, P. (2002) 'Management of infertility.' *British Medical Journal 325*, 7354, 28–32.

Collins, J. (1990) *Infertility: A Comprehensive Text.* New York, NY: McGraw-Hill/Appleton & Lange.

Crha, I., Hruba, D., Ventruba, P., Fiala, J., Totusek, J., and Visnova, H. (2003) 'Ascorbic acid and infertility treatment.' *Central European Journal of Public Health 11*, 2, 63–67.

Curtin, S.C., Abma, J.C., Ventura, S.J., and Henshaw, S.K. (2013) 'Pregnancy rates for U.S. women continue to drop.' *NCHS Data Brief 136*, 1–8.

De Vet, A., Laven, J., de Jong, F., Themmen, A., and Fauser, B. (2002) 'Antimullerian hormone serum levels: a putative marker for ovarian aging.' *Fertility and Sterility 77*, 357–362.

Derbyshire, E. (2007) 'Dietary factors and fertility in women of childbearing age.' *Nutrition & Food Science 37*, 2, 100–104.

Dunson, D., and Baird, D. (2004) 'Increased infertility with age in men and women.' *Obstetrics & Gynaecology 103*, 1, 51–56.

Gameiro, S.I., Canavarro, M.C., and Boivin, J. (2013) 'Patient centred care in infertility health care: direct and indirect associations with wellbeing during treatment.' *Patient Education and Counselling 93*, 3, 646–654.

Grodstein, F., Goldman, M., and Cramer, D. (1994) 'Infertility in women and moderate alcohol use.' *American Journal of Public Health 84*, 1429–1432.

Johnson, M., and Everitt, B. (2000) *Essential Reproduction*, 5th ed. Oxford: Blackwell Science.

Kennedy, H., and Griffin, M. (1998) 'Enabling conception and pregnancy: midwifery care of women experiencing infertility.' *Journal of Nurse-Midwifery 43*, 3, 190–207.

Leridon, H. (2004) 'Can assisted reproduction technology compensate for the natural decline in fertility with age? A model assessment.' *Human Reproduction 19*, 7, 1548–1553.

Lim, S., and Tsakok, M. (1997) 'Age-related decline in fertility: a link to degenerative oocytes.' *Journal of Fertility and Sterility 68*, 265–271.

Magarelli, P., Pearlstone, A., and Buyalos, R. (1996) 'Discrimination between chronological and ovarian age in infertile women aged 35 years and older: predicting pregnancy using basal follicle stimulating hormone, age and number of ovulation induction/ intra-uterine insemination cycles.' *Human Reproduction 11*, 6, 1214–1219.

Mello, N. (1988) 'Effects of alcohol abuse on reproductive function in women.' *Recent Developments in Alcoholism 6*, 253–276.

Mosher, W., and Pratt, W. (1990) *Fecundity and Infertility in the United States, 1965–1988. Advanced Data from Vital and Health Statistics.* Hyattsville, MD: National Centre for Health Statistics.

Nafee, T., Farrell, W., Carroll, W., Fryer, A., and Ismail, K. (2008) 'Epigenetic control of fetal gene expression.' *BJOG: An International Journal of Obstetrics & Gynaecology 115*, 2, 158–168.

National Institute for Health and Clinical Excellence (NICE) (2004) *Fertility: Assessment and Treatment for People with Fertility Problems.* London: Royal College of Obstetricians and Gynaecologists Press.

Nicolle, L., and Woodriff-Beirne, A. (2010) *Biochemical Imbalances in Disease.* London: Singing Dragon.

Office for National Statistics (ONS) (1997) *Birth Statistics for England and Wales.* Series FM1 No. 26. London: Stationery Office.

Office for National Statistics (ONS) (2004) *Birth Statistics: Review of the Registrar General on Births and Patterns of Family Building in England and Wales.* Series FM1 No. 31. London: Stationery Office.

Piette, C., De Mouzon, J., Bachelot, A., and Spira, A. (1990) 'In-vitro fertilization: influence of women's age on pregnancy rates.' *Human Reproduction 5*, 1, 56–59.

Rashidi, B., Montazeri A., Ramezanzadeh, F., Shariat, M., Abedinia, N., and Ashrafi, M. (2008) 'Health-related quality of life in infertile couples receiving IVF or ICSI treatment.' *Biomedcentral Health Services Research 8*, 186.

Rowe, T. (2006) 'Fertility and a woman's age.' *Journal of Reproductive Medicine 51*, 3, 157–163.

Shepperson Mills, D., and Vernon, M.W. (2002) *Endometriosis: A Key to Healing and Fertility Through Nutrition.* London: Thorsons.

Szmelskyj, I., and Aquilina, L. (2014) 'Acupuncture during ART.' In A. Szmelskyj (ed.) *Acupuncture for IVF and Assisted Reproduction. An Integrated Approach to Treatment and Management.* London: Churchill Livingstone.

Taylor, A. (2003) 'ABC of subfertility. Extent of the problem.' *British Medical Journal 23*, 327, 434–436.

Templeton, A., Morris, J., and Parslow, W. (1996) 'Factors that affect outcome of in-vitro fertilisation treatment.' *Lancet 348*, 9039, 1402.

Van Rooij, I., Broekmans, F., Scheffer, G., Looman, C., Habbema, J., de Jong, F., Fauser, B., Themmen, A., and Te Velde, E. (2005) 'Serum antimüllerian hormone levels best reflect the reproductive decline with age in normal women with proven fertility: a longitudinal study.' *Fertility and Sterility 83*, 4, 979–987.

Visser, J., de Jong, F., Laven, J., and Themmen, A. (2006) 'Anti-Müllerian hormone: a new marker for ovarian function.' *Reproduction 131*, 1–9.

Wallace, W., and Kelsey, T. (2010) 'Human ovarian reserve from conception to the menopause.' *PLoS ONE 5*, 1, e8772.

Westphal L., Polan, M., Trant, A., and Mooney, S. (2004) 'A nutritional supplement for improving fertility in women: a pilot study.' *The Journal of Reproductive Medicine 49*, 4, 289–293.

Zegers-Hochschild, F., Mansour, R., Ishihara, O., Adamson, G.D., de Mouzon, J., Nygren, K.G., and Sullivan, E.A. (2014) 'International Committee for Monitoring Assisted Reproductive Technology: world report on assisted reproductive technology, 2005.' *Fertility and Sterility 101*, 2, 366–378.

# Chapter 1

# Preparing for Fertility Treatment

*Justine Bold BA (Hons), PgCHE, Dip BCNH, NTCC, CNHC Senior Lecturer Institute of Health & Society, University of Worcester, UK*

## 1. Introduction

This chapter is designed to give both health professionals and patients insights into the experience of infertility and assisted reproductive techniques (ART) and the many ways they can affect those undergoing fertility treatment. The experience of infertility is also touched on in the following chapter, where different types of ART are introduced and two patient stories are presented.

The chapter provides a deeper focus on helping people better understand the experience of fertility treatment and what wider research tells us from a global perspective. It also aims to provide practical tips for coping with the treatment. It has been written as a result of a personal experience of infertility, recurrent pregnancy loss and multiple ART cycles, whilst using the author's experience as an academic and researcher to present information and review some of the evidence.

Health professionals and complementary practitioners working with infertile couples or individuals need an understanding of the process itself and to appreciate the various ways it can impact on emotions and day-to-day living. Sensitivity and empathy will also undoubtedly be required through contact with the patients and clients, together with an awareness of the ins and outs of inter-professional working and boundaries of practice. If you are about to embark on treatment yourself or with your partner, it is hoped that the information presented here might help you to manage your own expectations as well as those of the people around you and so be useful in helping you through each stage of the journey and treatment.

## 2. Infertility and the ART/IVF experience
### 2.1 The experience of infertility

It is very difficult for anyone who hasn't been through infertility and fertility treatment to understand the experience and the many effects it can have on the individuals concerned. Ried and Alfred (2013) explain that infertility is a 'lonely' journey, despite the fact that it is now increasingly common, with as many as 15 per cent of couples being affected. Greil (1997) reports on research findings from qualitative data analysis showing that infertility is particularly 'devastating' for women. Men are more likely to be affected by the distress of their partner and the way this impacts upon the relationship (Shapiro 2009), but a male factor can also negatively impact on self-esteem and male identity. However, research tells us that it may not affect all men in this respect; for example, Fisher, Baker and Hammarberg (2010) report results of a study in Australia showing that only 10 per cent of men in their sample associated being a father as a factor confirming their masculinity.

### BOX 1.1 EFFECTS OF INFERTILITY OR
··· INVOLUNTARY CHILDLESSNESS ·······························

The most frequently mentioned effects are distress, raised depression and anxiety levels, lowered self-esteem, feelings of blame and guilt, somatic complaints, and reduced sexual interest.

(Van Balen and Bos 2009)

·············································································

Research on the experience of infertility for women in the UK has pinpointed loneliness as a key feature, in contrast to women in USA, who did not report this and were more likely to be using peer support as a management strategy (Allan 2007). Other more recent research in the UK has identified that many of those who experience infertility report it as a factor that disrupts normal life and state that life is 'on-hold' (Cunningham 2014). A diagnosis of infertility can cause a response similar to bereavement (Christie 1997). Any patient struggling to come to terms with the effects on mood of this diagnosis might benefit from being informed of this, as well as being made aware of appropriate avenues of support.

There are not many studies on infertility and its psychosocial consequences, but some analysis does exist of the social and cultural consequences of involuntary childlessness or infertility in what the researcher called 'poor resource areas' of the world – essentially developing countries. A summary of the results of this research is presented in Box 1.2. The researchers used Interpretative Phenomenological Analysis (IPA); an approach (qualitative in nature) that is used in psychology to understand lived experience and what it means to people. The findings indicate that infertility in some parts of the world can have numerous far-reaching effects beyond the immediate emotional sphere, affecting factors such as a person's legal position, marriage and right of inheritance. These can obviously further impact upon a person's emotional state and sense of wellbeing. This is supported by findings from other studies. For example, a cross-sectional study from Iran pinpoints some of the consequences of infertility in more traditional societies (Direkvand-Moghadam, Delpisheh and Direkvand-Moghadam 2014), and reports that infertility is often cited as reason for divorce.

### BOX 1.2 SOCIAL AND CULTURAL CONSEQUENCES ··· OF INFERTILITY IN POOR RESOURCE AREAS ················

*Community effects*

▶ Loss of status

▶ Ridicule, insults and verbal abuse

▶ Stigmatisation or marginalisation

> ▶ Isolation and exclusion from ceremonies and social gatherings

> ▶ Physical abuse perpetrated by community members.

*Economic and in-law effects*

> ▶ Cost of treatment

> ▶ No economic security, including no care in old age, no economic support from others, unable to find work, no connections and restricted land use

> ▶ Harassment, pressure and rejection by in-laws

> ▶ Exploitation and abuse perpetrated by in-laws.

*Legal and family aspects*

> ▶ Inheritance restrictions affecting property and burial rights

> ▶ Marital instability, including fear of the husband taking a second wife or divorcing the childless woman or the husband actually having a second wife

> ▶ Divorce, including also expulsion from the home and physical abuse and violence perpetrated by the partner.

*Religious and spiritual effects*

> ▶ Effects perceived by self on religious obligation

> ▶ Being accused of witchcraft or 'evil eye'

> ▶ Being a person who brings sickness and disaster to area.

(Adapted from Van Balen and Bos 2009)

## 2.2 Pregnancy and pregnancy loss after ART

Other research on pregnancy loss after fertility treatment identifies the taboo nature of the issue (Freda, Devine and Semelsberger 2003). Bansen and Stevens reported on the 'hush surroundings' of miscarriage as far back as 1992, and sadly it seems there has been little change in many cultures. It has been recognised for some time that the development of a major depressive disorder after miscarriage is more common in childless women (Neugebauer *et al.* 1997), while other research on pregnancy after ART has demonstrated that women with

IVF pregnancies experience high levels of anxiety in pregnancy and about survival of the baby during childbirth (McMahon *et al.* 1997).

## 2.3 Impacts on quality of life, relationships and sex

Studies also indicate that women experiencing infertility report negative impacts on quality of life as a result of experiencing high levels of distress, guilt, grief and frustration (Ried and Alfred 2013). Other research in Germany has demonstrated negative impacts on self-esteem, relationships with partners and sexual activity (Wischmann *et al.* 2014). The researchers report a loss of spontaneous sexual activity, with women in particular reporting a decline in sexual activity and reduced sexual desire after an infertility diagnosis, whilst men undergoing ART experience a higher level of sexual problems such as premature ejaculation and erectile dysfunction when compared with the general populus (Wischmann *et al.* 2014).

## 2.4 Religion

In addition to cultural factors there are also religious perspectives to take into account with differing views on some aspects of ART, especially egg and sperm donation, surrogacy or advanced technologies such as pre-implantation genetic diagnosis (PGD) or developments such as three-person IVF (which has just been given the go-ahead in the UK). There are many ethical and moral issues surrounding these areas and a religion may view these in a particular way. Religious faith, prayer and circles of support may be beneficial to individuals but being at odds with one's faith and its established view on an aspect of fertility treatment might only compound an already stressful situation, especially if the treatment represents the only route to a viable pregnancy. Further information about religious perspectives and assisted reproduction can be found in Schenker (2005).

## 2.5 Effects of undergoing ART

Fertility treatment is recognised as being stressful for patients, but it is now widely accepted that patients undergoing treatment do have different emotional responses and that these variations in the response may be related to both the development of psychiatric problems and outcomes of fertility treatment itself (Rockliff *et al.* 2014). For example, self-criticism and escapist coping strategies are associated with distress, whilst social support lessens this (Rockliff *et al.* 2014). In addition, some aspects of fertility treatment, especially recognised complications such as ovarian hyperstimulation syndrome (OHSS), are known to cause additional pressures. For example, research in China pinpointed factors such as traumatisation from being required to stay in hospital and the way that this impacts on family life (Chang and Mu 2008).

For those who get a positive outcome and go on to have a healthy pregnancy and delivery, ART is a positive life-changing event, even if it is stressful to go through at the time. However, treatment failure remains on average around 75 per cent per cycle and it must be remembered that failure can also cause acute clinical depression (Chochovski, Moss and Charman 2013). Those undergoing ART report high levels of depression and anxiety disorders (Chiaffarino *et al.* 2011). Acute clinical depression may have many impacts on quality of life as well as affecting an individual's or a couple's ability to undergo further fertility treatment. It is therefore perhaps not surprising that since the passing of the Human Fertilisation & Embryology Act in 1990, clinics in the UK have been required by law to offer counselling. Other countries have similar guidelines specifying that psychological support has to be offered as a part of treatment itself. For example, in Australia this was initially introduced in the propagation bill of 1992 (Poehl *et al.* 1999). Counselling support should be offered within country-specific relevant professional frameworks by staff registered or chartered with appropriate professional bodies.

## 3. Effects of psychological interventions on fertility treatment outcome

Hämmerli, Znoj and Barth (2009) reported results from a meta-analysis on psychological interventions for infertile patients, finding that interventions had a positive impact on pregnancy rates. If this finding was accepted widely it would be big news; there is, however, still some debate about the evidence. The University of York (UK) Centre for Reviews and Dissemination reviewed the meta-analysis for the National Institute of Health Research in 2012, stating: 'despite the absence of clinical effects on mental health measures, psychological interventions were found to improve some patients' chances of becoming pregnant, but more randomised controlled trials (RCTs) were needed. The authors' cautious conclusions reflected the data presented, but the potential for various biases in the review means that their reliability is unclear.'

Caution is therefore required when examining the findings; however, it would suggest that patients undergoing fertility treatment would be wise to utilise any psychological interventions such as counselling offered by the clinics treating them. Often these are bundled into the overall treatment price, but research presented in Chapter 2 demonstrates that some patients may not realise this and may not book in for counselling sessions. Hence, health professionals and complementary practitioners alike are encouraged to stress with patients the importance and potential benefits of psychological interventions in terms of supporting the medical treatment. Patients not receiving any psychological support should also be encouraged to explore other sources of support offered professionally and through their family and friends. In the UK, the British Infertility Counselling Association has a list of specialist fertility counsellors on their website (www.bica.net).

## 4. Stress, distress and treatment outcome

It has been recognised that many patients find the experience of fertility treatment one of the most stressful experiences of their lives. This has been widely reported in the literature (Freeman *et al.* 1987; Eugster and Vingerhoets 1999; Cousineau and Domar 2007). Health professionals must also remember that the wait for commencement of treatment itself is associated with anxiety (Facchinetti, Tarabusi and Volpe 2004). Stress impacts negatively on reproduction in many ways (most notably gonadotrophin-releasing hormone [GnRH] is inhibited) – these mechanisms are explored more fully in Chapter 11. The key question for patients to consider is whether this impacts upon the chance of success of fertility treatment.

It seems from research that not all patients respond in the same way to the stress of undergoing treatment (Rockliff *et al.* 2014). Factors such as physical variations in response to stress and the treatment itself, personality type, relationship with spouse and a person's coping strategies (and whether they are adaptive or maladaptive) all influence this. With such variation in response it is important for individuals to be encouraged to communicate about all aspects of fertility treatment and their own specific needs for support. Many patients report the need for extra emotional support during the two-week wait after treatment has been completed (Skiadas *et al.* 2011). During this time they wait to undertake either a pregnancy test or a blood test to determine the outcome. Professionals working in this area need to be aware of how other supportive therapies and approaches can fit into an overall treatment strategy and be mindful of the importance of stress management and relaxation throughout the pre-treatment period, the treatment itself, and the two-week wait for the results as well as the period after the results are known. It is important to remember that therapies or approaches that work generally to relieve stress can be beneficial to people undergoing fertility treatment or recovering from a negative result. Complementary therapies such as reflexology or acupuncture and evidence surrounding their use are explored in other chapters within this book. There is also a consideration of yoga as a relaxation tool and support to fertility treatment.

## 5. Overview of psychological interventions

There are many types of psychological interventions offered by clinics and specialist service providers. Some of these are discussed here.

### 5.1 Supportive group interventions

Many clinics and some charities offer access to peer support groups and promote these. Meetings can be face-to-face and provide those undergoing treatment with a chance to meet others also undergoing ART. A facilitator may be present to guide discussion. This may help those undergoing fertility treatment to feel less isolated and provide an opportunity for discussion. Research confirms that group psychotherapy leads to reduced anxiety (de Liz and Strauss 2005). It is also established that men respond to group counselling, especially when offered as a part of the ART (Furman *et al.* 2010).

## BOX 1.3 PATIENT PERSPECTIVE ON COUNSELLING AS PART OF FERTILITY TREATMENT

'I had to have counselling after our first IVF cycle failed. I was just so convinced it would work, I was totally destroyed when it failed. I couldn't function. I cried all day; it was like I was in a dream. The body played a cruel trick on me as I had felt sick for a week before doing the pregnancy test and my breasts felt huge so I was utterly convinced I was pregnant. I had even ordered some maternity clothes from an online shop. I had also worked out what the baby's due date would be and their star sign. What I fool I was. I cannot believe I did that, but I did. I was so taken up in the dream; convinced it had worked. When I did the test and it was negative I couldn't believe it. Reality hit so very hard and I stopped functioning.

'The negative result meant all three embryos were dead and gone...and any chance we had was over. I struggled to eat, to clean, to get dressed. I slept a lot and couldn't go to work. I struggled with everything. I ripped the maternity clothes up when they arrived and threw them in the bin. Disgusted with myself and angry with my body for failing me again, I felt like a freak and was worried about how I would ever return to work or be strong enough to have another go at treatment.

'Eventually I realised I needed help and I saw a counsellor in the clinic. She was fantastic, she helped me to understand that what I was experiencing was normal. She said all my feelings were to be expected given the circumstances, and that I had formed emotional relationships with the three embryos, imagined they were my babies and bonded with them, so when the cycle failed, it's a bereavement three times over. She explained how bereavement affects some people. She likened it to a wave, a tide that comes in and out – and that the time between tides eventually gets longer; this helped me see it as a process that I had to go through to get strong enough to face treatment again. It took a long time though, a very long time to be ready and be able to start again and face the chance of it failing again, knowing I'd have to pick myself up if it didn't.'

## 5.2 Psychotherapeutic interventions

Interventions such as psychotherapy, counselling, cognitive behavioural therapy (CBT), couples therapy or sexual counselling may have roles through many areas of fertility treatment. Individual psychotherapy helps reduce anxiety associated with infertility (de Liz and Strauss 2005). The researchers report that the effects of this have been demonstrated on depressive symptoms six months after cessation of the therapy itself. Research also demonstrates that CBT works at various stages of the fertility treatment process to help manage both anxiety and depressive symptoms and additionally that it helps manage stress through the course of treatment itself (Tarabusi, Volpe and Facchinetti 2004). Mitsi and Efthimiou (2014) report that CBT is superior to other psychotherapeutic investigations during several stages of the fertility treatment; they also cite reports that CBT can enhance the pregnancy rate though urge caution owing to methodological issues with the studies. Other studies have demonstrated CBT's positive effect on both the hormonal response to stress and associated cardiovascular parameters in women waiting for commencement of IVF treatment (Facchinetti *et al.* 2004). Articles on developing optimal standards of care for the future refer to the need to prioritise psychological interventions (Gameiro, Boivin and Domar 2013). It is also important to remember that specialist counselling may be needed in circumstances where genetic issues are identified, so couples undergoing PGD may need specialist support.

## 5.3 Mind/body approaches

Hypnosis/hypnotherapy and mindfulness are used by some as adjuncts to fertility treatment. Research demonstrates that both approaches have a role in supporting those going through fertility treatment cycles. Research findings from a study undertaken in 2006 demonstrate that hypnosis may improve the cycle outcome (Levitas *et al.* 2006). In this study, the researchers compared 98 IVF cycles where hypnosis was performed during the embryo transfer with 96 cycles without hypnosis. After statistical analysis they report significant improvements with hypnosis, with a clinical pregnancy rate of 53 per cent in the hypnosis group (52 clinical pregnancies) compared with 30.2 per cent in the control group (29 clinical pregnancies). Galhardo, Cunha and Pinto-Gouveia (2013) report a clinical controlled study on the benefits of a ten-week group programme Mindfulness-Based Program for Infertility (MBPI). They compared a group receiving the intervention with a group who did not. Those receiving the programme attended for two hours, with men in the group attending three sessions. Women who attended the programme 'revealed a significant decrease in depressive symptoms, internal and external shame, entrapment, and defeat', so the researchers conclude that the results suggest that the MBPI is an effective psychological intervention to support those undergoing ART.

## 5.4 Education interventions

These would include interventions providing information on skills such as stress management, relaxation and problem solving. Boivin (2003) reports that education interventions using skills-based approaches such as stress management and relaxation techniques have more beneficial impact on a range of measures/outcomes compared with counselling solely encouraging emotional expression about infertility.

The author has developed a set of tips for those embarking on treatment, as shown in Box 1.4. These are practical in nature and it is hoped that those going through treatment will find them of some use.

### BOX 1.4 PRACTICAL TIPS ON PREPARING FOR
··· AND COPING WITH FERTILITY TREATMENT ····················
*Ask questions*

Patients should always voice any concerns or queries they have with the professionals responsible for their fertility treatment and with any other health professionals supporting medical treatments. Patients should remember that it is their body and their money (if they are paying for treatment) and not be afraid to ask questions.

### Do some reading and research

Being more informed can help make the process less daunting and can help patients find the most appropriate treatments.

### Ideally allow three months preparation for a treatment cycle

If time allows, this would be ideal to encourage healthy egg and sperm formation. It must be recognised, though, that this is not always possible, for example if sperm or eggs are frozen in advance of cancer treatments or if a woman is already over 40 years of age and timing is critical.

### When preparing for treatment, consider changes that can be managed without extra stress

Preparing for treatment, losing weight, eating more healthily, and reducing alcohol and smoking can add extra stress to an already difficult situation. Change has to be managed positively, supported and organised at an appropriate pace for the individual. People should be reminded that change is a process and should be encouraged to own this process, setting their own goals throughout (we know that self-efficacy and regulation are effective ways of changing health-related behaviours).

### Think about nourishment

Think about nourishment, both physical and emotional. The basic area to concentrate upon physically is on eating nutritious foods, a starting point being eating plenty of vegetables and fruits of all colours every day. Aim for 400g or more a day in total (that's five 80g portions) and eat fresh nuts and seeds such as walnuts, brazil nuts, almonds and pumpkin seeds. Also consume fish (both oily and white fish), whole grains and vegetable proteins such as legumes. Emotional nourishment can obviously take many forms, for example hobbies and contact with family, friends, nature and animals.

## Manage stress before treatment and during treatment

Managing stress can help people get through treatment. Relaxation, yoga and meditation can all be useful in this regard. Complementary therapies can also be helpful.

## Be flexible about timings during the course of fertility treatment

Fertility treatment takes time and can be quite physically demanding and many patients struggle to plan this into their lives, balancing it with employment and the ongoing need to earn (this is especially important for those funding private treatment). Patients should be encouraged to understand that treatment cycle duration is difficult to predict as most fertility treatment cycles progress according to follicular development and individual responses to drugs can vary. Many undergo treatment in holidays, some are signed-off work by doctors, some undergo treatment whilst still working; wherever possible, flexibility should be encouraged in terms of cycle planning and patients should be encouraged to discuss this with those around them, especially in a professional context. Patients would do well to be aware that treatment often doesn't go to plan, and dates are rarely fixed.

Patients should also try to find out if an employer has a policy relating to fertility treatment, and to explore options such as unpaid leave. Patients should also aim to understand relevant legislation in their country. For example in the UK, employers must not record sickness time related to a pregnancy as normal sickness. This can be useful for women to know if they experience pregnancy loss after fertility treatment. The medications can also affect mood and there may be surgical procedures (surgical sperm recovery, cyst aspiration and egg collection). So an individual's ability to work may be affected and it is important for individuals to consider this.

### Use all the resources of clinics

If counselling is part of the package, patients should be encouraged to use it!

### Communicate

Patients may feel very isolated during treatment, so communication with others also undergoing treatment can be a helpful tool to combat this. Patients should explore support groups and online sources of support. They may also find it helpful to write a treatment diary.

### Prepare for test day

Encourage patients to prepare for test day, considering where they will be and whether there will be any support around them should the result be negative. Perhaps a patient can plan ahead to spend the day with a partner or close friend or family member? An activity such as a shopping trip, or visit to a gallery or café, might be a positive distraction.

### Build recovery time into cycle planning wherever possible

If a patient is embarking on fertility treatment for another time after a failed treatment or a pregnancy loss, they should be encouraged to think about time for both physical and emotional recovery.

·················································································

## References

Allan, H. (2007) 'Experiences of infertility: liminality and the role of the fertility clinic.' *Nursing Inquiry 14*, 2, 132–139.

Bansen, S.S., and Stevens, H.A. (1992) 'Women's experiences of miscarriage in early pregnancy.' *Journal Nurse-Midwifery 37*, 2, 84–90.

Boivin, J. (2003) 'A review of psychosocial interventions in infertility.' *Social Science Medicine 57*, 12, 2325–2341.

Chang, S.N., and Mu, P.F. (2008) 'Infertile couples' experience of family stress while women are hospitalized for ovarian hyperstimulation syndrome during infertility treatment.' *Journal of Clinical Nursing 17*, 4, 5318.

Chiaffarino, F., Baldini, M.P., Scarduelli, C., Bommarito, F., *et al.* (2011) 'Prevalence and incidence of depressive and anxious symptoms in couples undergoing assisted reproductive treatment in an Italian infertility department.' *European Journal of Obstetrics & Gynaecology & Reproductive Biology 158*, 2, 235–241.

Chochovski, J., Moss, S.A., and Charman, D.P. (2013) 'Recovery after unsuccessful in vitro fertilization: the complex role of resilience and marital relationships.' *Journal of Psychosomatic Obstetrics and Gynaecology 34*, 3, 1228.

Christie, G. (1997). 'Grief management in infertile couples.' *Journal of Assisted Reproduction and Genetics 14*, 189–191.

Cousineau, T.M., and Domar, A.D. (2007) 'Psychological impact of infertility.' *Best Practice & Research Clinical Obstetrics and Gynaecology 21*, 293–308.

Cunningham, N. (2014) 'Lost in transition: women experiencing infertility.' *Human Fertility (Camb.) 17*, 3, 154–158.

de Liz, T.M., and Strauss B. (2005) 'Differential efficacy of group and individual/couple psychotherapy with infertile patients.' *Human Reproduction 20*, 5, 1324–1332.

Direkvand-Moghadam, A., Delpisheh, A., and Direkvand-Moghadam, A. (2014) 'Effect of infertility on the quality of life, a cross-sectional study.' *Journal of Clinical and Diagnostic Research 8*, 10, OC13–OC15.

Eugster, A., and Vingerhoets, A.J.J.M. (1999) 'Psychological aspects of in vitro fertilisation.' *Social Science Medicine 48*, 575–589.

Facchinetti, F., Tarabusi, M., and Volpe, A. (2004) 'Cognitive-behavioral treatment decreases cardiovascular and neuroendocrine reaction to stress in women waiting for assisted reproduction.' *Psychoneuroendocrinology 29*, 2, 162–173.

Fisher, J.R., Baker G.H., and Hammarberg, K. (2010) 'Long-term health, well-being, life satisfaction, and attitudes toward parenthood in men diagnosed as infertile: challenges to gender stereotypes and implications for practice.' *Fertility Sterility 94*, 2, 574–580.

Freda, M.C., Devine, K.S., and Semelsberger, C. (2003) 'The lived experience of miscarriage after infertility.' *The American Journal of Maternal/Child Nursing 28*, 1, 16–23.

Freeman, E.W., Rickels, K., Tausig, J., Boxer, A., Mastrionni, L., and Tureck, R. (1987) 'Emotional and psychosocial factors in follow-up of women after IVF-ET treatment, a pilot investigation.' *Acta Obstetricia Et Gynecologica Scandinavica 66*, 517–521.

Furman, I., Parra, L., Fuentes, A., and Devoto, L. (2010) 'Men's participation in psychologic counseling services offered during in vitro fertilization treatments.' *Fertility Sterility 94*, 4, 1460–1464.

Galhardo, A., Cunha, M., and Pinto-Gouveia, J. (2013) 'Mindfulness-Based Program for Infertility: efficacy study.' *Fertility Sterility 100*, 4, 1059–1067.

Gameiro, S., Boivin, J., and Domar, A. (2013) 'Optimal in vitro fertilization in 2020 should reduce treatment burden and enhance care delivery for patients and staff.' *Fertility Sterility 100*, 2, 302–309.

Greil, A.L. (1997) 'Infertility and psychological distress: a critical review of the literature.' *Social Science Medicine 45*, 11, 1679–1704.

Hämmerli, K., Znoj, H., and Barth, J. (2009) 'The efficacy of psychological interventions for infertile patients: a meta-analysis examining mental health and pregnancy rate.' *Human Reproduction Update 15*, 3, 279–295.

Levitas, E., Parmet, A., Lunenfeld, E., Bentov, Y., Burstein, E., Friger, M., and Potashnik, G. (2006) 'Impact of hypnosis during embryo transfer on the outcome of in vitro fertilization-embryo transfer: a case-control study.' *Fertility Sterility 85*, 5, 1404–1408.

McMahon, C.A., Ungerer, J.A., Beaurepaire, J., Tennant, C., and Saunders, D. (1997) 'Anxiety during pregnancy and fetal attachment after in-vitro fertilization conception.' *Human Reproduction 12*, 1, 176–182.

Mitsi, C., and Efthimiou, K. (2014) 'Infertility: psychological-psychopathological consequences and cognitive-behavioural interventions.' *Psychiatriki 24*, 4, 293–302. [In Greek, Modern.]

National Institute of Health Research (2012) The University of York (UK) Centre for Reviews and Dissemination. Available at www.ncbi.nlm.nih.gov/pubmedhealth/ PMH0027057, accessed on 18 May 2015.

Neugebauer, R., Kline, J., Shrout, P., Skodol, A., *et al.* (1997) 'Major depressive disorder in the 6 months after miscarriage.' *Journal of American Medical Association 277*, 5, 383–388.

Poehl, M., Bichler, K., Wicke, V., Dorner, V., and Feichtinger, W. (1999) 'Clinical assisted reproduction psychotherapeutic counseling and pregnancy rates in in vitro fertilization.' *Journal of Assisted Reproduction and Genetics 16*, 6, 302–305.

Ried, K., and Alfred, A. (2013) 'Quality of life, coping strategies and support needs of women seeking Traditional Chinese Medicine for infertility and viable pregnancy in Australia: a mixed methods approach.' *Bio Med. Central Womens Health 13*, 17.

Rockliff, H.E., Lightman, S.L., Rhidian, E., Buchanan, H., Gordon, U., and Vedhara, K. (2014) 'A systematic review of psychosocial factors associated with emotional adjustment in in vitro fertilization patients.' *Human Reproduction Update 20*, 4, 594–613.

Schenker, J.G. (2005) 'Assisted reproductive practice: religious perspectives.' *Reproductive Bio Medicine Online 10*, 3, 310–319.

Shapiro, C.H. (2009) 'Therapy with infertile heterosexual couples: it's not about gender— or is it?' *Clinical Social Work Journal 37*, 140–149.

Skiadas, C.C., Terry, K., De Pari, M., Geoghegan, A., *et al.* (2011) 'Does emotional support during the luteal phase decrease the stress of in vitro fertilization?' *Fertility Sterility 96*, 6, 1467–1472.

Tarabusi, M., Volpe, A., and Facchinetti, F. (2004) 'Psychological group support attenuates distress of waiting in couples scheduled for assisted reproduction.' *Journal of Psychosomatic Obstetrics and Gynaecology 25*, 3–4, 273–279.

Van Balen, F., and Bos, H.M.W. (2009) 'The social and cultural consequences of being childless in poor-resource areas.' *Facts, Views & Vision in ObGyn 1*, 2, 106–121.

Wischmann, T., Schilling, K., Toth, B., Rösner, S., *et al.* (2014) 'Sexuality, self-esteem and partnership quality in infertile women and men.' *Geburtshilfe Frauenheilkd 74*, 8, 759–763.

# Chapter 2

# Introduction to Assisted Conception

*Karen Veness*

## 1. Introduction

Some readers will already be familiar with the various types of fertility treatments available. Yet despite their differences, they are often simply referred to generically as IVF or in vitro fertilisation, which does little to help patients understand which specific treatment might be best for them. If you are a patient considering fertility treatment, it is hoped that this chapter might give you a clearer insight into the options available. If you are a health professional sitting across the table from someone struggling to conceive, their hope for a family may well rest in your hands. It is vital to remember that, for the patient, this is far from just a treatment protocol to be followed, and the emotional impact of infertility may be far harder for them to deal with than the physical processes involved. An infertility diagnosis of any kind is crippling: sensitivity and empathy should be at the forefront of patient contact as you tread the fine line between hope and expectation.

With regard to the funding situation, this chapter looks at the UK only. In other countries without social medical funding, the industry may be entirely privately funded; even in countries providing government assistance in a similar way to the National Health Service

(NHS) in the UK, the guidelines vary and are beyond the remit of the UK regulatory authorities.

It takes just one sperm and one egg to create a new life, yet the miracle of making babies sometimes needs a little help from outside nature. And that help – and hope – can come with a very high financial *and* emotional price tag. Getting pregnant can be much harder than you might think – and if you're having trouble or your patients are having trouble, you or they are not alone. Looking at figures from the Human Fertilisation and Embryology Authority (2013) – the UK's independent regulator overseeing the use of gametes and embryos in fertility treatment and research – we know that an estimated one in seven heterosexual couples in the UK today has difficulty conceiving. That means that in the UK, more than three million people will, at some point, face the agony of infertility, robbing them of the free choice to plan their family.

The Human Fertilisation and Embryology Authority (HFEA)'s latest report on fertility treatment (2013) reveals a continuing rise in the overall number of IVF cycles in the UK, with more undertaken in 2013 than ever before. IVF-conceived babies now account for around 2 per cent of all babies born in the UK. The report covers treatment cycles and outcomes for treatments started in 2012 and 2013 and how these coincide with short- and long-term trends. In 2013, 49,636 women had a total of 64,600 cycles of IVF and 2379 women had a total of 4611 cycles of donor insemination (DI), representing an increase in both categories from the previous year. Overall, the HFEA reports that success rates have remained constant at around 25 per cent (2013). A range of useful links to the HFEA website is given in the References for this chapter.

The UK's only national charity dedicated to helping couples struggling to conceive is Infertility Network UK, which works to provide a mass of up-to-date information and support to guide everyone through the whole minefield of infertility. Its website (www.infertilitynetworkuk.com) is an excellent resource for health professionals and patients alike, and a range of useful links to this website is also given in the References for this chapter.

If you or your patients are struggling to conceive, the absolute priority *must* be to see a doctor as soon as possible, because a referral will be required for any investigations or treatment.

When all you want is a baby, no price can seem too high, but there are huge variations in treatment options and costs. So before we begin to look at possible treatment options, it is vital to understand how infertility treatment is funded. In the UK a patient may be eligible for some treatment on the NHS, depending on where they live, but it is very complicated. The criteria for who, and what treatment, is funded by the NHS vary enormously. A GP, local Clinical Commissioning Group (CCG) or Health Board will be able to advise on local funding arrangements. To find out more, patients should start by asking their GP. Infertility Network UK's website (2015) also offers information about localised funding.

## 2. After diagnosis – what next?

The pain and shock of getting a diagnosis of infertility leaves people confused and desperate to find a solution. There is a mass of information out there on clinics and treatment options, and it can seem impossible to make immediate sense of it all without some independent help and guidance.

For many people forced to pay for treatment, the level of expenditure is not directly proportional to achieving success. Today, more than 30 years after the world's first 'test tube baby', Louise Brown, was born in Oldham, successful IVF remains as much of a lottery as ever with success rates varying between clinics, and wide fluctuations in treatment costs. Infertility is very much an industry in its own right: HFEA figures (2013) show that in the UK in 2013, 78 licensed clinics performed IVF treatment – and there are many more clinics based overseas. It is very hard to compare 'like for like', as the bare statistics often only tell half the story.

Every clinic has its own website, and every clinic will be painting the best possible picture of its services. If a patient has to pay for treatment, there is no such thing as an 'average cost' for treatment because private clinics are free to set their own prices. Making accurate comparisons between clinics is always going to be difficult as the success rates of one clinic may vary from another due to a range of factors, most notably the precise medical history of the patients being treated. Lord Winston, the Labour peer who helped pioneer the development of fertility medicine within the NHS, has been vocal in his criticism of the IVF 'industry', referring to it in *The Independent* (Connor 2014) as 'an unregulated "jungle" being driven by profit, often at the expense of patients'. The same article also referred to his deep concern about the commercialisation of a sector where people can pay thousands of pounds for each treatment cycle, irrespective of whether they succeed in having a baby.

So choosing a clinic is a clearly an important decision – but where do patients in the UK start? A good source of impartial information on clinics is, once again, the industry's independent regulator, the HFEA.

The HFEA (2013) database holds detailed information about all UK licensed fertility treatments and any births associated with them since 1991. The information published by the HFEA has been verified; as well as data about success rates, the 'Choose a Fertility Clinic' section also explains what the statistics mean and the degree of confidence with which comparisons can be made. It is a rich resource for prospective patients when researching clinics and the treatment they provide, and each year around 60,000 new treatment cycles are recorded and validated. But it is important not to rely solely on published success rates because:

- they do not reflect the possible differences in the patients who go to different clinics.

- they do not reflect the fact that different clinics choose to treat some patients – but not others.

- they do not reflect individual circumstances and all the possible factors that might affect treatment prospects.

An increasing number of UK patients are choosing to travel abroad for fertility treatment, often because of lower treatment costs, and many patients report positive experiences of their experience overseas.

However, the HFEA licenses and regulates clinics in the UK only: it has no jurisdiction overseas. The level of legal or regulatory standards of clinics in overseas countries can vary greatly and not all countries will have organisations equivalent to the HFEA. Some places have no specific laws or regulations relating to assisted reproductive services. Yet many couples have overseas clinics to thank for their miracle babies and are happy to share their positive experiences. Infertility Network UK (2015) also has a patient factsheet on what to think about when considering treatment overseas.

## 3. What are the options?

The birth of Louise Brown led to the coining of the phrase 'test tube baby', and IVF has become a catch-all description to explain the process of assisted conception. Yet IVF is just one piece of a complex jigsaw of assisted conception techniques available today. Although the number of cycles performed annually shows no signs of slowing down, it is important to remember that assisted conception, in any form, is not an easy route to parenthood, and nor is it any kind of guarantee of a successful outcome. The decision about what fertility treatment might best suit a patient's circumstances will be taken after detailed discussions with the medical team at the chosen clinic, and there may well be more than one option available. There are many complex reasons for infertility and, therefore, many possible treatment options, which is why decisions can only be taken after careful evaluation of a couple's medical history.

Types of infertility treatment include in vitro fertilisation (IVF), intracytoplasmic sperm injection (ICSI), intrauterine insemination (IUI) and donor insemination (DI). However, medical advances have created other options. Clinics may also offer a variety of extra tests and techniques, and very often they will come at extra cost. When you're trying to have a baby, hope can have a very high price tag. The HFEA website (2015) has detailed information about all assisted reproduction options.

### 3.1 In vitro fertilisation (IVF)

In simple terms, IVF treatment involves the fertilisation of an egg – or eggs – outside the body. The treatment can be performed using a patient's own eggs and sperm, or using either donated sperm or donated eggs, or both. IVF techniques vary according to individual circumstances and the approach of the clinic. Before any treatment starts, various consent forms are usually completed and blood tests are undertaken to screen for infections such as HIV, hepatitis B, hepatitis C and human T cell lymphotropic virus (HTLV) I and II. A clinic may recommend IVF if:

- a patient has been diagnosed with unexplained infertility
- the fallopian tubes are blocked
- other techniques such as fertility drugs or IUI have not been successful
- the male partner has fertility problems but which are not severe enough to require ICSI
- frozen sperm is being used in treatment and IUI is not suitable
- donated eggs or frozen eggs are being used in treatment
- the embryos are being tested to avoid passing on a genetic condition.

## 3.2 In vitro maturation (IVM)

In the IVM process, eggs are removed from the ovaries when they are still immature. They are then matured in the laboratory before being fertilised. The difference between IVM and conventional IVF is that the eggs are immature when they are collected. This means that a patient won't need to take as many drugs before the eggs can be collected as with conventional IVF, when mature eggs are collected. A clinic may recommend IVM:

- if a patient is at risk of developing ovarian hyperstimulation syndrome (OHSS). This is a potentially dangerous complication from taking fertility drugs and women with polycystic ovary syndrome (PCOS) are particularly at risk of developing this complication.
- where the cause of a couple's infertility has been identified as being male factor only.

## 3.3 Intracytoplasmic sperm injection (ICSI)

ICSI treatment involves the injection of a single sperm directly into the egg using a specially prepared needle. With ICSI, very few sperm are required and, as the process involves the penetration of the sperm into the egg, the penetrative ability of the sperm is no longer a factor. ICSI is recommended:

- in severe cases of male infertility
- where there has been no fertilisation following IVF treatment previously.

## 3.4 Physiological intracytoplasmic sperm injection (PICSI)

PICSI is a scientific technique sometimes used in ICSI. It is yet another advancement in the field of fertility treatment, and one that remains a subject of considerable discussion. PICSI selects sperm according to how well they bind to the hyaluronan around an egg cell (called hyaluronic acid) through a test called a Hyaluronan Binding Assay. Its effect has yet to be fully established.

## 3.5 Intracytoplasmic morphologically selected sperm injection (IMSI)

IMSI is a technique where sperm samples are examined under a microscope which is many times more powerful than normal ICSI microscopes. This technique enables the medical team to choose the best quality sperm to inject into the patient; it is recommended for couples whose sperm samples are unusually low or highly abnormal.

## 3.6 Intrauterine insemination (IUI)

IUI involves a laboratory procedure to separate fast-moving sperm from more sluggish or non-moving sperm. The fast-moving sperm are then placed into the woman's womb close to the time of ovulation when the egg is released from the ovary in the middle of the monthly cycle.

## 3.7 Donor insemination (DI)

DI uses sperm from a donor to help the woman become pregnant. Sperm donors are screened for sexually transmitted diseases and some genetic disorders. In DI, sperm from the donor is placed into the neck of the womb (cervix) when the woman ovulates.

## 3.8 Assisted zona hatching (AZH)

Before an embryo can attach to the wall of the womb, it has to break out or 'hatch' from its outer layer, the zona pellucida. It has been suggested that making a hole in, or thinning, this outer layer may help embryos to hatch – but please be aware that the NHS guideline on fertility, issued by NICE, says: 'Assisted hatching is not recommended because it has not been shown to improve pregnancy rates' (NICE 2013).

## 3.9 Pre-implantation genetic diagnosis (PGD)

This treatment enables people with an inheritable condition in their family to avoid passing it on to their children. It involves checking the genes and/or chromosomes of embryos created through IVF. PGD can be used to test for virtually any genetic condition where a specific gene is known to cause that condition, for example cystic fibrosis or Huntington's disease. It is currently approved to screen for over 250 genetic conditions; to see the types of conditions that may be tested for, see the HFEA website. A specialist may recommend PGD if:

- previous pregnancies have been terminated because of a serious genetic condition
- a couple already have a child with a serious genetic condition
- there is a family history of a serious genetic condition
- there is a family history of chromosome problems.

## 3.10 Reproductive immunology (RI)

This is a service offered by a few fertility clinics in the UK. It includes a range of tests and treatment to do with the patient's immune system in pregnancy. There is currently much debate about the role of the immune system in promoting – or preventing – a healthy pregnancy. This is discussed in more detail in Chapters 8 and 9.

### 3.11 Donated eggs or embryos (DE)

If a patient is unable to conceive using their own eggs, an egg donated by another woman can be combined with sperm. The resulting embryo is then implanted in the uterus. A donated embryo can be used in the same way.

### 3.12 Elective single embryo transfer (eSET)

Women who have a good chance of becoming pregnant and have several embryos available may choose to have only one embryo transferred in order to reduce the risk of a multiple pregnancy. This is known as elective single embryo transfer, or eSET. Clinics in the UK are required to limit the number of embryos transferred in order to reduce the chance of a multiple birth. For women under the age of 40 years, one or two embryos can be transferred in a treatment cycle. For women aged 40 years or over, a maximum of three embryos can be transferred. Remaining embryos may be frozen for future IVF attempts if they are suitable.

### 3.13 Surrogacy

Surrogacy is when another woman carries and gives birth to a baby for a couple who want to have a child. The HFEA does not regulate surrogacy and strongly recommends that people seek further advice before choosing to go ahead with this option.

## 4. England: a 'postcode lottery'

In England, fertility services are commissioned locally by GP-led groups known as Clinical Commissioning Groups (CCGs). There are 211 of these decision-making bodies across England and, although it is the duty of local commissioners to try to provide services in line with the latest guideline published by the government body National Institute for Health and Care Excellence (NICE), many local commissioners simply do not follow the NICE guideline because it is not legally binding. Quite simply, this means that the availability of fertility services in England varies widely and arbitrarily depending simply on where patients live – the infamous 'postcode lottery' approach to treatment, which has caused untold heartache for thousands of couples who find themselves unable to access the NHS treatment they should be entitled to.

Broadly speaking, the most recent NICE Clinical Guideline on Fertility (2013) recommends that women aged up to and including 39 should have access to three full cycles of IVF/ICSI treatment. It also recommends that women aged between 40 and 42 who have never had IVF treatment, and do not have a low ovarian reserve, should be able to access one full cycle of IVF/ICSI. But in reality, cash-strapped funders are often minded to set their own local criteria; this leaves many couples outside the net with no option other than to fund treatment privately. And HFEA figures – again from its 2013 report – show that a minority of IVF treatment cycles (41.3%) were funded by the NHS in 2013. The majority (58.7%) were privately funded. Fertility Fairness (2014) has campaigned for more than 20 years for people to have equal access to NHS-funded infertility treatment, yet its research in 2014, which is published on its website, shows that more than 80 per cent of CCGs in England are still failing to provide the recommended number of cycles NICE recommends. In Scotland, all 14 Health Boards offer up to two cycles of IVF/ICSI to eligible women who meet the standard access criteria (Infertility Network UK 2014). Similarly in Wales, all seven Health Boards offer up to two cycles of IVF/ICSI to eligible women who meet the standard access criteria (Infertility Network UK 2014). In Northern Ireland, eligible women are offered just one cycle of IVF/ICSI (Infertility Network UK 2014). So, because where a patient lives will ultimately determine what NHS treatment they may be offered, if any, an understanding of the specific rules and criteria and NICE guidelines can help a patient better access the treatment they are entitled to.

## 5. Patient experience of infertility and assisted reproduction

Many people would argue that the emotional challenges of infertility are by far the most difficult to overcome. It is hard to put into words the devastating impact delivered by an infertility diagnosis. It's a heart-stopping moment to realise that the cosy family life you imagined may be out of reach. Many couples find themselves putting their lives on hold whilst living in month-to-month cycles of hope and disappointment that revolve around clinic appointments, tests and medication. The sorrow, anger and frustration that can come with prolonged fertility problems invade every area of life, shattering self-confidence, straining friendships and testing the most stable relationships.

Chapter 1 has already provided an overview of the research on the impact of infertility. In brief, several studies have investigated the relationship between infertility and psychological distress, and the majority of these studies have reported a high prevalence of anxiety, mood disorders and depressive symptoms in infertile women. For example, results from a large population study of 98,000 women by Baldur-Felskov *et al.* (2012) showed that childless women with fertility problems were at an 18 per cent higher risk of hospitalisation for psychiatric disorders, thus adding an important component to the counselling of women with fertility problems.

In the UK, all licensed clinics have a responsibility to offer counselling, but a joint survey carried out in 2014 by the British Infertility Counselling Association (BICA) and patient charity Infertility Network UK found that one-third of the infertility patients who responded were not offered any counselling by their clinics (BICA 2014). The online survey showed that 33 per cent of the respondents had not been offered any counselling and 20 per cent said they were not even aware that counselling was available at their clinic. By failing to offer counselling to their patients, some of these infertility clinics are breaching their licence conditions, as the HFEA Code of Practice clearly states that the offer of counselling by licensed clinics is a statutory legal requirement. The HFEA clearly sets out exactly when and how clinics are meant to offer counselling – yet from the survey responses it is apparent that this guidance is either insufficient or has simply not been followed. Of those patients who were aware of counselling, the majority (61%) felt that the potential benefits of having counselling were not made clear to them.

Speaking at the time, Ruth Wilde, the outgoing chair of BICA, said:

> Counselling is an integral part of infertility treatment, not a luxury, and clinics have a duty of care to their patients and the HFEA makes it clear that the offer of counselling is a mandatory part of this care in a defined set of circumstances. Infertility is an extremely stressful procedure with huge potentially long-term emotional consequences and patients should expect to have access to counselling support as part of this process. The issue is not simply about patients being made aware of counselling, it is about how it is offered and the value and emphasis attributed to it. The survey reflects what we as practitioners know, but clinics and clinicians sometimes fail to understand – that it is not just about offering counselling as a box-ticking exercise, but about communicating the reasons and benefits for having it. There is support out there: BICA seeks to continually raise the standard of support offered to people affected by fertility issues and involuntary childlessness and to help them access the right help. Everyone having licensed treatment should be able to see an infertility counsellor through his or her clinic.

For more on specialist infertility counsellors in the UK visit www.bica.net.

··· BOX 2.1 MY STORY ·················································································

'As the mother of two much-longed-for daughters myself, I know what it feels like to desperately covet the "F" word: family. The desire to have your own family changes your view on life in a way you won't believe possible, and one that you will never forget. Family is just a word. But it's the password to a precious exclusive, members-only club where there is no guarantee of getting in. For me, like so many others, IVF simply changed my life. Without this most life-changing advance in medical science – which has happened well within my own lifetime – my husband and I would just be two more people desperately hoping for the miracle of a baby son or daughter. We would not have our own family and that little word would forever drive a stake through our hearts.

'Instead, we have two amazing daughters who make our lives complete with their fun, laughter and love. They give us permission to use that incredibly powerful word – family – when I describe to others who were are. Back in 1996, shortly after our wedding, we discovered I had one blocked fallopian tube, and the second was partially blocked. An undetected burst appendix when I was only 23 had wreaked havoc on my delicate tissues and now threatened our future. This discovery – and the heartache that followed as we realised were unlikely to have children on our own – was simply devastating.

'We had taken for granted that we would be able to choose when to start a family. That we could plan and have a free choice. Infertility robbed us of that free choice, as it does for millions of people all over the world today. We became a statistic: one of the 1 in 7. Yuk. Grief, anger and sadness were new – and commonplace – emotions as we watched close friends and relatives conceive with ease. How I hated the false smiling through tears as new babies were proudly displayed. And passed round! I had to hold them!

'New and destructive feelings seeped through my skin as I struggled to feel kindness when I really only felt displeasure. Displeasure at their happiness. It is impossible to accurately describe the feelings of grief, loss and desperation. I hated all these new parents with their little bundles: their new families and the new and amazing futures that lay ahead for them. With our hopes in tatters, we were forced down a path of protocol, process and drugs in our bid to have a child. The IVF clinic at our local hospital – Queens Medical Centre in Nottingham – became our second home. After what seemed like an endless cycle of injections and scans, a few precious embryos were created. Hope lay before us, suspended in a glass dish. And from those precious embryos our first daughter Holly was born in June 1998. Georgia was born 14 months later in August 1999. Incredibly, Georgia was conceived naturally – but in reality, medicine has delivered both our daughters. People tell me that they feel stigmatised because of their infertility, that it is still a taboo subject, spoken about in hushed voices, making them feel that somehow they have failed. Infertility can be devastating and it's time we openly acknowledged that. We all know that it's good to talk – so let's talk more about it and bring infertility out of the closet.'

················································································

## ··· BOX 2.2 JESSICA HEPBURN'S STORY ····························

Theatre producer Jessica Hepburn was diagnosed with unexplained infertility in her thirties and has since become a veteran of the fertility world, having endured 11 rounds of fresh and frozen IVF at numerous clinics, which have resulted in several miscarriages but sadly, as yet, no baby.

'I was 34 and running a London theatre when I decided to start a family. I thought that making the decision to fit a baby into my busy life was the hard part. I was wrong. After a year of having sex to schedule, my partner and I were diagnosed with "unexplained infertility" and so began our eight-year journey to have a child (and we're still counting).

'Over the last eight years I have been to lots of different clinics, had every test known to woman and doctor, and been through multiple rounds of IVF. Like many women I have also gone to alternative – and sometimes absurd – lengths to understand my infertility, from visiting a psychic tarot card reader to attending an intense therapeutic process to discover whether my "inner child" has anything to do with it (!). I have also faced the heartbreak of several miscarriages and a life-threatening ectopic pregnancy.

'For a long time I went through treatment in secrecy as I felt so sad and ashamed about what my body couldn't do, but shortly after I turned 40 I started writing about my experiences. In spring 2014, my book was published (Hepburn 2014) and since then my life has changed completely.

'I have spoken out about my story and the fertility industry as a whole; going public has helped me tremendously, and I hope that it has helped other women to feel less alone. I write a regular column for *Fertility Road* magazine and a blog and I am constantly amazed by how many people are affected by infertility in some way. I am passionate about raising awareness of the emotional effects of infertility; championing equality of access to treatment; improving patient care; and encouraging more understanding and research into the causes of infertility. I hope my book will provide solace and advice to other women going through the same thing. I also want to campaign to change some of the really hard and unsaid things about the fertility industry today including the terrible environment of some clinics and the ubiquity of IVF as a solution to fertility problems when it isn't always the answer. I also want to open up the conversation about what happens next if it doesn't end up working out, because maybe it won't.'

## 6. Concluding remarks

Back in 1965, the 18th World Health Assembly recognised that building a family should be the free choice of the individual couple. The World Health Organisation (WHO) recognises infertility as a physical illness that requires treatment (2015). And in parts of the world today, reproduction is an obligation, not a choice: failure to reproduce devastates communities – Larsen *et al.* (2010) suggest that the necessity for a woman to have a child remains basic in sub-Saharan Africa. Motherhood continues to be a defining factor in an individual's treatment by others in the community, in her self-respect and in her understanding of what it means to be a woman. The achievement of motherhood represents a milestone for many women as it confers on them an adult identity and represents normative fulfilment of what is considered by many to be female destiny.

## References

Baldur-Felskov, B., Kjaer, S., Albieri, V., Steding-Jessen, M., *et al.* (2012) *Hospitalizations for Psychiatric Disorders in Women with Fertility Problems – A Large Danish Register-based Cohort Study.* European Society of Human Reproduction and Embryology. Available at www. eshre.eu/~/media/emagic%20files/Press%20room/Annual%20meeting/Istanbul/ Abstract%20Baldur.pdf, accessed on 18 May 2015.

British Infertility Counselling Association (BICA) (2014) *Infertility Network UK Counselling Survey Findings*. Available at www.bica.net/news/91/bica-infertility-network-uk-counselling-survey-findings, accessed on 18 May 2015.

Connor, S. (2014, 15 June) 'Lord Winston criticises "jungle" world of British fertility treatment.' *The Independent*. Available at www.independent.co.uk/news/science/lord-winston-criticises-jungle-world-of-british-fertility-treatment-9537859.html, accessed on 18 May 2015.

Fertility Fairness (2014) *IVF Provision in England*. Available at www.fertilityfairness.co.uk/nhs-fertility-services/ivf-provision-in-england, accessed on 18 May 2015.

Hepburn, J. (2014) *The Pursuit of Motherhood*. Leicester: Matador.

Human Fertilisation and Embryology Authority (2015) *An Estimated One in Seven Couples Have Difficulty Conceiving*. Available at www.hfea.gov.uk/fertility.html, accessed on 18 May 2015.

Human Fertilisation and Embryology Authority (2015) *Assisted Hatching*. Available at www.hfea.gov.uk/assisted-hatching.html, accessed on 18 May 2015.

Human Fertilisation and Embryology Authority (2015) *Considering Fertility Treatment Abroad: Issues and Risks*. Available at www.hfea.gov.uk/fertility-clinics-treatment-abroad.html, accessed on 18 May 2015.

Human Fertilisation and Embryology Authority (2013) *Fertility Treatment in 2013 – Trends and Figures*. Available at www.hfea.gov.uk/docs/HFEA_Fertility_Trends_and_Figures_2013.pdf, accessed on 18 May 2015.

Human Fertilisation and Embryology Authority (2015) *How to Research Clinics and What to Expect*. Available at www.hfea.gov.uk/fertility-clinic-guide.html, accessed on 18 May 2015.

Human Fertilisation and Embryology Authority (2015) *PGD Conditions Licensed by the HFEA*. Available at http://guide.hfea.gov.uk/pgd, accessed on 18 May 2015.

Human Fertilisation and Embryology Authority (2015) *Treatment and Storage Options*. Available at www.hfea.gov.uk/IVF.html, accessed on 18 May 2015.

Infertility Network UK (2015) *Current Criteria for Publicly Funded Fertility Treatment In Northern Ireland*. Available at www.infertilitynetworkuk.com/nhs_funding_2/nhs_funding_in_northern_ireland, accessed on 18 May 2015.

Infertility Network UK (2015) *Factsheet, Treatment Overseas*. Available at www.infertilitynetworkuk.com/uploaded/Fact%20Sheets/Treatment%20Overseas%202014.pdf, accessed on 18 May 2015.

Infertility Network UK (2015) *NHS Funding for Fertility Treatment in Scotland*. Available at www.infertilitynetworkuk.com/nhs_funding_2/nhs_funding_in_scotland, accessed on 18 May 2015.

Infertility Network UK (2015) *NHS Funding in Wales*. Available at www.infertilitynetworkuk.com/nhs_funding_2/nhs_funding_in_wales, accessed on 18 May 2015.

Infertility Network UK (2015) *NHS Funding*. Available at www.infertilitynetworkuk.com/nhs_funding_2, accessed on 18 May 2015.

Infertility Network UK (2015) *Welcome to Infertility Network UK*. Available at www.infertilitynetworkuk.com, accessed on 18 May 2015.

Larsen, U., Hollos, M., Obono, O., and Whitehouse, B. (2010) 'Suffering infertility: the impact of infertility on women's life experiences in two Nigerian communities.' *Journal of Biosocial Science 42*, 787–814.

National Institute for Health and Care Excellence (2013) *Fertility: Assessment and Treatment for People with Fertility Problems*. Available at www.nice.org.uk/guidance/cg156/resources/updated-nice-guidelines-revise-treatment-recommendations-for-people-with-fertility-problems, accessed on 18 May 2015.

World Health Organisation (2015) *Sexual and Reproductive Health*. Available at www.who.int/reproductivehealth/topics/infertility/definitions/en, accessed on 18 May 2015.

# Chapter 3

# Obesity, Body Mass Index, Associated Factors and Their Effect on Fertility

*Susan Bedford BSc (Hons), PGCE, MSc (Nut. Th), mBANT, CNHC*

## 1. BMI, obesity and factors associated with obesity

The aim of this chapter is to consider the effect and consequences of body mass index (BMI) and obesity on fertility. Obesity in women is on the increase in the western world, and is a cause for concern in many countries. In the USA it is estimated that almost a quarter of women of reproductive age have a BMI greater than 30 (Vahratian 2009) and obesity is estimated to affect more than one-third of all US adults (Flegal *et al.* 2010). This situation can potentially impact on reproductive health in a number of ways. An increase in body weight and fat tissue is associated with an imbalance of hormones, especially in fertile women. This can involve androgens, oestrogens and overall their carrier protein, sex hormone-binding globulin (SHBG) (Pasquali *et al.* 2003). SHGB is a glycoprotein that binds to androgens and oestrogens (sex hormones). Oestradiol and testosterone circulate in the bloodstream, attached mostly to SHBG. Therefore the availability of sex hormones is influenced by the level of SHBG; the higher the level of SHBG, the fewer unbound hormones there will be available (Hammond 2011). Changes in SHBG concentrations lead to a change of androgen and oestrogen transport to target tissues (Hammond 2011). The way in which body fat is distributed in the body can also regulate androgen production and metabolism to a large extent, and has also been shown substantially to affect SHBG concentrations (Pasquali *et al.* 1990). Women with central obesity have higher testosterone production rates compared with those with peripheral obesity (peripheral obesity is the accumulation of excess fat in the buttocks, hips and thighs) (Kirschner *et al.* 1990).

## 2. Body mass index
### 2.1 Effect of high and low BMI on fertility

BMI is the calculation of a person's height-to-weight ratio, the simplest expression for this being weight (kg) divided by height squared ($m^2$). A BMI score below 18.5 means that a person is more than likely to be underweight, a score of 18.5–24.9 indicates a healthy weight, a score of 25–29.9 is above the ideal range and a score of 30 or more indicates obesity (NHS Choices 2014a). Excessive body weight can lead to significant effects on health including cardiovascular disease, diabetes and infertility (Brannian 2011). It is, however, important to view each case individually and be aware that BMI does have some limitations. For example, some individuals with a high muscle mass may have a high BMI even though they have a low body fat content. If a woman is overweight or underweight this may affect fertility and success with assisted reproductive techniques (ART) (Davies 2006; Norman and Clark 1998; Winter *et al.* 2002). However, the findings from research on underweight women are generally more variable when compared with those in relation to obese women (Fedorcsak *et al.* 2004), where more consistency exists. The sections below will review some of the evidence relating to weight and BMI in more detail.

### 2.2 Effect of low BMI on female fertility

A low BMI may reduce female sex hormone levels and, as a result, affect menstrual periods and increase the risk of miscarriage (Wentz 1980). It may also increase the risk of complications arising during fertility treatment. However, this is not a consistent view as some authors have found no links between being underweight (except in relation to anovulation and anorexia) and reproduction, including ART such as IVF (Roth, Grazi and Lobel 2003). Various studies and research over the years have suggested that there is a relationship between low body weight, strenuous exercise and infertility in women, with improvement in fertility rates associated with a reduction in exercise and some weight gain (Bolúmar *et al.* 2000; Grodstein, Goldman and Cramer 1994; Hassan and Killick 2004).

## 2.3 Effect of high BMI on female fertility

Obese women are less likely to become pregnant through IVF and assisted reproduction (Crosignani *et al.* 1994; Zaadastra, Seidell and Van Noord 1993). A BMI of over 30 (considered obese) has been shown to affect fertility and success at assisted reproduction by affecting ovulation and response to fertility treatment in terms of poor response to the stimulation drugs. This in turn may reduce pregnancy rates (Fedorcsak *et al.* 2004; Veleva *et al.* 2008). Some research studies have discovered that obese and morbidly obese (an individual is considered morbidly obese if he or she is 100 pounds over his/her ideal body weight, has a BMI of 40 or more, or 35 or more and experiencing obesity-related health conditions such as high blood pressure or diabetes) women have half the chance of conceiving with IVF compared with women with a normal BMI range (Wang, Davies and Norman 2002; Wittemer *et al.* 2000). However, other studies found BMI and increased weight to have no impact on IVF success and outcome (Dechaud *et al.* 2006; Lashen *et al.* 1999; Metwally *et al.* 2007) but in morbidly obese women there can be an increased number of IVF cycles cancelled (Dokras *et al.* 2006).

In 2007 Maheshwari and Stofberg conducted a systematic review of the literature available on the effect of being overweight and obesity on ART and they discovered that with a BMI greater than 25, the pregnancy rate reduced in those undergoing ART such as IVF. The combined odds of pregnancy were 1.47 (95% Confidence Interval, CI: 1.20–1.80) for a woman with a BMI of 20–30kg/m² as compared with women with a BMI of greater than 30kg/m². The greater the BMI the more ovarian stimulation drugs were required and the higher the miscarriage rate was (Maheshwari and Stofberg 2007). They did, however, discover a number of limitations in the research regarding the effect of BMI and being overweight on IVF success including: different drug protocols being used from clinic to clinic and within the same clinic; differences in ages; and differences in the calculations of BMI and being 'overweight'. They also discovered that the amount of ovarian stimulation drugs being used at the beginning of treatment differed from clinic to clinic, as some based the amount on the female AMH (anti-Müllerian hormone) result or ovarian reserve whilst others used BMI and age to help calculate dosage. Maheshwari and Stofberg (2007) further found that differences in age were an identified limiting factor. It was concluded by the researchers that further studies are required, with the same starting point and measurements used to determine the real effect of BMI and weight on ART success.

## 2.4 BMI and age in female fertility

Age has also been identified as a factor to consider in relation to BMI. In a recent study conducted by Sneed *et al.* in 2008 which examined the effect of BMI on IVF success it was discovered that in younger patients a high BMI (>29) had a negative impact on IVF success, but in patients over 36 years of age it had little influence on success. Another study conducted by Loveland *et al.* in 2001, involving 139 women under 40 years old, found that IVF success is reduced in patients with a BMI greater than 25. Lintsen *et al.* (2005) found similar results. Overall, there is conflicting evidence from the research studies to date on the effect of BMI and assisted reproduction success. However, when the sample sizes of different studies are taken into account, the largest three studies seem to indicate that in those women with a BMI greater than 25 there is lower success rate at IVF (Fedorcsak *et al.* 2004; Lintsen *et al.* 2005; Loveland *et al.* 2001). Age is an important factor that must be taken into account. This is considered in further detail in Chapter 12.

## 2.5 BMI and male fertility

In men, excess weight may be linked with altered testosterone and oestradiol levels, poor semen quality and infertility (Hinz, Rais-

Bahrami and Kempkensteffen 2010). In those who are overweight (BMI 25–30) and obese (BMI >30), there is a relationship between the degree of excessive weight and poor quality and quantity of sperm. In a study conducted in 2007 by Nguyen *et al.*, it was discovered that there was a trend of increased infertility with increased male BMI. After adjusting for the woman's BMI, coital frequency and the ages and smoking habits of both partners, the odds ratio for infertility was 1.20 (increasing odds) for overweight men (BMI 25–29.9; 95% CI = 1.04–1.38) and 1.36 for obese men (BMI 30–34.9; 95% CI = 1.13–1.63) relative to men with low–normal BMI (20.0–22.4). When BMI was divided into eight categories, there was a trend of increased infertility with increased male BMI. The effect of BMI in men was nearly identical when coital frequency was not included, indicating that the effect is not mediated by sexual dysfunction in heavier men. The researchers also concluded that further research was required to discover if weight loss in these men improved their fertility. In a study of 91 male Japanese workers, Ohwaki and Yano (2009) found an increased incidence of not fathering a child per year of marriage with increasing male BMI.

The effect of male obesity on the outcome of fertility treatment has been studied infrequently. Bakos *et al.* (2011) researched the effect of male obesity on the outcome of fertility treatment in couples undergoing IVF. In this study including 305 couples undergoing an initial IVF treatment, the effect of male obesity on embryo quality and pregnancy rate was analysed. Men with a normal BMI were found to have a higher sperm concentration than overweight, obese and morbidly obese men. Morbidly obese men had a higher rate of the use of ICSI for fertilisation. After treatment, there was a higher rate of blastulation (this is the process following the morula and precedes the gastrulation). Cleavage results in a blastula consisting of about 128 cells in couples with normal weight men when compared with those with obese and severely obese men. They also report a linear reduction in chemical and clinical pregnancy rates, and live-birth rates with increasing BMI in the male partners.

## 2.6 Guidance

The National Institute for Health and Care Excellence (NICE 2013) provides guidelines in relation to fertility, obesity and also low body weight in the UK. The main guidelines (current as at time of writing) are listed in Table 3.1.

### Table 3.1 Current NICE guidelines in relation to fertility, obesity and low body weight

**Obesity**

Women who have a BMI of 30 or over should be informed that they are likely to take longer to conceive (2004, amended 2013).

Women who have a BMI of 30 or over and who are not ovulating should be informed that losing weight is likely to increase their chance of conception (2004, amended 2013).

Women should be informed that participating in a group programme involving exercise and dietary advice leads to more pregnancies than weight loss advice alone (2004).

Men who have a BMI of 30 or over should be informed that they are likely to have reduced fertility (2004, amended 2013).

**Low body weight**

Women who have a BMI of less than 19 and who have irregular menstruation or are not menstruating should be advised that increasing body weight is likely to improve their chance of conception (2004).

## 2.7 BMI and polycystic ovary syndrome (PCOS)

Many women diagnosed with PCOS have difficulty controlling their weight and thus often have a higher BMI. In this section issues relating to PCOS and BMI will be explored, as these can impact on their fertility. Weight loss in women with PCOS has been shown to improve fertility, insulin resistance and psychological symptoms, even when BMI remains above 24.9 (Teede, Deeks and Moran 2010).

Losing weight has been found to improve ovulation, pregnancy rates and outcomes (NICE 2013). The clinical presentation of PCOS may include menstrual irregularities, signs of androgen excess (such as alopecia, acne, hirsutism) and obesity. Insulin resistance and elevated serum luteinising hormone (LH) levels are also common features in PCOS (Zisser 2007). In women with PCOS, an increased risk of miscarriage was found in research conducted by Hamilton-Fairley *et al.* (1992) if the women were moderately overweight (BMI 25–27.9).

## 2.8 Effect of visceral adiposity on fertility

Visceral fat, as opposed to subcutaneous fat found under the skin, is located in the abdominal cavity (visceral fat surrounds vital organs such as the kidneys and liver). Visceral fat cells are larger than subcutaneous, are more metabolically active and produce inflammatory cytokines (Wisee 2004). Continual production of cytokines can lead to chronic inflammation and chronic diseases. Researchers have found that visceral fat secretes a protein called retinol-binding protein 4 (RBP4) that has been shown to have a detrimental effect and increase resistance to insulin (Kotnik, Fischer-Posovszky and Wabitsch 2011). Adipose tissue is loose connective tissue composed of adipocytes. Its main function is to store energy in the form of fat. It also insulates the body and acts not only as a fat reservoir, but also as a reservoir for immune cells. Macrophages, neutrophils, and T and B cells (which help protect the body as part of our immune system) can all be located in these fat stores (Kanneganti and Deep Dixit 2012).

Visceral fat, when produced in excess, can also contribute to fertility issues as it can lead to an increase in the amount of oestrogen in the body (Sikaris 2004). In women, excess visceral fat may lead to irregular ovulation, endometriosis and PCOS (Faloia *et al.* 2004; Moran *et al.* 2010). There are some lifestyle factors that may lead to an increase in visceral fat. These include stress, poor diet, over-consumption of alcohol, lack of exercise, a diet high in sugar and processed foods, and a lack of sleep (Kanneganti and Deep Dixit 2012). All these factors are explored further in this book. Cortisol (a steroid hormone released in response to stress) can cause visceral fat deposition due to high stress. Cortisol levels can also increase due to ageing and the counterbalancing levels of oestrogens along with a testosterone drop. As a result, chronically high cortisol levels can lead to a variety of conditions such as insulin resistance or reduced immune function (Sears 2005).

## 3. How does obesity affect fertility?

Obesity affects fertility in a number of ways. Research has shown that obese women who do become pregnant have an increased risk of miscarriage, pre-eclampsia, gestational diabetes, and congenital defects in offspring (Jungheim and Moley 2010).

Obesity is thought to affect egg and embryo quality (Carrell *et al.* 2001; Ramsay, Greer and Sattar 2006) and is also thought to increase the risk of an early miscarriage after IVF treatment (Fedorcsak *et al.* 2000; Wang *et al.* 2002). Excess weight is thought to affect how the ovaries function and the ability to conceive, due to changes in hormones and metabolism, such as high oestrogen production, altered steroid metabolism, reduced availability of gonadotrophin-releasing hormone (GnRH), and changes in the way in which insulin is secreted and acts on other adipose hormones such as leptin (Budak *et al.* 2006; Fedorcsak *et al.* 2004; Gesink Law, Maclehose and Longnecker 2007; Pasquali *et al.* 2003). It has been found that throughout assisted reproduction procedures in obese women, higher levels of gonadotrophin drugs are required to stimulate the ovaries to produce adequate numbers of eggs for collection (Fedorcsak *et al.* 2001; Fedorcsak *et al.* 2004; Loveland *et al.* 2001). Amounts of gonadotrophins need to be raised as BMI increases in both long and short stimulation IVF protocols (Butzow *et al.* 1999; Loh, Wang and Mattheus 2002).

### 3.1 Oestrogen dominance and role of oestrogen metabolites (hydroxyoestrogens)

Oestrogens are necessary and vital hormones that are involved in many processes within the body. Oestrogen is needed in the natural form by the body as it is involved in sexual maturation, ovulation and regulating the menstrual cycle. Oestrogen is produced mainly in the ovaries in women in the form of oestradiol (E2). It is also produced in the peripheral tissue in the form of oestrone (E1). Androgens are converted into the forms of E1 and E2 by the enzyme aromatase. An increase in aromatase can cause oestrogen production in women and men to increase (Nelson and Bulun 2001). Obesity can lead to oestrogen dominance in the body due to the fact that fat cells are able to release pro-inflammatory signals that may increase the activity of the enzyme aromatase (Yang *et al.* 2010). However, oestrogen and compounds of oestrogen can be found in the environment as well. They can be found in water, air, food, medications, hormone replacement therapy (HRT), the contraceptive pill and plastic residues to name a few examples (Simonich and Hites 1995). They are also available in synthetic and natural sex hormones, such as the contraceptive pill and HRT. Too much exposure to this 'extra' oestrogen can therefore disrupt the working of other hormones within the body, particularly progesterone (Crowther 2008). Some synthetic oestrogens have the ability to occupy and block the receptor sites of natural oestrogen produced in the body and thus affect its usual role of action (Goldzieher and Castracane 2008).

## 3.2 What is oestrogen dominance and what are its effects?

Oestrogen dominance occurs when there is too much oestrogen in the body or an imbalance between oestrogen and other hormones such as progesterone (Crowther 2008). There are a number of lifestyle factors that may lead to oestrogen dominance (see Table 3.2). Oestrogen dominance significantly increases cancer risk, alters brain neurotransmitters, contributes to infertility, and can also affect mood (Shepherd 2001). If a person is overweight, fat tissue increases levels of aromatase that turns testosterone to oestrogen (Carreau *et al.* 2003). Oestrogen causes fat to accumulate, mainly around the abdomen, hips and thighs, leading to central obesity. Obesity can alter the metabolism of oestrogen resulting in oestrogen metabolites. Women who are overweight or obese are thus more exposed to these than women of a normal weight or those who are underweight (Kirschner *et al.* 1990).

## Table 3.2 Factors that may contribute to oestrogen dominance (adapted from Kaur Dharam, Dapylak-Arhanic and Dean 2005)

| Factor | Example(s) |
| --- | --- |
| Stress | High cortisol levels can lead to low progesterone levels |
| Diet | High glycaemic index foods |
| | Foods containing high hormone levels such as meats, dairy and poultry |
| | Excess saturated fat |
| Dysbiosis (intestinal) | Intestinal parasites |
| Sugar imbalances | Insulin resistance – anovulation |
| | Low SHBG |
| Environmental toxins | Heavy metals |
| | Dioxins |
| Reduced oestrogen detoxification | Obesity |

### 3.3 Oestrogen dominance in men

In males, a greater amount of body fat, especially around the waist and chest, causes testosterone to be converted to oestrogen, irreversibly, due to the action of aromatase, thus reducing testosterone levels (Glass 1994; Svartberg, von Muhlen and Sundsfjord 2004). Gynaecomastia (an enlargement of male breast tissue) is seen with an altered oestrogen/testosterone balance and signals oestrogen excess (Glass 1994).

### 3.4 Dietary and lifestyle approaches to reduce oestrogen dominance

Optimum oestrogen metabolism can be supported with good nutrition in order to aid efficient metabolism and detoxification (Hofmekler and Osborn 2007) (see Table 3.3). Boosting the intake of cruciferous vegetables such as broccoli, kale, cabbage and cauliflower, containing the phytonutrients diindolylmethane (DIM) and sulfurophane, in the diet may help to break down oestrogens to non-toxic forms. Oestrogen is eliminated by the body by it binding with glucuronic acid in the liver, where it is then excreted through the bile and eliminated via the colon. Beta-glucuronidase, an enzyme produced by the colonic microflora, is capable of cleaving oestrogen from the glucuronic acid, making it possible for the oestrogens to be reabsorbed (O'Connor 2013). High-circulating free oestradiol and overactivity of the beta-glucuronidase enzyme (as seen in dysbiosis) amplifies oestrogen excess. Potent, multistrain probiotics and dietary fibre reduce elevated beta-glucuronidase activity by working to restore the balance of microflora (O'Connor 2013).

Too much saturated fat in the diet can also affect the way in which oestrogen is reabsorbed from the bowel into the body due to an increase in beta-glucuronidase levels (Goldin 1982). It is wise to decrease the consumption of saturated fats and increase sources of monounsaturated fat and polyunsaturated fat (particularly omega-3) consumed. In the UK the guidance is that the average man should eat no more than 30g of saturated fat per day and the average woman no more than 20g per day (NHS Choices 2014b). A study found that vegetarian women had half the levels of free circulating oestrogen of omnivores due to consuming less saturated fat in the diet (Goldin 1982). Certain foods (see Chapter 11, Section 6 on endocrine disruptors) such as soy, beer (alcohol), liquorice, clover and some foods in plastic increase the amount of oestrogen in the body and therefore should be avoided (Tarr-Kent 2013).

### 3.5 Cruciferous vegetables and oestrogen

Consuming cruciferous vegetables may also assist in the reduction of oestrogen because certain vegetables such as cabbage, broccoli and Brussels sprouts contain a compound called indole-3-carbinol that increases the body's ability to break down oestrogen and reduce the amount in circulation (Hofmekler and Osborn 2007). There are supplemental forms of the phytochemicals indole-3-carbinol (I3C) and 3,3'-DIM available, and these are an area of active interest due to their role in oestrogen metabolism. There are mixed opinions on their use and research is still continuing regarding the benefits and safety of supplemental use (Mathrick 2010; Minich and Bland 2007).

## 3.6 Other useful supplements in oestrogen dominance

Foods rich in methionine, including beans, legumes, onion and garlic, also assist in the breakdown of oestrogen (Mathrick 2010). (However, care must be taken with supplementation of methionine due to the fact that it may be converted to homocysteine – it is therefore important to ensure that the diet contains other methyl donors such as B6, B12 and folic acid to help prevent this.) They will also aid the methylation of oestrogen. Methylation involves a chemical reaction where the liver breaks down oestrogen (oestradiol) into a less potent form (oestriol) (Murray, Granner and Mayes 1996). In studies it has been discovered that soluble fibre can help with the removal of oestrogen due to its ability to bind oestrogen in the digestive tract, as a result reducing the amount of free oestradiol in circulation (Shultz and Howie 1986).

## 3.7 Micronutrients and other supplements and oestrogen dominance

Ensuring adequate vitamin E in the diet, by supplementation if necessary, may help reduce oestrogen levels and aid oestrogen detoxification (Hall 2001). Vitamins B12, B6 and folate are also important in oestrogen detoxification as they act as cofactors to the enzymes involved in the process (Hall 2001). A reduced level of B vitamins can lead to an increase in circulating oestrogen, thus raising levels (Hall 2001). Good sources are oatmeal, walnuts, legumes and chicken. Magnesium is also important as it promotes oestrogen detoxification by promoting methylation and glucuronidation, both of which are key oestrogen detoxification pathways (Muneyvirci-Delale, Naxharaju and Altura 1998).

## 3.8 Phytoestrogens

Phytoestrogens (oestrogen-like chemicals found in plant foods such as beans, seeds and grains) have competing claims of having both beneficial and adverse effects in the body (Patisaul and Jefferson 2010), but it is thought that they may be useful in that they have the ability to prevent the oestrogens produced in the body from binding to their receptor sites. They are also involved in slowing down the conversion of androgens to oestrogen that normally occurs in fatty tissue, and they can make oestrogen relatively unavailable by increasing the levels of oestrogen's carrier protein, SHBG (Blondel 2011). When more oestrogen is bound to SHBG, less is available to bind to oestrogen receptors. Examples of foods that contain include phytoestrogens include soy, fennel, alfalfa and a large range of grains and seeds.

### Table 3.3 Dietary recommendations to reduce oestrogen dominance (adapted from Slater 2012)

| Food Group | Foods to include | Foods to exclude |
|---|---|---|
| Legumes | All legumes and legume products, especially organic non-GMO soy products | None |
| Vegetables | All, especially cruciferous and sea vegetables (various seaweeds) | None |
| Fruits | All whole and dry fruits, especially citrus | None |
| Grains | All whole grains and whole-grain products, especially rye | Non-whole grains, refined flours, refined flour products |
| Nuts/seeds | All nuts and seeds and their butters, especially flaxseeds, walnuts and pumpkin seeds – raw form only | None |

| | | |
|---|---|---|
| Fish | All, especially cold water fish: salmon, sardines, tuna, halibut are an excellent source of omega-3 fatty acids | Salted or cured fish |
| Eggs | From organically raised hens | Non-organic eggs |
| Poultry/meat | Meat – organic meats and poultry | Non-organic meats and poultry, salted and cured meats |
| Dairy | Organic dairy products and soy, nut- and grain-based dairy substitutes | Non-organic dairy products |
| Oils | Organic cold-pressed, unrefined, seed and nut oils, especially flaxseed, walnut, sesame and olive oil | Refined vegetable oils, butter, lard, margarine, shortening and saturated or hydrogenated fats |
| Beverages | Mineral or filtered water; herbal tea; fresh fruit juice | Alcohol, coffee |
| Sweeteners | Brown rice syrup, fruit sweetener, molasses, stevia | Refined or artificial sweeteners |
| Spices and herbs | Especially nutmeg, anise, thyme, sage, fennel, caraway, turmeric and fresh lemon and lime juice | Chocolate (due to high sugar content), high sodium foods and salt |

## BOX 3.1 DIETARY CHECKLIST TO HELP
··· BALANCE OESTROGEN IN THE BODY ··························

- ▶ Keep saturated fats to a minimum. Instead, try to consume monounsaturated/beneficial omega-3 polyunsaturated fats. Some good sources are oily fish, nuts and cold pressed oils.

- ▶ Drink 6–8 glasses of still water each day.

- ▶ Eat some quality protein daily. Good sources include organic/free range eggs, lentils, beans, fish, low fat dairy foods and chicken.

- ▶ Include plenty of complex carbohydrates in the diet wherever possible. Good sources are vegetables, fruit, whole-grains, beans and lentils.

- ▶ Ensure that ample food sources of vitamin E, B12, B6, folate and magnesium are included in the diet, such as sweet potato, eggs, beans, broccoli, nuts, seeds and wholegrains.

- ▶ Increase consumption of cruciferous vegetables such as broccoli, Brussels sprouts, cabbage, cauliflower, kale and watercress.

## 3.9 Wider effects of oestrogen dominance

If the hormonal balance in the body is affected then there can be a wider knock-on effect on other systems in the body. Oestrogen dominance can affect the fine working of the delicate hormonal system and affect the functioning and balance of the thyroid gland and also the adrenal gland.

## 3.10 Thyroid hormones

The thyroid gland is located at the base of the neck and produces the hormone thyroxine that helps to regulate the metabolic rate and is also important in balancing other hormones in the body (Friedman 2005). The pituitary gland in the brain produces thyroid-stimulating hormone (TSH). In response the thyroid gland produces thyroid hormones. The two main thyroid hormones produced are triiodothyronine (T3) and thyroxine (T4). A high proportion of T4 is converted into the more active T3 inside the cells of the body (Brownstein 2004). Each cell in the body possesses receptors for thyroid and cortisol hormones and, thus, these regulate heart rate, blood pressure, body temperature, weight, metabolism and growth (Borowski 2012).

Thyroid function can be affected by a variety of factors such as infections, high stress levels, autoimmune disorders, exposure to toxins (such as heavy metals and pesticides) and other hormone imbalances such as high prolactin levels and oestrogen dominance (Slater 2012). Sometimes oestrogen dominance can be mistaken for hypothyroidism leading to an individual taking medication unnecessarily instead of correcting the oestrogen imbalance or excess (Brownstein 2004). Oestrogen dominance can affect the balance of the thyroid gland as it can impact on conversion of T4 into T3 thyroid hormone and result in low T3 levels (Lam and Lam 2012).

### 3.11 Adrenal glands

When the adrenal glands are stressed there is a greater need for cortisol that serves to reduce progesterone levels in the body, due to the fact that progesterone is used to make more cortisol, and thus meaning there is less progesterone in circulation to balance out oestrogen levels. It is therefore often the case that correction of oestrogen dominance can help restore adrenal gland balance and help normalise progesterone levels.

## 4. Hyperinsulinism, hyperandrogenism, hyperleptinaemia, anovulation and their effect on fertility

There are some important pathophysiological features often associated with obesity and its related conditions such as PCOS. These are hyperinsulinaemia, functional hyperandrogenism and anovulation (Poretsky *et al.* 1999). Hyperleptinaemia also presents as a factor and the way in which these features may impact on fertility will be considered below.

## 4.1 Hyperinsulinaemia

Hyperinsulinaemia is a condition where higher levels of insulin than normal circulate in the blood, relative to the level of glucose (Ferry 2010). It is often associated with obesity, high blood pressure, glucose intolerance and dyslipidaemia (often known collectively as metabolic syndrome) (Matsuzawa, Fanahashi and Nakamura 1999). Hyperinsulinaemia can be triggered by obesity with visceral fat accumulation (Jensen 2008). It can have a number of effects on fertility such as reduced embryo quality and reduced implantation rates, and is also thought to amplify PCOS symptoms (Cano et al. 1997; Jakubowicz et al. 2001). Furthermore, it is thought that the rate of early pregnancy loss is higher in women with PCOS than in normal women (Jakubowicz et al. 2002). Hyperinsulinaemia affects granulosa cells in small follicles and theca cells, which can lead to anovulation (Sakumoto et al. 2010). PCOS has a complex aetiology but many women with PCOS have insulin resistance, in which the body cannot use insulin efficiently (Teede et al. 2010). Increased levels of androgens can affect ovulation and menstrual cycles in many women with PCOS. In research conducted by Poretsky et al. (1999) it was discovered that women with PCOS are often hyperinsulinaemic and the degree of hyperandrogenism may be positively and significantly correlated with that of hyperinsulinaemia. PCOS causes hormonal imbalances, including elevated testosterone (male hormone) and oestrogen (female hormone) levels (Azziz, Carmina and Dewailly 2006; Moran et al. 2010).

## 4.2 Effect of a high carbohydrate diet on other reproductive hormones

An increase in high glycaemic index carbohydrate foods in the diet increases insulin production, which causes the amount of testosterone produced by the ovaries to rise and this decreases globulin concentrations (Marsh and Brand-Miller 2005). The higher levels of testosterone affect the pituitary ovarian axis causing luteinising hormone (LH) levels to increase (Apter 1997). This can affect ovulation in that an egg may not be released from the ovary (Doufas and Mastorakos 2000). This situation can affect the response to the follicle-stimulating drugs used during IVF and thus affect the number of eggs collected for potential fertilisation, ultimately affecting success (Butzow *et al.* 1999; Fedorcsak *et al.* 2004). Reducing the amount of carbohydrate food eaten can cause a reduction in testosterone levels and fasting insulin concentrations, decreased hyperlipidaemia and increased SHBG concentrations (Pasquali *et al.* 1989).

## 4.3 Hyperandrogenism

Hyperandrogenism is a condition in which there are excess levels of male sex hormones (androgens) found in women or men. This can lead to a number of symptoms such as:

- obesity
- acne
- increased growth of body hair
- infertility
- irregular menstrual cycles
- deepening of voice
- reduced size of uterus.

A common cause of hyperandrogenism is polycystic ovary syndrome (PCOS) where the ovaries produce excesses of male hormone and do not ovulate regularly. Being obese can influence hyperandrogenism and has been linked to subfertility and disruption of the menstrual cycle. In studies it has been found that consuming a diet that is high in saturated fat and low in fibre is often associated with PCOS (Azziz *et al.* 2006). Obesity causes hyperinsulinaemia and insulin resistance, which in turn may cause an increase in the amount of insulin available to the ovarian tissue and this may cause an increase in excess androgen synthesis to occur (Poretsky and Kalin 1987). In women with PCOS, the rise in androgens, along with an increase in insulin and LH, often leads to premature luteinisation and follicular arrest. PCOS is thought to be caused by a combination of several factors/diseases which can be influenced by obesity. Weight loss has shown to improve hyperandrogenism and in some cases may encourage spontaneous ovulation (Hunter and Garvey 1998).

## 4.4 Anovulation (in obesity)

Anovulation is the failure of the ovary to release ova over a period of time generally exceeding three months. The normal functioning ovary releases one ovum every 25–28 days (Davis and Segars 2009). Anovulation in obesity results from excess androgens and oestrogen causing decreased progesterone (Zhang, Stern and Rebar 1984). Anovulation plays a large role in the various imbalances and dysfunctions of PCOS. In many but not all patients with PCOS, insulin insensitivity and obesity are seen. Half of PCOS patients are obese (Broekmans et al. 2006). Women with PCOS who are obese are more likely to show symptoms of excess androgens and be anovulatory (Franks, Stark and Hardy 2008). This can be explained by the fact that an excess of adipose tissue causes an increase in peripheral conversion of androgens to oestrone, inhibiting ovulation at the hypothalamus as a result. As discussed previously, elevated insulin levels play a role in hyperandrogenaemia and anovulation. Obese women with PCOS have a higher incidence of insulin resistance than obese patients without PCOS. Weight loss of 5–10 per cent of body weight in obese patients will increase ovulation, with a 50 per cent return to ovulation and a 33 per cent pregnancy rate within six months (Davis and Segars 2009). If weight loss alone is not successful, then the drug clomiphene citrate may often be considered as a treatment option (Cristello et al. 2005).

## 4.5 Other causes of anovulation

There are other causes of anovulation, a few examples of which are premature ovarian failure (POF), menopause, low body weight, anorexia, breast feeding and thyroid issues.

## 4.6 Hyperleptinaemia

Leptin is a hormone associated with numerous effects including appetite control, inflammation, and decreased insulin secretion (Ghanayem et al. 2010). It is made by fat cells and regulates the amount of fat stored in the body by adjusting the hunger sensation and energy expenditure levels of the body. Serum leptin levels are linked to the amount of fat tissue in the body (Moschos, Chan and Mantzoros 2002). When the amount of fat stored in the body reaches a certain level then the hunger sensation is reduced and leptin is secreted into the bloodstream where it activates receptors in the hypothalamus, known as leptin receptors. As a result energy expenditure is increased (Brennan and Mantzoros 2006).

In obese women leptin resistance increases, which in turn leads to hyperleptinaemia. The state of hyperleptinaemia affects fertility in a number of ways. High levels of leptin seem to affect the ovaries directly, leading to a lack of eggs or no egg being released; this greatly affects fertility and thus will reduce success at IVF and assisted reproduction (Budak *et al.* 2006; Moschos *et al.* 2002). High levels of leptin can affect the action of follicle-stimulating hormone (FSH) in the ovary, affecting how many follicles may mature, and so affecting IVF success (Agarwal *et al.* 1999). It has also been linked with stimulating LH production, thus affecting ovulation and, in turn, success at IVF (Pasquali 2006; Yu *et al.* 1997). Leptin levels and BMI are now being used in some IVF clinics to predict possible success at IVF, as the higher the leptin concentrations in the blood, the greater the effect is on reduction of egg quality and early embryonic development, and thus the lower the success at IVF (Brannian *et al.* 2001; Clarke and Henry 1999). However, other researchers in a recent study have found there to be no correlation between leptin levels and IVF success (Almog *et al.* 2010). A study conducted in mice demonstrated that leptin was nearly five times higher in obese mice than lean mice, and that the higher leptin levels corresponded to five times lower fertility in the obese mice (Ghanayem *et al.* 2010). It has also been discovered that leptin can affect ovulation independently of androgen or insulin level (Barash, Cheung and Weigle 1996).

## 5. Concluding remarks

Fertility can be negatively affected by obesity. In women, early onset of obesity favours the development of menstrual irregularities, chronic oligo-anovulation and infertility in adults. Obesity in women can also increase risk of miscarriages and impair the outcomes of ART and pregnancy, when the BMI exceeds $30\text{kg}/\text{m}^2$. The main factors implicated in the association may be insulin excess and insulin resistance (Pasquali, Patton and Gambineri 2007) being linked to hormonal imbalances.

# References

Agarwal, S., Vogel, K., Weitsman, S., and Magoffin, D. (1999) 'Leptin antagonizes the insulin-like growth factor-I augmentation of steroidogenesis in granulosa and theca cells of the human ovary.' *Journal of Clinical Endocrinology and Metabolism 84*, 1072–1076.

Almog, B., Azem, F., Kapustiansky, R., Azolai, J., *et al.* (2010) 'Intrafollicular and serum levels of leptin during in vitro fertilization cycles: comparison between the effects of recombinant follicle-stimulating hormones and human menopausal gonadotrophin.' *Gynaecological Endocrinology 9*, 666–668.

Apter, D. (1997) 'Leptin in puberty.' *Clinical Endocrinology 47*, 175–176.

Azziz, R., Carmina, E., and Dewailly, D. (2006) 'Androgen Excess Society: position statement. Criteria for defining polycystic ovary syndrome as a predominantly hyperandrogenic syndrome: an Androgen Excess Society guideline.' *Journal of Clinical Endocrinology and Metabolism 91*, 4237–4245.

Bakos, H., Henshaw, R., Mitchell, M., and Lane, M. (2011) 'Paternal body mass index is associated with decreased blastocyst development and reduced live birth rates following assisted reproductive technology.' *Fertility and Sterility 95*, 5, 1700–1704.

Barash, I., Cheung, C., and Weigle, D. (1996) 'Leptin is a metabolic signal to the reproductive system.' *Endocrinology 137*, 3144–3147.

Blondel, J. (2011) *The Natural PCOS Diet – A Naturopath's Easy Step-by-Step Guide to Overcoming PCOS*. E-book. Available at www.natural-hormone-health.com/the-natural-PCOS-diet.html, accessed on 19 May 2015.

Bolúmar, F., Olsen, J., Rebagliato, M., Sáez-Lloret, I., and Bisanti, L. (2000) 'Body mass index and delayed conception: a European Multicenter Study on Infertility and Subfecundity.' *American Journal of Epidemiology 151*, 1072–1079.

Borowski, T. (2012) *Thyroid Function Imbalance*. Available at www.nutritionalvalues.co.uk/thyroid.php, accessed on 19 May 2015.

Brannian, J. (2011) 'Obesity and fertility.' *South Dakota Journal of Medicine 64*, 251–254.

Brannian, J., Schmidt, S., Kreger, D., and Hansen, K. (2001) 'Baseline non-fasting serum leptin concentration to body mass index ratio is predictive of IVF outcomes.' *Human Reproduction 16*, 9, 1819–1826.

Brennan, A., and Mantzoros, C. (2006) 'Drug insight: the role of leptin in human physiology and pathophysiology–emerging clinical applications.' *Nature Clinical Practice Endocrinology & Metabolism 2*, 6, 318–327.

Broekmans, F., Knauff, E., Laven, J., Eijkemans, M., and Fauser, B. (2006) 'PCOS according to the Rotterdam consensus criteria.' *British Journal of Obstetrics and Gynaecology 113*, 1210.

Brownstein, D. (2004) *Overcoming Thyroid Disorders*. West Bloomfield, MI: Medical Alternatives Press.

Budak, E., Fernández, M., Bellver, J., Cerveró, A., Simón, C., and Pellicer, A. (2006) 'Interactions of the hormones leptin, ghrelin, adiponectin, resistin and PYY3-36 with the reproductive system.' *Fertility and Sterility 85*, 1563–1581.

Butzow, T., Moilanen, J., Lehtovirta, M., Tuomi, T., *et al.* (1999) 'Serum and follicular fluid leptin during in vitro fertilization: relationship among leptin increase, body fat mass, and reduced ovarian response.' *Journal of Clinical Endocrinology & Metabolism 84*, 9, 3135–3139.

Cano, F., Garcia-Velasco, J., Millet, A., Remohi, J., Simon, C., and Pellicer, A. (1997) 'Oocyte quality in polycystic ovaries revisited: identification of a particular subgroup of women.' *Journal of Assisted Reproduction and Genetics 14*, 254–261.

Carreau, S., Lambard, S., Delalande, C., Denis-Galeraud, I., Bilinska, S., and Bourguiba, S. (2003). 'Aromatase expression and role of estrogens in male gonad: a review.' *Reproductive Biology and Endocrinology 1*, 35.

Carrell, D., Jones, K., Peterson, C., Aoki, V., Emery, B., and Campbell, B. (2001) 'Body mass index is inversely related to intrafollicular hCG concentrations, embryo quality and IVF outcome.' *Reproductive Biomedicine Online 3*, 109–111.

Clarke, I., and Henry, B. (1999*)* 'Leptin and reproduction.' *Reviews of Reproduction 4*, 48–55.

Cristello, F., Cela, V., Artini, P., and Genazzani, A. (2005) 'Therapeutic strategies for ovulation induction in infertile women with polycystic ovary syndrome.' *Gynaecological Endocrinology 21*, 6, 340.

Crosignani, P., Ragni, G., Parazzini, F., Wyssling, H., Lombroso, G., and Perotti, L. (1994) 'Anthropometric indicators and response to gonadotrophin for ovulation induction.' *Human Reproduction 9*, 420–423.

Crowther, P. (2008) 'Food for thought: oestrogen dominance.' *Positive Health 151*, 1.

Davies, M. (2006) 'Evidence for effects of weight on reproduction in women.' *Reproductive Biomedicine Online 12*, 552–561.

Davis, J., and Segars, J. (2009) *Menstruation and Menstrual Disorders: Anovulation.* The Global Library of Women's Medicine. Available at www.glowm.com/section_view/heading/Menstruation%20and%20Menstrual%20Disorders:%20Anovulation/item/295, accessed on 19 May 2015.

Dechaud, H., Anahory, T., Reyftmann, L., Loup, V., Hamamah, S., and Hedon, B. (2006) 'Obesity does not adversely affect results in patients who are undergoing in vitro fertilization and embryo transfer.' *European Journal of Obstetrics and Gynaecology and Reproductive Biology 127*, 88–93.

Dokras, A., Baredziak, L., Blaine, J., Syrop, C., Van Voorhis, B., and Sparks, A. (2006) 'Obstetric outcomes after *in-vitro* fertilization in obese and morbidly obese women.' *Obstetrics and Gynaecology 180*, 61–69.

Doufas, A., and Mastorakos, G. (2000) 'The hypothalamic-pituitary-thyroid axis and the female reproductive system.' *Annals of the New York Academy of Sciences 900*, 1, 65–76.

Faloia, E., Canibus, P., Gatti, C., Frezza, F., *et al.* (2004) 'Body composition, fat distribution and metabolic characteristics in lean and obese women with polycystic ovary syndrome.' *Journal of Endocrinological Investigation 27*, 5, 424–429.

Fedorcsak, P., Dale, P., Storeng, R., Ertzeid, G., *et al.* (2004) 'Impact of overweight and underweight on assisted reproduction treatment.' *Human Reproduction 19*, 11, 2523–2528.

Fedorcsak, P., Storeng, R., Dale, P., Tanbo, T., and Abyholm, T. (2000) 'Obesity is a risk factor for early pregnancy loss after IVF or ICSI.' *Acta Obstetricia et Gynecologica Scandinavica 79*, 43–48.

Fedorcsak, P., Storeng, R., Tanbo, T., and Abyholm, T. (2001) 'The impact of obesity and insulin resistance on the IVF or ICSI in women with polycystic ovarian syndrome.' *Human Reproduction 6*, 1086–1091.

Ferry, R. (2010) *Hyperinsulinism.* Available at www.emedicine.medscape.com/article/921258-followup, accessed on 19 May 2015.

Flegal, K., Carroll, M., Ogden, C., and Curtin, L. (2010) 'Prevalence and trends in obesity among US adults, 1999–2008.' *Journal of the American Medical Association 303*, 235–241.

Franks, S., Stark, J., and Hardy, K. (2008) 'Follicle dynamics and anovulation in polycystic ovary syndrome.' *Human Reproductive Update 14*, 4, 367.

Friedman, M. (2005) *Fundamentals of Naturopathic Endocrinology.* Toronto, Ontario: Canadian College of Naturopathic Medicine Press.

Gesink Law, D., Maclehose, R., and Longnecker, M. (2007) 'Obesity and time to pregnancy.' *Human Reproduction 22*, 414–420.

Ghanayem, B., Bai, R., Kissling, G., Travlos, G., and Hoffler, U. (2010) 'Diet-induced obesity in male mice is associated with reduced fertility and potentiation of acrylamide-induced reproductive toxicity.' *Biology of Reproduction 82*, 96–104.

Glass, A. (1994) 'Gynecomastia.' *Endocrinology and Metabolism Clinics of North Americas 23*, 4, 825–837.

Goldin, B. (1982) 'Estrogen patterns and plasma levels in vegetarian and omnivorous women.' *New England Journal of Medicine 307*, 1542–1547.

Goldzieher, J., and Castracane, V. (2008) 'Physiology and mechanisms of action of steroids.' *The Global Library Of Women's Medicine*, 1756–2228.

Grodstein, F., Goldman, M., and Cramer, D. (1994) 'Infertility in women and moderate alcohol use.' *American Journal of Public Health 84*, 1429–1432.

Hall, D. (2001) 'Nutritional influences on estrogen metabolism.' *Applied Nutritional Science Reports 1*, 1–8.

Hamilton-Fairley, D., Kiddy, D., Watson, H., Paterson, C., and Franks, S. (1992) 'Association of moderate obesity with a poor pregnancy outcome in women with polycystic ovary syndrome treated with low dose gonadotrophin.' *British Journal of Obstetrics and Gynaecology 99*, 128–131.

Hammond, G. (2011) 'Diverse roles for sex hormone-binding globulin in reproduction.' *Biology of Reproduction 85*, 3, 431–441.

Hassan, M., and Killick, S. (2004) 'Negative lifestyle is associated with a significant reduction in fecundity.' *Fertility and Sterility 81*, 384–392.

Hinz, S., Rais-Bahrami, S., and Kempkensteffen, C. (2010) 'Effect of obesity on sex hormone levels, antisperm antibodies, and fertility.' *Urology 76*, 4, 851–856.

Hofmekler, O., and Osborn, R. (2007) *The Anti-Estrogenic Diet: How Estrogenic Foods and Chemicals Are Making You Fat and Sick.* Berkeley, CA: North Atlantic Books.

Hunter, S., and Garvey, W. (1998) 'Insulin action and insulin resistance: diseases involving defects in insulin receptors, signal transduction, and the glucose transport effector system.' *American Journal of Epidemiology 105*, 331–345.

Jakubowicz, D., Iuorno, M., Jakubowicz, S., Roberts, K., and Nestler, J. (2002) 'Effects of metformin on early pregnancy loss in the polycystic ovary syndrome.' *Journal of Clinical Endocrinology and Metabolism 87*, 524–529.

Jakubowicz, D., Seppala, M., Jakubowicz, S., Rodriguez-Arms, O., et al. (2001). 'Insulin reduction with metformin increases lutealphase serum glycodelin and insulin-like growth factor-binding protein 1concentrations and enhances uterine vascularity and blood flow in the polycysticovary syndrome.' *Journal of Clinical Endocrinology and Metabolism 86*, 1126–1133.

Jensen, H. (2008) 'Role of body fat distribution and the metabolic complications of obesity.' *Journal of Clinical Endocrinology and Metabolism 93*, 11, 57–63.

Jungheim, E., and Moley, K. (2010) 'Current knowledge of obesity's effects in the pre- and periconceptional periods and avenues for future research.' *American Journal of Obstetrics and Gynaecology 203*, 525–530.

Kanneganti, T., and Deep Dixit, V. (2012) 'Immunological complications of obesity.' *Nature Immunology 13*, 707–712.

Kaur Dharam, S., Dapylak-Arhanic, M., and Dean, C. (2005) *The Complete Guide to Natural Medicine.* Toronto, Ontario: Robert Rose.

Kirschner, M.A., Samojlik, E., Drejka, M., Szmal, E., Schneider, G., and Ertel, N. (1990) 'Androgen-estrogen metabolism in women with upper body versus lower body obesity.' *Journal of Clinical Endocrinology and Metabolism 70*, 473–479.

Kotnik, P., Fischer-Posovszky, P., and Wabitsch, M. (2011) 'RBP4: a controversial adipokine.' *European Journal of Endocrinology 165*, 703–711.

Lam, L., and Lam, D. (2012) *Estrogen Dominance: Hormonal Imbalance of the 21st Century*. Loma Linda, CA: Adrenal Institute Press.

Lashen, H., Ledger, W., Bernal, A. and Barlow, D. (1999) 'Extremes of body mass do not adversely affect the outcome of superovulation and in-vitro fertilization.' *Human Reproduction 14*, 712–15.

Lintsen, A., Pasker-de Jong, P., de Boer, E., Burger, C., *et al.* (2005) 'Effects of subfertility cause, smoking and body weight on the success rate of IVF.' *Human Reproduction 20*, 1867–1875.

Loh, S., Wang, J., and Mattheus, C. (2002) 'The influence of body mass index, basal FSH and age on the response to gonadotrophin stimulation in non-polycystic ovarian syndrome patients.' *Human Reproduction 17*, 1207–1211.

Loveland, J., McClamrock, H., Malinow, A., and Sharara, F. (2001) 'Increased body mass index has a deleterious effect on in vitro fertilization outcome.' *Journal of Assisted Reprododuction and Genetetics 18*, 382–386.

Maheshwari, A., and Stofberg, L. (2007) 'Effect of overweight and obesity on assisted reproductive technology – a systematic review.' *Human Reproduction Update 13*, 433–444.

Marsh, K., and Brand-Miller, J. (2005) 'The optimal diet for women with polycystic ovary syndrome?' *British Journal of Nutrition 94*, 2, 154–165.

Mathrick, S. (2010) *Oestrogendetox*. Available from www.sparklewell.com.au/2012/12/oestrogen-detox, accessed on 19 May 2015.

Matsuzawa, Y., Fanahashi, T., and Nakamura, T. (1999) 'Molecular mechanism of metabolic syndrome X: contribution of adiposcyte-derived bioactive substances.' *Annals of the New York Academy of Sciences 892*, 146–154.

Metwally, M. and Ledger, W. (2009) 'The impact of obesity on female reproductive function.' *Obesity Reviews 8*, 6, 515–23.

Minich, M., and Bland, S. (2007) 'A review of the clinical efficacy and safety of cruciferous vegetable phytochemicals.' *Nutrition Reviews 65*, 6, 259–267.

Moran, L., Misso, M., Wild, R., and Norman, R. (2010) 'Impaired glucose tolerance, type 2 diabetes and metabolic syndrome in polycystic ovary syndrome: a systematic review and meta-analysis.' *Human Reproduction Update 16*, 4, 347–363.

Moschos, S., Chan, J., and Mantzoros, C. (2002) 'Leptin and reproduction: a review.' *Fertility and Sterility 77*, 433–444.

Muneyvirci-Delale, O., Nacharaju, V., and Altura, B. (1998) 'Sex steroid hormones modulate serum ionized magnesium and calcium levels throughout the menstrual cycle in women.' *Fertility and Sterility 69*, 5, 958–962.

Murray, R., Granner, D., and Mayes, P. (1996) *Harper's Biochemistry* (24th edition). Stamford, CT: Appleton & Lange.

Nelson, L., and Bulun, S. (2001) 'Estrogen production and action.' *Journal of American Acadamy of Dermatology 453*, S116–S124.

Nguyen, R., Wilcox, A., Skjaerven, R., and Baird, D. (2007) 'Men's body mass index and infertility.' *Human Reproduction 22*, 9, 2488–2493.

NHS Choices (2014a) *Eat Less Saturated Fat*. Available at www.nhs.uk/Livewell/Goodfood/Pages/Eat-less-saturated-fat.aspx, accessed on 19 May 2015.

NHS Choices (2014b) Available at www.nhs.uk/Livewell/loseweight/Pages/BodyMassIndex, accessed on 10 February 2014.

NICE (2013) *Fertility – Assessment and Treatment For People With Fertility Problems*. Available at www.nice.org.uk/guidance/CG156, accessed on 19 May 2015.

Norman, R., and Clark, A. (1998) 'Obesity and reproductive disorders: a review.' *Reproduction Fertility and Development 10*, 55–63.

O'Connor, L. (2013) *Oestrogen excess.* Available at www.natureandhealth.com.au/news/ gynae-sos, accessed on 19 May 2015.

Ohwaki, K., and Yano, E. (2009) 'Body mass index as an indicator of metabolic disorders in annual health checkups among Japanese male workers.' *Industrial Health 47*, 6, 611–616.

Pasquali, R. (2006) 'Obesity and androgens: facts and perspectives.' *Fertility and Sterility 85*, 5, 1319–1340.

Pasquali, R., Antenucci, D., Casimirri, F., Venturoli, S., and Paradisi, R. (1989) 'Clinical and hormonal characteristics of obese amenorrheic, hyperandrogenic women before and after weight loss.' *Journal of Clinical Endocrinology and Metabolism 68*, 173–179.

Pasquali, R., Casimirri, F., Plate, L. and Capelli, M. (1990) 'Characterization of obese women with reduced sex hormone-binding globulin concentrations.' *Hormone and Metabolic Research 22*, 303–306.

Pasquali, R., Patton, L., and Gambineri, A. (2007) 'Obesity and infertility.' *Current Opinion in Endocrinology Diabetes Obesity 14*, 6, 482–487.

Pasquali, R., Pelusi, C., Genghini, S., Cacciari, M., and Gambineri, A. (2003) 'Obesity and reproductive disorders in women.' *Human Reproduction Update 4*, 359–372.

Patisaul, H., and Jefferson, W. (2010) 'The pros and cons of phytoestrogens.' *Frontiers in Neuroendocrinology 31*, 4, 400–419.

Poretsky, L., and Kalin, M. (1987) 'The gonadotropic function of insulin.' *Endocrine Reviews 8*, 132–141.

Poretsky, L., Cataldo, N., Rosenwaks, Z., and Giudice, L. (1999) 'The insulin related ovarian regulatory system in health and disease.' *Endocrine Reviews 20*, 535–582.

Ramsay, J., Greer, I., and Sattar, N. (2006) 'Obesity and reproduction.' *British Medical Journal 333*, 1159–1162.

Roth, D., Grazi, R., and Lobel, S. (2003) 'Extremes of body mass index do not affect first-trimester pregnancy outcome in patients with infertility.' *American Journal of Obstetrics and Gynaecology 188*, 1169–1170.

Sakumoto, T., Tokunaga, Y., Tanaka, H., Nohara, M., *et al.* (2010). 'Insulin resistance/ hyperinsulinemia and reproductive disorders in infertile women.' *Reproductive Medicine and Biology 9*, 185–190.

Sears, B. (2005) *The Anti-Inflammation Zone.* New York, NY: HarperCollins.

Shepherd, J. (2001) 'Effects of Estrogen on Cognition, Mood, and Degenerative Brain Diseases.' *Journal of the American Pharmacists Association 41*, 2.

Shultz, T., and Howie, B. (1986) 'In vitro binding of steroid hormones by natural and purified fibers.' *Nutrition and Cancer 8*, 2, 141–147.

Sikaris, K. (2004) 'The clinical biochemistry of obesity.' *Clinical Biochemist Reviews 25*, 3, 165–181.

Simonich, S., and Hites, R. (1995) 'Global distribution of persistent organochlorine compounds.' *Science 269*, 1851–1854.

Slater, C. (2012) *A Symphony Uncovered. The Endocrine Dance.* University of Natural Medicine. Available at http://universitynaturalmedicine.org, accessed on 19 May 2015.

Sneed, M., Uhler, M., Grotjan, H., Rapisarda, J., Lederer, K. and Beltsos, A. (2008) 'Body mass index: impact on IVF success appears age-related.' *Human Reproduction 23*, 8, 1835–1839.

Svartberg, J., von Muhlen, D., and Sundsfjord, J. (2004) 'Waist circumference and testosterone levels in community dwelling men. The Tromso study.' *European Journal of Epidemiology 19*, 657–663.

Tarr-Kent, L. (2013) *Estrogenic foods to avoid.* Available at www.livestrong.com/article/70189-estrogenic-foods-avoid, accessed on 19 May 2015.

Teede, H., Deeks, A., and Moran, L. (2010) 'Polycystic ovary syndrome: a complex condition with psychological, reproductive and metabolic manifestations that impacts on health across the lifespan.' *Biomedcentral Medicine 8*, 41.

Vahratian, A. (2009) 'Prevalence of overweight and obesity among women of childbearing age: results from the 2002 National Survey of Family Growth.' *Maternal and Child Health Journal 13*, 268–273.

Veleva, Z., Tiitinen, A., Vilska, S., Hyden-Granskog, C., *et al.* (2008) 'High and low BMI increase the risk of miscarriage after IVF/ICSI and FET.' *Human Reproduction 23*, 4, 878–884.

Wang, J., Davies, M., and Norman, R. (2002) 'Obesity increases the risk of spontaneous abortion during infertility treatment.' *Obesity Research 10*, 551–554.

Wentz, A. (1980) 'Body weight and amenorrhea.' *Obstetrics and Gynaecology 56*, 482–487.

Winter, E., Wang, J., Davies, M., and Norman, R. (2002) 'Early pregnancy loss following assisted reproductive technology treatment.' *Human Reproduction 17*, 3220–3223.

Wisee, B. (2004) 'The inflammatory syndrome: the role of adipose tissue cytokines in metabolic disorders linked to obesity.' *American Society of Nephrology 15*, 2792–2800.

Wittemer, C., Ohl J., Bailly, M., Bettahar-Lebugle, K., and Nisand, I. (2000) 'Does body mass index of infertile women have an impact on IVF procedure and outcome?' *Journal of Assisted Reproduction and Genetics 17*, 547–552.

Yang, H., Youm, Y., Vandanmagsar, B., Ravussin, A., *et al.* (2010) 'Obesity increases the production of proinflammatory mediators from adipose tissue T cells and compromises TCR repertoire diversity: implications for systemic inflammation and insulin resistance.' *Journal of Immunology 185*, 3, 1836–1845.

Yu, W., Kimura, M., Walczewska, A., Karanth, S., and McCann, S. (1997) 'Role of leptin in hypothalamic-pituitary function.' *Proceedings of the National Academy of Sciences USA 94*, 3, 1023–1028

Zaadastra, B., Seidell, J., and Van Noord, P. (1993) 'Fat and female fecundity: prospective study of effect of body fat distribution on conception rates.' *British Medical Journal 306*, 484–487.

Zhang, Y., Stern, B., and Rebar R. (1984) 'Endocrine comparison of obese menstruating and amenorrheic women.' *Journal of Clinical Endocrinology and Metabolism 58*, 1077.

Zisser, H. (2007) 'Polycystic ovary syndrome and pregnancy: is metformin the magic bullet?' *Diabetes Spectrum 20*, 2, 85–89.

# Chapter 4

# Introduction to Female Factors in Infertility and Pregnancy Loss

*Justine Bold BA (Hons), PgCHE, Dip BCNH, NTCC, CNHC Senior Lecturer Institute of Health & Society, University of Worcester, UK*

## 1. Introduction

This chapter gives a brief overview of the main female fertility issues and their wider context and explains how we have approached these in the book, as many are explored in depth in other chapters. For example, in Chapter 3 factors such as obesity and the underpinning hormonal imbalances and effects on both female and male fertility are reviewed. In terms of female fertility, this is very relevant regarding management of polycystic ovary syndrome (PCOS) and readers should consult that chapter for a more detailed analysis of the imbalances and their pathophysiology. Other chapters investigate other areas relevant to female fertility. As endometriosis is such a significant cause of female fertility issues a specific chapter has been devoted to it (see Chapter 5). Chapters 8 and 9 look at how the immune system impacts fertility, Chapter 10 outlines how nutritional deficiencies may affect fertility, Chapter 11 focuses on lifestyle factors such as sleep, smoking, exercise and endocrine-disrupting chemicals, and in Chapter 12 factors affecting women trying to conceive over the age of 40 are considered.

The anatomy and physiology of the female reproductive tract and hormonal control of the menstrual cycle will not be reviewed in this chapter as some is explored in the other chapters and there is not sufficient space in this book to include another detailed presentation.

## 2. Main issues

Many women are affected by specifically female fertility issues; for example, in the USA an estimated 6.1 million women aged 15–44 have difficulty getting or staying pregnant (Office on Women's Health 2012). Some of the leading causes include PCOS, uterine myomas (fibroids), premature ovarian failure (POF), pelvic inflammatory disease (PID), other tubal problems and genetic issues as well as cancer treatment. Some of these will now be reviewed briefly providing an overall context and key information about factors such as epidemiology, medical diagnosis and treatment and key considerations for an integrated approach.

### 2.1 PCOS

PCOS is the most common endocrine disorder and is one of the leading causes of anovulatory infertility in women (Farshchi *et al.* 2007). Its prevalence is estimated at 5–10 per cent in young reproductive-age women but there are variations in some specific groups (Ehrmann 2005). For example, there is an increased prevalence in Asians in the UK and in the black population of the USA (Farshchi *et al.* 2007). If the European Society for Human Reproduction and Embryology/American Society for Reproductive Medicine criteria are used the estimated prevalence could be as high as high as 15–20 per cent (Sirmans and Pate 2014). It usually develops around the onset of menarche (menstruation) but polycystic ovaries (PCO) have been found in girls as young as six (Bridges *et al.* 1993).

PCOS has a complex pathophysiology involving both the glycoprotein sex hormone-binding globulin (SHBG), which acts as a carrier for sex steroids, and the protein insulin-like growth factor 1 (IGF1). Sex steroids circulate in the bloodstream attached mostly to SHBG and research confirms that lower levels of SHBG are associated with PCOS and metabolic syndrome (Chen *et al.* 2006) as well as being associated with markers for cardiovascular disease. For example, lower SHBG levels are inversely associated with C-reactive protein (Joffe *et al.* 2005). (Refer to Chapter 3 for more details about SHBG.)

It is therefore perhaps not surprising that PCOS is associated with many health problems, including an elevated cardiovascular (CVD) risk with both dyslipidaemia and hypertension and hormonally responsive cancers in later life (Ehrmann 2005). Women with PCOS also have an increased risk of ovarian hyperstimulation syndrome (OHSS) when undergoing fertility treatment (Banker and Garcia-Velasco 2015) and need very careful monitoring during ovarian stimulation.

Risk factors for the development of PCOS include:

- Obesity (this is covered in Chapter 3).

- Insulin resistance – this can be present in normal weight individuals with PCOS as well as in overweight women (Farshchi *et al.* 2007). The related hormonal imbalances such as hyperinsulinaemia and hyperleptinaemia are also covered in Chapter 3.

- Metabolic syndrome and diabetes mellitus Type 2 are also risk factors, as is inflammation (Kalgaonkar *et al.* 2011). Malin *et al.* (2015) have conducted research that demonstrates that systemic inflammation involving mono-nuclear cell activation and nuclear factor kappa b is involved in pancreatic beta cell dysfunction in PCOS; even though the research is small-scale, they conclude that inflammation may play a role in impairing insulin release prior to the development of overt hyperglycaemia. (See Chapter 3, Section 2.8, for further information on the links between visceral fat and inflammation.)

The signs and symptoms of PCOS are varied and a woman may not experience all of them simultaneously. They include:

- chronic anovulation (Vuguin 2010)

- clinical and/or biochemical hyperandrogenism (Vuguin 2010); this causes problems such as hirsutism – see Chapter 3 for more on this

- skin problems (e.g. acne and brown patches known as acanthosis nigricans)

* depression

* abdominal/central obesity (increased waist-to-hip ratio >0.85).

### BOX 4.1 PCOS DIAGNOSIS AND
··· DIAGNOSTIC CRITERIA ·············································

▶ Oligomenorrhea (infrequent or light periods) or amenorrhoea (absence of periods) associated with anovulation (this is where ovulation does not occur so no oocyte is released).

▶ Hyperandrogenaemia.

▶ Abnormal ovarian ultrasound 12 or more follicles in each ovary 2–9mm or increased ovarian volume.

▶ Increased luteinising hormone (LH) with increased LH/follicle-stimulating hormone (FSH) ratio.

(Farshchi et al. 2007)

Medical management of PCOS is via using drugs such as metformin, androgen blockers, clomiphene citrate and hormone agonists; and surgical procedures such as laparoscopic ovarian drilling (where ovarian tissue implicated in androgen production is removed). This procedure is used where women are unresponsive to the drug clomiphene citrate (Mitra, Nayak and Agrawal 2015).

It is estimated that at least 50 per cent of patients with PCOS are overweight (Gambineri et al. 2002). In such cases integrated approaches would include nutritional support focusing on weight loss and management. Exercise is also key in the management of PCOS as it can help improve insulin sensitivity (see Chapter 11 for further information, specifically Box 11.1, which outlines the benefits of exercise in PCOS). Other dietary support strategies to be considered in an integrated approach include sugar reduction and blood sugar balancing (for example by increasing fibre intake to improve satiety) as well as increasing nutrient density, in particular the consumption of B vitamins (as many of these are involved in carbohydrate metabolism). Omega-3 fatty acids may be helpful as they can help reduce inflammation, and animal studies have demonstrated improvements in insulin sensitivity (Neschen *et al.* 2007). See also Chapter 3, Section 2.7, BMI and PCOS for more on weight, body mass index (BMI) and PCOS.

In terms of other dietary approaches, cinnamon can be a useful addition to the diet as polyphenols within it have been shown to improve insulin sensitivity (Anderson 2008). It may also be a good idea to miminise intake of dairy foods as these are known to increase levels of insulin-like growth factor 1 (IGF-1) within the body, which appears to be associated with insulin resistance and hirsutism (Çakir *et al.* 2014). Moreover, it has been suggested that acne (which is often present in PCOS) is an IGF-1 'mediated disease' (Melnik and Schmitz 2009). As the signs of PCOS can cause problems such as hirsutism, psychotherapeutic interventions should be explored to provide support where self-esteem is affected. Other complementary therapies may also play a role in the ongoing management; a case study on the supporting role of acupuncture in PCOS is presented later in this book (see Chapter 13, Section 4.1).

## 2.2 Myomas (fibroids)

Myomas (sometimes known as leiomyomas or fibroids) are solid uterine tumours (Wallach and Vlahos 2004), generally benign, varying in size from very small to melon-sized. They are the most common solid pelvic tumours in women (Grabo *et al.* 1999). Up to 40 per cent of women are believed to be affected, with higher incidence in some groups. Myomas are believed to affect more African American women, and prevalence also increases with age (Evans and Brunsell 2007). There are different types, depending on where and how they grow. Intra-cavity fibroids grow inside the uterine cavity, submucous fibroids grow partially in the cavity and partially in the wall of the uterus, intramural fibroids grow within the wall, and subserous fibroids are on the outside wall of the uterus (Healthline 2015). Pedunculated fibroids can be attached either to the inside or outside wall and are characterised by a stalk (Healthline 2015). They usually require treatment if they are growing large enough to cause pressure on other organs, such as the bladder, or if they are rapidly increasing in size or causing abnormal bleeding or causing problems with embryo implantation. The causes are not fully understood but oestrogen is considered the primary stimulus. It has been suggested that unopposed oestrogen (sometimes referred to as oestrogen dominance) may increase the risk of myomas (Chiaffarino *et al.* 1999) – see Chapter 3, Section 3.1, for more about this.

Signs and symptoms of fibroids can include abdominal pressure and pain, painful intercourse, frequent urination, fatigue (anaemia from heavy bleeding) and infertility (Evans and Brunsell 2007), but most cases are asymptomatic. The main symptom is heavy prolonged periods with potential anaemia. If fibroids are pedunculated, they can twist, causing complications; and large fibroids can enlarge/distort the womb, making implant of a fertilised egg impossible. Fibroids generally shrink in the menopause (NHS 2014a). Diagnosis is normally via non-invasive transvaginal ultrasonography or magnetic resonance imaging (MRI). MRI offers very accurate means of diagnosis but is more costly (Evans and Brunsell 2007). Fibroids may also be diagnosed after surgical investigations including sonohysterography or hysteroscopy. Various drug treatments are offered, including the levonorgestrel intrauterine system (LNG-IUS) that releases progesterone slowly into the uterus to help manage heavy bleeding (NHS 2014a). Other hormonal medications include the contraceptive pill, non-steroidal anti-inflammatory drugs (NSAIDs) and oral norethisterone (NHS 2014a). Surgical procedures may be operative and used to offer women medical treatment such as myomectomy. Other techniques include uterine artery embolisation and ablation (Grabo *et al.* 1999).

Generally, the medical approach is to monitor, including monitoring haemoglobin (Hb) and ferritin, and treat only if causing a problem. Surgical removal may involve hysterectomy; obviously, this is not desirable if a woman is still trying to conceive. Fibroids are the reason behind approximately 30 per cent of hysterectomies (Evans and Brunsell 2007). Nutritional approaches would be to support the regulation of oestrogen in the body, ongoing weight management and strategies to optimise liver function, especially supporting the pathways (sulphation and glucuronidation) involved in oestrogen conjugation, avoiding oestrogenic foods and environmental oestrogens. General dietary improvement, reducing meat and saturated fat whilst increasing vegetables, fish and legumes, may be beneficial as women with myomas reported more frequent consumption of beef, other red meat and ham, and less frequent consumption of green vegetables, fruit and fish (Courtney 2006). Isoflavonoids available through vegetable and fruit intake have moderate oestrogenic activity and may therefore compete with other stronger endogenous oestrogens. (Refer to the discussion in Chapter 3 for more about oestrogen dominance.)

Chapter 10 contains an overview of the evidence in terms of nutrition. In brief, a sensible dietary approach would be to manage weight and minimise the following:

- Alcohol (regarding supporting liver health as the liver is so important in metabolism).

- Animal fats and dairy foods (regarding liver function and weight management – given these foods are fatty and calorific and adipose tissues can produce oestrogen).

- Ready-made meals in plastic containers (regarding possible exposure to endocrine-disrupting chemicals).

- Pesticides and herbicides (again regarding endocrine disrupters).

- Refined foods and sugars (regarding weight management).

## 2.3 Premature ovarian failure (POF)

This is when menopause occurs before the age of 40, and is believed to affect one per cent of women (Sherman 2000). Hormone replacement therapy (HRT) is recommended until the natural age of menopause. Often no cause is found, but cases fall into two broad types: follicle depletion or follicle malfunction (Lash and Nelson 2009). Possible causes include chromosome abnormalities such as the mutation causing fragile X syndrome (Sherman 2000). Fragile X syndrome is a genetic condition that can affect both males and females causing learning disabilities (The Fragile X Society 2014), but in females it is associated with POF, though not all women with the mutation will develop POF (Lash and Nelson 2009)). Other causes of POF include autoimmune problems such as autoimmune oophoritis (Lash and Nelson 2009) and hormonal problems such as hypothyroidism, Addison's disease (Lash and Nelson 2009) and diabetes and FSH receptor abnormalities. Additionally, metabolic galactosaemia is also implicated in POF's development as galactose and its metabolites may be toxic to the ovaries (Fridovich-Keil *et al.* 2011). In females with galactosaemia lifelong dietary restrict of galactose is recommended (Fridovich-Keil *et al.* 2011).

Signs and symptoms of POF are the same as those of menopause and include hot flushes, insomnia, irritability, depression, poor memory, joint pains, low libido and vaginal dryness. A woman with POF who wishes to have a child may need to be counselled regarding use of donor eggs, adoption or surrogacy. Nutritional strategies to support POF include the consumption of fermented soya products such as tempeh or miso to bolster phytoestrogen intake. As the colonic flora biotransform plant polysaccharides, releasing lignases and isoflavones, the gut flora also play a role in metabolising these valuable phytochemicals, so strategies to support gut function could be considered.

## 2.4 Pelvic inflammatory disease (PID) and tubal problems

Upper genital tract infections can affect the endometrium, the fallopian tubes causing salpingitis and the pelvic peritoneum causing peritonitis. These infections usually result from ascending spread of lower genital tract infections caused by factors such as sexually transmitted infections (STI) or infections from surgery or pregnancy loss. Tubal problems may be associated with ectopic pregnancy, where an embryo implants in the fallopian tube. This can be life-threatening and cause serious complications such as such as pain, bleeding and haemorrhage as there is a risk of rupture and severe blood loss. Intervention is required to end the pregnancy (obviously distressing under any circumstances, but where a woman is pregnant after fertility treatment the emotional implications are considerable – see Chapter 1 for more details about pregnancy loss after infertility). In this scenario, intervention to end the pregnancy can be surgical or pharmacological. If it is diagnosed early, drug treatment may be used to end the pregnancy. Sometimes an ovary or fallopian tube may be lost, causing further problems with fertility.

The most common risk factors for PID include bacterial infections such as *Neisseria gonorrhoeae*, *Chlamydia trachomatis* and other bacterial species found in the vagina, particularly *Bacteroides*, anaerobic gram-positive cocci (*peptostreptococci*), *E. coli* and *Mycoplasma hominis*.

*Chlamydia trachomatis* is the most common sexually transmitted pathogen worldwide (Malhotra *et al.* 2013); it is often asymptomatic and so passed on. Refer to Chapter 9 where a case study involving silent *Chlamydia trachomatis* is presented.

Psychotherapeutic interventions may be key in an integrated approach to help a woman recover from a failed pregnancy or loss of an ovary or fallopian tube. Other approaches in the integrated management would be to support the immune system and wound healing processes in the body. See Chapter 10 on nutrition and dietary factors.

## 2.5 Cancer treatment

Cancer treatments such as chemotherapy or radiotherapy can cause infertility, depending on the types of therapy offered. Oocyte and embryo cryopreservation (freezing and banking) are used wherever possible to preserve fertility. The American Society of Clinical Oncology stated in 2006:

> Oncologists should address the possibility of infertility with patients treated during their reproductive years and be prepared to discuss possible fertility preservation options or refer appropriate and interested patients to reproductive specialists. Clinician judgment should be employed in the timing of raising this issue, but discussion at the earliest possible opportunity is encouraged. Sperm and embryo cryopreservation are considered standard practice and are widely available; other available fertility preservation methods should be considered investigational and be performed in centers with the necessary expertise. (Lee *et al.* 2006)

At the time of writing this chapter, the world's first baby has recently been born from a transplanted womb, so it is important to remember that scientific developments are rapid and can provide hope to many individuals. Where it has not been possible to preserve fertility, patients may need to explore options around the use of donor gametes, adoption or surrogacy.

## 2.6 Other problems with female fertility

There are many other problems with female fertility but unfortunately there is not space in this chapter to cover them all. One of these problems is Asherman's syndrome (AS), which is intrauterine adhesions or scarring characterised by the formation of adhesions inside the uterus and/or the cervix. Women with AS may experience primary and secondary infertility or miscarriage (Conforti *et al.* 2013) as well as menstrual problems such as scanty menstrual periods or amenorrhoea where periods are absent altogether (Yasmin, Nasie and Noorani 2007). In many cases the front and back walls of the uterus stick to one another and this can cause problems with implantation or with repeated fertility treatment failure. Scientific literature has reported sub-cellular modifications to organelles such as ribosomes and mitochondria as well as vascular abnormalities (Conforti *et al.* 2013). Hysteroscopy is used to diagnose and treat the condition (Yasmin *et al.* 2007), though some researchers report a lack of consensus regarding ongoing management (Conforti *et al.* 2013). Psychotherapeutic interventions may be important in an integrated approach, especially if there have been several failed pregnancies. Healthy eating and weight management would also be encouraged.

Other problems include ovarian cysts, which can be a cause for surgical removal of ovarian tissue, thus reducing fertility potential, or even causing the surgical removal of the ovary (oophorectomy). Most ovarian cysts are benign, but a few may become malignant. There are two main types of cyst: functional and pathological (NHS 2014b). Functional cysts form from either the collapsed follicle after an ova has been released or form when the ova is not properly released (NHS 2014b); they can cause pain but often disappear on their own. Pathological cysts are abnormal cell growths (NHS 2014b). Cysts may occur as a result of ovarian stimulation in fertility treatment. Psychotherapeutic interventions may be important in an integrated approach, especially if a woman has lost an ovary or has diminished fertility potential. Healthy eating and weight management would also be encouraged.

There are also other genetic problems such as Turner syndrome, which affects one in 2000 girls, where part of the X chromosome is missing (NHS 2013). There are many other types of chromosomal abnormalities that affect women (some of these are detailed in Chapter 6 on male factor infertility as they affect both genders – see Section 6.7 for further information). Patients may need to be counselled regarding use of donor eggs, adoption or surrogacy.

## References

Anderson, R.A. (2008) 'Chromium and polyphenols from cinnamon improve insulin sensitivity.' *Proceedings of the Nutrition Society 67*, 1, 48–53.

Banker, M., and Garcia-Velasco, J.A. (2015) 'Revisiting ovarian hyper stimulation syndrome: towards OHSS free clinic.' *Journal of Human Reproductive Sciences 8*, 1, 13–17.

Bridges, N.A., Cooke, A., Healy, M.J., Hindmarsh, P.C., and Brook, C.G. (1993) 'Standards for ovarian volume in childhood and puberty.' *Fertility & Sterility 60*, 456–460.

Çakir, E., Topaloğlu, O., Çolak Bozkurt, N., Karbek Bayraktar, B., *et al.* (2014) 'Insulin-like growth factor 1, liver enzymes, and insulin resistance in patients with PCOS and hirsutism.' *Turkish Journal of Medical Sciences 44*, 5, 781–786.

Chen, M.J., Yang, W.S., Yang, J.H., Hsiao, C.K., Yang, Y.S., and Ho, H.N. (2006) 'Low sex hormone-binding globulin is associated with low high-density lipoprotein cholesterol and metabolic syndrome in women with PCOS.' *Human Reproduction 21*, 9, 2266–2271.

Chiaffarino, F., Parazzini, F., La Vecchia, C., Chatenoud, L., Di Cintio, E., and Marsico, S. (1999) 'Diet and uterine myomas.' *Obstetrics & Gynaecology 94*, 3, 395–398.

Conforti, A., Alviggi, C., Mollo, A., De Placido, G., and Magos, A. (2013) 'The management of Asherman syndrome: a review of literature.' *Reproductive Biology Endocrinology 11*, 118.

Courtney, H. (2006) *500 of the Most Important Health Tips You'll Ever Need* (New edition). London: Cico Books.

Ehrmann, D.A., (2005) 'Polycystic Ovary Syndrome.' *New England Journal of Medicine, 352*, 1223.

Evans, P., and Brunsell, S. (2007) 'Uterine fibroid tumors: diagnosis and treatment.' *American Family Physician 75*, 10, 1503–1508.

Farshchi, H., Rane, A., Love, A., and Kennedy, R.L. (2007) 'Diet and nutrition in polycystic ovary syndrome (PCOS): pointers for nutritional management.' *Journal of Obstetrics and Gynaecology 27*, 8, 762–773.

Fridovich-Keil, J.L., Gubbels, C.S., Spencer, J.B., Sanders, R.D., Land, J.A., and Rubio-Gozalbo, E. (2011) 'Ovarian function in girls and women with GALT-deficiency galactosemia.' *Journal of Inherited Metabolic Disease 34*, 2, 357–366.

Gambineri, A., Pelusi, C., Vicennati, V., Pagotto, U., and Pasquali, R. (2002) 'Obesity and the polycystic ovary syndrome.' *International Journal of Obesity and Related Metabolic Disorders 26*, 7, 883–896.

Grabo, T.N., Stewart Fahs, P., Nataupsky, L.G., and Reich, H. (1999) 'Uterine myomas: treatment options.' *Journal of Obstetric, Gynecologic, & Neonatal Nursing 28*, 23–31.

Healthline (2015) *Types of Fibroids*. Available at www.healthline.com/health/uterine-fibroids#Overview1, accessed on 19 May 2015.

Joffe, H.V., Ridker, P.M., Manson, J.E, Cook, N.R., Buring, J.E., and Rexrode, K.M. (2005) 'Sex hormone-binding globulin and serum testosterone are inversely associated with C-reactive protein levels in postmenopausal women at high risk for cardiovascular disease.' *Annals of Epidemiology 16*, 105–112.

Kalgaonkar, S., Almario, R.U., Gurusinghe, D., Garamendi, E.M., Buchan, W., Kim, K., Karakas, S.E. (2001) 'Differential effects of walnuts vs. almonds on improving metabolic and endocrine parameters in PCOS.' *European Journal of Clinical Nutrition* 65, 3, 386–93.

Lash, M., and Nelson, L.M. (2009) 'Primary ovarian insufficiency (aka premature menopause).' *American Society For Reproductive Medicine 17*, 2 May.

Lee, S.J., Schover, L.R., Partridge, A.H., Patrizio, P., *et al.* (2006) 'American Society of Clinical Oncology recommendations on fertility preservation in cancer patients.' *Journal of Clinical Oncology: Official Journal of the American Society of Clinical Oncology 24*, 18, 2917–2931.

Malhotra, M., Sood, S., Mukherjee, A., Muralidhar, S., and Bala, M. (2013). 'Genital *Chlamydia trachomatis*: an update.' *Indian Journal of Medical Research 138*, 3, 303–316.

Malin, S.K., Kirwan, J.P., Sia, C.L., and Gonzalez, F. (2015) 'Pancreatic β-cell dysfunction in polycystic ovary syndrome: role of hyperglycemia-induced nuclear factor-κB activation and systemic inflammation.' *American Journal of Physiology Endocrinology and Metabolism 308*, 9, E770–777.

Melnik, B.C., and Schmitz, G. (2009) 'Role of insulin, insulin-like growth factor-1, hyperglycaemic food and milk consumption in the pathogenesis of acne vulgaris.' *Experimental Dermatology 18*, 10, 833–841.

Mitra, S., Nayak, P.K., and Agrawal, S. (2015). 'Laparoscopic ovarian drilling: an alternative but not the ultimate in the management of polycystic ovary syndrome.' *Journal of Natural Science, Biology, and Medicine 6*, 1, 40–48.

National Health Service (2013) *Turner Syndrome*. Available at www.nhs.uk/Conditions/Turners-syndrome/Pages/Introduction.aspx, accessed on 19 May 2015.

National Health Service (2014a) *Fibroids Treatment*. Available at www.nhs.uk/Conditions/Fibroids/Pages/Treatment.aspx, accessed on 19 May 2015.

National Health Service (2014b) *Ovarian Cyst – Causes*. Available at www.nhs.uk/Conditions/Ovarian-cyst/Pages/Causes.aspx, accessed on 19 May 2015.

Neschen, S., Morino, K., Dong, J., Wang-Fischer, Y., *et al.* (2007) 'N-3 fatty acids preserve insulin sensitivity in vivo in a PPAR{alpha}-dependent manner.' *Diabetes*. Available at http://diabetes.diabetesjournals.org/content/56/4/1034.full, accessed on 19 May 2015.

Office on Women's Health (2012) *Infertility Factsheet*. Washington: Office on Women's Health. Available at www.womenshealth.gov/publications/our-publications/fact-sheet/infertility.html, accessed on 19 May 2015.

Sherman, S.L. (2000) 'Premature ovarian failure in the fragile X syndrome.' *American Journal of Medical Genetics 97*, 3, 189–1 94.

Sirmans, S.M., and Pate, K.A. (2014) 'Epidemiology, diagnosis, and management of polycystic ovary syndrome' *Clinical Epidemiology 6*, 1–13.

The Fragile X Society (2014) *Fragile X Syndrome*. Available at www.fragilex.org.uk/#!syndrome/cndc, accessed on 19 May 2015.

Vuguin, P.M. (2010) 'Interventional studies for polycystic ovarian syndrome in children and adolescents.' *Ped Health 4*, 1, 59–73.

Wallach, E.E. and Vlahos, N.F. (2004) 'Uterine myomas: an overview of development, clinical features and management.' *Obstetrics & Gynaecology 104*, 2, 393–406.

Yasmin, H., Nasir, A., and Noorani, K.J. (2007) 'Hystroscopic management of Ashermans syndrome.' *Journal of the Pakistan Medical Association 57*, 11, 553–555.

# Chapter 5

# Endometriosis

*Dian Shepperson Mills Cert. Ed., BSc Nutrition,*
*BA Education and Psychology, Dip ION*
*Nutritional Therapy, MA, Health Education*
*(Preconceptional Nutrition and Medical Ethics)*

## 1. Introduction

Endometriosis is an enigma, a disease affecting some women during their reproductive years. Prevalence is on a par with asthma, eczema and diabetes, affecting millions of women worldwide. With taboos around menstruation and pain, publicity is low. For many women it is agonising and life-changing. The mystery remains why some women with small patches of endometriosis have severe pain, whilst others develop huge endometriosis implants yet have no pain. More research is required to ascertain how endometriosis implants affect digestion, immune, nervous and endocrine systems. The endometrial implants produce proteins and chemicals (ENDO I and ENDO II, oestrogen and inflammatory prostaglandins PGE2), and these have systemic effects within the body. Implants may be shallow or deep-infiltrating endometriosis (DIE), forming large blood-filled cysts (endometriomas) on/in the ovaries, adhesions pull organs out of place. Orthodox medical treatments use pharmaceutical drugs and surgery. This chapter explores research into the effects of lifestyle and diet upon development and perpetuation of endometriosis. Case studies are also examined to see how changes in dietary consumption of anti-inflammatory foods and nutrients may alter the pain pathways, having beneficial effects upon fertility.

## 2. Endometriosis – what it is and how it affects fertility

Endometriosis affects an estimated 176 million women of reproductive age worldwide and at least 2 million women in the UK (Adamson, Kennedy and Hummelshoj 2010). It is described by Giudice (2010), as an inflammatory condition characterised by lesions of endometrial-like tissue outside the uterus and is associated with pelvic pain and infertility. There is as yet no known cure for endometriosis – the triggers are not understood. Symptoms may begin as soon as menstruation starts. Research is ongoing to discover markers to highlight commonalities in women with the disease. Studies show that the youngest known case was nine years old, the oldest 76 years old (Laufer and Ballweg 2003). Many teenagers have stage 1 or 2 disease (Laufer, Gitein, and Bush *et al.* 1997) however, Roman (2010) found that endometriosis of any stage, I to IV, can be present during adolescence.

### Table 5.1 The American Society for Reproductive Medicine (ASRM) staging system developed in 1992

| | |
|---|---|
| **Stage I**<br>**Minimal** | Small spots of endometriosis, filmy adhesions |
| **Stage II**<br>**Mild** | Small spots of endometriosis, filmy adhesions, small cysts |
| **Stage III**<br>**Moderate** | Larger endometriosis implants, more extensive areas, deep infiltrating endometriosis 3cm deep, organs stick together with dense adhesions. |
| **Stage IV** | The womb, ovaries, bowel and bladder are covered with implants, the abdomen may fill with blood from implants, the organs are adhered together, known as a frozen pelvis |

Women with endometriosis often display a range of pelvic–abdominal-pain symptoms, e.g. painful periods (dysmenorrhoea), painful intercourse (dyspareunia), heavy menstrual bleeding, non-menstrual pelvic pain, pain at ovulation, pain with defecation (dyschezia) and urination (dysuria) as well as chronic fatigue, noted in research conducted by Kennedy and Bergqvist (2005) and Nnoaham and Hummelshoj (2011). Quality of life studies undertaken by Huntingdon and Gilmour (2005), show that symptoms of endometriosis impact on many aspects of a woman's life, including work and education, relationships and social functioning.

## 3. Causes

The causes are thought to be variable retrograde flow of menstrual blood was sited in 1860; other possible causes include immune system failure; viral infections or failure of the peritoneum epithelial tissue. It is therefore multifactorial and includes genetic factors, with possible epigenetic influences, perhaps promoted through environmental exposures to toxins (Nayyar and Bruner-Tran *et al.* 2007).

## 4. Family history

Reports suggest that endometriosis is five to nine times more likely in individuals from families with diagnosed cases. In addition, the disease is more severe and the symptoms more likely to begin at a younger age. These factors are often taken as evidence that the disease is genetic (Kennedy *et al.* 1995).

## 5. What is endometriosis? What are we trying to address?

Endometriosis is recognised as a disease that proliferates in the presence of oestrogen. It appears to be an inflammatory disease with immune system dysfunction, but more research is needed to confirm it as an autoimmune disease (Guo *et al.* 2009). The presence of inflammation may cause extreme pain and fatigue. Chemicals produced by endometriotic implants may compromise fertility. Endometriosis is seen to be more common in atopic/allergic women (Sinaii *et al.* 2002). Pain can reduce normal quality of life.

Researchers think that an imbalance in the three different types of prostaglandins may be one cause of endometriosis pain (Rock and Hurst 1990; Halme 1996, 1997). These studies show that women with severe period pain, infertility and endometriosis had raised levels of prostaglandins series 2 (PGE2 from arachidonic acid) in their peritoneal fluid, which could trigger inflammation – PGE2 appears to affect skin and mucous membranes, causing inflammatory irritable-bowel symptoms. Danish research has shown that women with endometriosis suffer a specific symptom correlation – 'visceral syndrome' – seen to be uncommon in women who do not have endometriosis (Nnoaham *et al.* 2011). The pain in women with endometriosis appears to be more severe than in women without the disease, in a study conducted by Nnoaham *et al.* (2011). In another study conducted by Hansen *et al.* (2014), of 610 women diagnosed with endometriosis in one group, plus 751 women in the control group (without endometriosis), results showed that the endometriosis group had pelvic pain unrelated to menstruation, that is, painful urination and bowel movements, irregular bleeding, constipation, diarrhoea, nausea, vomiting and fatigue. Five out of these seven symptoms were reported ten times more often in women with endometriosis compared with controls (22.7% vs. 2.2%) (Hansen *et al.* 2014). There are serious health consequences for women affected – many years of unbearable pain, reduced quality of life and lack of productivity (Simoens 2012).

High concentrations of prostaglandins at the wrong time could interfere with conception and may prevent fertilisation (Ylikorkala 1984). An excess of prostaglandins PGF2 and PGE2 could cause contractions that are too strong and expel the egg too quickly. Women with endometriosis have been shown, in research conducted by Tummon in 1987, to have smaller, but many more, follicles maturing at the time of ovulation than controls. Inappropriate concentrations of implant-produced prostaglandins could stimulate forced uterine contractions (cramps) at the time of embryo implantation and lead to early expulsion of the embryo (Ylikorkala 1984).

## 6. Oestrogen-dependent pain syndrome

Pam Stratton, Head of Women's Health at the National Institute of Health in the USA, believes that endometriosis is characterised by pelvic-abdominal pain and infertility (Stratton and Berkley 2011), and has elements of a pain syndrome with central-neurological-sensitisation (having some hallmarks of a neurological disorder). Endometriosis, especially deep infiltrating lesions, may be innervated. Endometriotic lesions create a chronic pain syndrome and, together with denervation and re-innervation, may result in accompanying changes in the central nervous system (central sensitisation) (Stratton and Berkley 2011). Meanwhile, Pabona *et al.* (2012) believe that endometriosis is a proliferative, oestrogen-dependent disorder (with growing evidence of progesterone resistance). Research by Osteen and Bruner-Tran at Vanderbilt University in 2014 suggests that environmental toxicants such as TCDD dioxin (2,3,7,8-tetrachlorodibenzo-p-dioxin) play a role in the development of endometriosis, affecting biological progress of the disease through their role as endocrine-disrupting compounds, and may be responsible for the progesterone resistance seen in the endometrium of the disease. Trials looked at mice exposed to TCDD, showing that it leads to progesterone-resistant phenotypes in adult animals that can persist for several generations (Nayyar *et al.* 2007). Indeed, Bruner-Tran, Yeaman *et al.* (2008) suggest that dioxins may promote inflammation-related development of endometriosis.

## 7. Infertility and endometriosis

Endometriosis is associated with infertility. Lessey (2011) states that there is a strong association between severity of disease and impact on fertility. This may be because of impaired fallopian tube and ovarian function, ovarian endometriomas, inflammation of the peritoneal pelvic cavity, with probable reduced egg quality and reduced receptivity within the womb endometrium to implantation (Lessey 2011). Endometriosis and adenomyosis (lesions occurring in the uterine-intramural-muscular layer) reduce the chance of success of assisted reproductive treatment (ART) (Barnhart *et al.* 2002; Maubon *et al.* 2010).

Newer IVF treatments include scratching the endometrium before implanting the embryo. Meta-analysis shows that this approach can improve pregnancy rates in cases of implantation failure (Potdar *et al.* 2012). An endometrial scratch creates a wound site with inflammation for a few days – it is thought that this clears necrotic tissue and bacteria and brings in growth factors. Nutrients essential for healing and rebuilding collagen include vitamins A, C and E, and trace elements such as zinc, iron, copper manganese and selenium (Stanner *et al.* 2009). These nutrients may well help the embryo implantation enzymes to work more efficiently.

The author's consultations with women diagnosed with endometriosis and infertility often reveal that these women have been trying to fall pregnant for up to twelve years or longer. Whilst successful careers progress, their sadness and despair with their infertility grows. Women feel anxious about their failure to fall pregnant, and as natural and IVF efforts falter, they often stop talking about trying at all. Month on month, no conception takes place, or they may suffer from early miscarriages. Sexual intercourse becomes a chore, lack of pregnancy causes monthly distress, and relationships struggle.

## 8. Conventional treatment options and their impact on pregnancy success

Patient surveys and studies in the literature consistently suggest that there is a delay between the onset of symptoms and a surgical diagnosis of 7–13 years (Arruda *et al.* 2003; Sinaii *et al.* 2002; Treloar *et al.* 2002; Hadfield *et al.* 1996). Hence it seems that obtaining a diagnosis of endometriosis is notoriously difficult worldwide, taking around ten years. Severe period pains are often seen as normal and many patients have informally reported to the author that health professionals seem unable to comprehend the severity of the pain caused by the internal bleeding into the peritoneal cavity from the endometriosis implants. (This can happen at any time of the month, not just at the menstrual cycle). The author's clinical experience is that some women have their most severe pains at ovulation or, when ovarian cysts rupture, the pain levels erupt as the bowel is hit by material from within the cyst, triggering acute abdominal spasms. Many women consulting the author have informally reported that Accident and Emergency departments have misdiagnosed the condition as appendicitis, cystitis, irritable bowel syndrome (IBS) or pelvic inflammatory disease (PID) and many women report being sent home with antibiotics instead of a correct diagnosis. Magnetic resonance imaging (MRI) scans are expensive, and ultra-sound scans only reveal large implants. Unless the GP or gynaecologist has extensive experience of endometriosis, then misdiagnosis is common in young teens and women. Endoscopies and colonoscopies come back negative and the women are deemed to have psychosomatic pains and are often put on antidepressants.

## 9. Gold-standard diagnosis

Surgical options are considered when drug treatments fail to solve the pain problem. Laparoscopy is the preferred gold-standard tool for diagnosis; however, laparotomies are now rarely done unless the endometriosis implants or adhesions are in awkward positions. Conservative surgery ensures preservation of the womb and ovaries. Laparoscopy normally involves day surgery. The surgeon enters through the umbilicus and carbon dioxide or nitric oxide gas is pumped in to extend the abdominal cavity to create space for visual identification of implants and adhesion sites, thus allowing for greater ease in moving the ovaries and uterus around in the space created. Laparoscopy allows the best visualisation of lesions, preferably with histological confirmation (in the absence of histological sampling, the false positive rate with laparoscopy visualisation alone may approach 50 per cent) (Wykes *et al.* 2004). Biopsies need to be taken during manual or robotic surgery to check for occult endometriosis, which is invisible to the eye.

After the operation there may be vaginal bleeding, and pains may increase if lasers or diathermy have been used to burn away the adhesions and implants. Some gynaecologists use micro-surgery, in which small cutting instruments are used rather than the burning away of tissue. Complications are around 5–10 per 10,000 (Chandler *et al.* 2001). The skilled endometriosis surgeon will be able to remove the endometriosis implants carefully without damaging surrounding healthy tissues. Ovarian tissue is particularly vulnerable to damage so micro-surgery or use of a laser is finer and causes less damage than diathermy. Adhesions can be removed – as when the ovary and bowel are impacted together.

IBS-type symptoms from adhesions and implants are severe. Intercourse may become painful as adhesions within a frozen pelvis solidify. Ovarian cysts can be drained, but the cyst core must be removed to prevent it refilling afterwards. DIE implants must be removed carefully by a skilled surgeon cutting along the plane of tissues. Adenomyosis (endometriosis within the uterus muscle) can be gently shaved. The skill of a specialist endometriosis surgeon is crucial, so there is need to check on their history and experience; in the UK it is a good idea to check whether the gynaecologist has attended conferences and training courses approved by the Royal College of Obstetrics and Gynaecology (RCOG). Endometriosis Centres of Expertise approved by the British Society of Gynaecological Endoscopy (BSGE) are now springing up.

CA125, a cancer tumour marker for the ovary, may also suggest the presence of endometriosis. Normal levels are below 30. When the reading is very high, cancer is suspected and the test HE4+ROMA should be performed to confirm ovarian carcinoma, as it is a more accurate marker than CA125 alone. HE4+ROMA is a calculated algorithm for pre- and post-menopausal risk of malignant disease (The Doctors Laboratory 2015).

## 10. Multidisciplinary network of endometriosis experts

Worldwide, endometriosis charities are requesting development of Centres of Expertise, as with cancer treatments, staffed by expertly skilled and specifically trained endometriosis surgeons, along with teams from several disciplines (gastroenterologists, dermatologists, immunologists, endocrinologists, neurologists, nutritional therapists, acupuncturists, herbalists and counsellors) to advise on informed choice and treatments. Endometriosis patients have unique case histories needing individualised care. Sometimes treatments require a long time, as health priorities evolve over time and as manifestations of endometriosis change. Women find that their symptoms change as different treatment options progress (D'Hooghe and Hummelshoj 2006).

## 11. Impacts of medication prescribed for endometriosis on fertility

Drug treatments include painkillers, oral contraceptive pills (OCPs), GnRH analogues and antagonists, uterine coils, contraceptive implants, aromatase inhibitors, antidepressants and epilepsy drugs used to dampen neural pains, muscle relaxants and antibiotics. Non-steroidal anti-inflammatory (NSAIDs) drugs such as ibruprofen and naproxen are seen as well-tolerated, low-cost drug treatments (Allen *et al.* 2009). NSAIDs are seen to trigger luteinised unruptured follicle (LUF) syndrome, which impairs ovulation. Research by Koninckx *et al.* (1980) has shown that in LUF syndrome, women will have the normal sequence of endocrine events and a normal menstrual period but their ovary will not release an egg. Steroid-hormone concentrations in peritoneal fluid are much lower after the ovulatory cycle, and this may facilitate the development of endometriosis (Koninickx *et al.* 1980). The British National Formulary (2004) suggests that long-term use of NSAIDs is associated with reduced female fertility, reversible on stopping treatment, advising that 'NSAIDs should not be given to women with fertility problems'. If women are in pain but trying to fall pregnant, they should avoid NSAIDs and ask their GP for a different painkiller. A combination of analgesics, such as paracetamol or opioid-tramadol, are reserved as second line treatment. Other gynaecologists suggest continuous use of the OCP, or the GnRH analogues such as Zoladex (Davis *et al.* 2007; Harada *et al.* 2008; Guzick *et al.* 2011; Vercellini *et al.* 2011). Long-term deprivation of oestrogen with GnRH analogues has serious implications for female health, and for bone density, cardiovascular and neurological systems, well-being and sexual health in particular (De Vas *et al.* 2010).

Use of traditional progestins (synthetic progesterone), medroxyprogesterone acetate, are suggested (Schlaff *et al.* 2006; Crosignani *et al.* 2006; Vercellini *et al.* 2006). Others consider norethisterone helpful in reducing endometriosis symptoms, and some feel that progestins and anti-progestins aid pain reduction (Vercellini *et al.* 2011; Brown *et al.* 2012).

The newer progestins for treatment of endometriosis, dienogest (Visanne), produce side-effects of breast tenderness, rashes, nausea and irritability (Strowitzki, Faustman *et al.* 2010; Momoeda *et al.* 2009; Kohler *et al.* 2010). Research showed that a 2mg dose per day of Dienogest effectively alleviated painful symptoms, reducing endometriotic lesions and improving quality of life (Schindler 2011; Strowitzki, Faustmann *et al.* 2010; Strowitzki, Marr *et al.* 2010; Petraglia *et al.* 2012). The Mirena and junior JayDee coils give a slow constant release of the progestin hormone levonorgestrel, remaining in place for three years, preventing pregnancy and controlling heavy periods.

Many painkillers are tested on males under laboratory conditions. Often women comment that painkillers dull them as a person whilst the pain stays. Trying to drive to work and hold down a full-time career during days of immense period pain whilst on medication affects concentration, so finding the correct painkillers may help maintain a career. Women often say 'What could we have been without endometriosis?' as regular cyclic menstrual pain affects career prospects and causes tribulation in relationships as sexual intercourse becomes painful.

## 12. Possible links between endometriosis and other conditions that affect fertility

Coeliac disease, thyroid problems and immune abnormalities are implicated in reduced fertility. Women diagnosed with coeliac disease may fall pregnant but have increased rates of miscarriage. Men with coeliac disease show reduced male hormone levels and reduced sperm count. Both have immunological and hormonal abnormalities (Jones 2006). Coeliac disease should be tested for and ruled out with infertility, as explored in Chapter 7.

A study by Marziali (2012) in Italy shows that painful symptoms of endometriosis decrease after 12 months on a gluten-free diet. Two hundred and seven patients entered the study, diagnosed with endometriosis and chronic pelvic pain. After 12 months, 75 per cent of the patients reported a statistically significant change in painful symptoms. Twenty-five per cent reported improvement of symptoms, and no patients reported worsening of pain (Marziali 2012). Research by Shepperson Mills (2011a) showed that 85 per cent of women whilst off wheat/gluten for three months reported that their endometriosis pain was reduced by fifty per cent.

Coeliac disease is triggered by a specific antigen, the gluten/gliadin protein, and zonulin is then expressed (Fasano *et al.* 2000; Fasano 2010). Zonulin regulates the permeability and integrity of the epithelial tissue in the body (Lu 2000). Gliadin affects zonulin expression even in people without the gene for coeliac disease (Drago *et al.* 2006).

There are 300 billion bacteria living inside our small intestinal gut flora and they collectively express 100-fold more genes than the human genome (Rabizadeh and Sears 2008). The Human Genome Project (Nicolle 2007) showed that man has 23,000 genes which we inherit from our parents, whilst the healthy gut flora passengers in our microbiome contain at least four million genes. Gut flora work constantly on our behalf, manufacturing vitamins B and K, preventing infections by building 80 per cent of immunoglobulins and aiding digestion. Damage to the gut membrane by gliadin alters the way gut flora behave. Research suggests that gut bacteria may even alter our brain chemistry, affecting moods and behaviour (Blaser and Falkow 2009). Healthy gut flora are crucial for oestrogen metabolism in the intestine and liver. Research by Khalili, a Harvard gastroenterologist, and colleagues (Khalili *et al.* 2013) suggests that in susceptible women with high-risk genes, taking the contraceptive pill triples the risk of Crohn's disease, in one in every 650 people; the OCP is taken by 3.5 million women at present in Britain. The change in a woman's sex hormone profile can make the gut lining more permeable and reduce levels of 'friendly' bacteria in the intestines, thus disrupting immune system function. If women have these genes they should be advised not to take the OCP. This study looked at 1500 women, one-third of whom had Crohn's disease, with malabsorption of nutrients affecting reproduction. Small bowel gut-flora produces 80 percent of all the immunoglobulin-producing cells in the body: healthy flora is the largest immune organ in the body (Shanahan 1994).

··· BOX 5.1 FOODS TO SUPPORT GUT FLORA ·····················

▶ Avocado

▶ Raw coconut cream

▶ Flaxseeds

▶ Sauerkraut

▶ Chicory

▶ Jerusalem artichokes

▶ Fresh vegetable juice

▶ Blueberries

▶ Cucumber

▶ Tomatoes

▶ Live kefir and yoghurt

▶ Coconut kefir.

Body fat cells, ovaries and adrenal glands produce oestrogen. Healthy gut flora and liver enzymes break down the used oestrogen into a safe form ready to be bound to soluble fibre such as oats (wheat is insoluble fibre) within the gut. Safe forms of oestrogen can be excreted from the body within stools. Blood-levels of oestrogen are affected by activity of bacterial enzymes in the intestine and drop significantly when activity is reduced (Gorbach and Goldin 1992). If oestrogen remains in the body it can cause havoc. Eating green leafy vegetables (containing indoles) and soluble fibres (oats and vegetable fibres) helps reduce levels. Oestrogen excess acutely inhibits the rate of thyroxine release from the thyroid in adults, but any effect appears to be transient (Gambert 1991). Testing for thyroid disease seems to be warranted in all women and men with unexplained infertility (Weetman 1997). Autoimmune thyroid diseases are thought to be involved in infertility and thyroid antibodies are used to predict women at risk for early miscarriage (Singh *et al.* 1995; Jones 2006; Ciacci *et al.* 1996). Thyroid peroxide antibodies (TPO-Ab) are the main antibody indicators of possible thyroid disease and their appearance usually precedes the development of thyroid disorders (Dayan 2001).

Hypothyroidism is a significant risk factor for infertility, especially in women with endometriosis (Poppe and Velkeniers 2002). High or normal thyroid hormone is protective against cancer, while low thyroid hormone is thought to invite it. High oestrogen invites cancer (and endometriosis), whereas normal oestrogen lessens its development (Fredericks 1989). Oestrogen and thyroxine (built from iodine) have to be in balance in the body. Eating iodine contained in some fish or seaweed in a healthy diet is important as it is a precursor to thyroxine production and so is vital for thyroid function. Foods containing goitrogens should be eaten cooked if diagnosed as hypothyroid.

## BOX 5.2 ANTI-THYROID FOODS –
··· GOITERGENS – HIGH OXALATES ·····························

Soya and wheat are both phyto-oestrogens and in excess imbalance thyroxine. Eat the following vegetables and fruits cooked to reduce the goitergen effect if diagnosed as hypothyroid: cabbage, broccoli, Brussels sprouts, turnips, kale, spinach, peaches and pears.

(Shepperson Mills and Vernon 2002)

Excessive thyroid production is found in 4.2 per cent of people with coeliac disease and underactivity of the thyroid gland is found in 13 per cent of coeliac patients (Glinoer et al. 1994; Collin et al. 1994; Cuoco et al. 1999). Some researchers recommend all autoimmune-thyroid patients be routinely screened for coeliac disease as there appears to be an overlap (Glinoer et al. 1994; Collin et al. 1994; Cuoco et al. 1999). Correct treatment (avoiding gluten) lowers inflammatory responses and antibody levels, reducing inflammation in the thyroid and the gut (Counsell et al. 1994).

Oestrogen has profound effects on the body and the menstrual cycle. It causes the womb lining to thicken and can prolong menstruation time. It stimulates the nervous system causing copper levels to increase and zinc to decrease, and it stimulates high corticosteroid levels (Lee 1994). It stimulates breast tissue and is linked to breast and uterine cancer when unopposed at high levels (Grant 1994) causing body fat deposits to increase and impairing blood sugar control. High oestrogen reduces thyroxine hormone and may produce a hypothyroid state. Bifidobacteria encourage oestrogen clearance by inhibiting an enzyme known as beta glucoronidase. When high this encourages the deactivated safe oestrogen to become reactivated so that it can be sent back into circulation (this is not good with endometriosis). In this scenario acidophilus use seems to be helpful (Shepperson-Mills and Vernon 2002).

## 13. Effects of lifestyle factors on endometriosis

Physical activity may increase levels of sex hormone-binding globulin (SHBG) (An et al. 2000) or lower luteal oestrogen (Tworoger et al. 2007) and reduce insulin resistance (Stoll 2000). Exercise is very important to reduce oestrogen levels (An et al. 2000; Tworoger et al. 2007; Stoll 2000). Movement tones muscles, keeps heart and lungs fit, massages the digestive tract and ensures lymph circulates, keeping the immune system healthy. Exercise raises levels of endorphins (brain chemicals which are natural painkillers) helping elevate mood (Granges and Littlejohn 1993). There are many other benefits of exercise: for example, walking or swimming helps muscles increase the number of mitochondria (organelles which make energy) (Clayton 2004; Shepperson-Mills and Vernon 2002). The content of mitochondria improves with exercise (Elizabeth et al. 2006). A British Medical Journal study found that if patients with chronic fatigue started slowly with just 5 to 15 minutes of walking, 5 days a week, they tolerated it well (Fulcher and White 1997), this might be helpful advice to those with endometriosis. Exercise is discussed in further detail in Chapter 11.

## 14. Dioxins and subfertility

Reducing toxic exposures is crucial to reduce onset of endometriosis. Toxic effects of dioxins and PCBs, phthalates and bisphenol A (BPA) are well known endocrine-disruptors, damaging the embryo, foetus and newborns, and women with endometriosis (Birnbaum 1994; Nayyar et al. 2007). Endocrine-disrupting chemicals (phthalates, BPA, dioxins, PCBs) settle into body fat cells, causing inflammation in endometriosis (Bruner-Tran, Yeaman et al. 2008). Mammals are very sensitive to toxicants during their development. Simple dietary modifications, including essential omega-3 fatty acids, reduced the impact of TCDD on progesterone-receptor expression, improving pregnancy outcomes (Bruner-Tran, Crispens *et al.* 2008).

TCDD-concentrations in the breast milk of women in Belgium are among the highest in the world (WHO Environmental series 1992) (Koninickx *et al.* 1994). The association between human endometriosis and PCBs was first suggested by Gerhard and Runnebaum (1992). The 2001 study demonstrated both elevated serum TCDD and elevated serum triglycerides in monkeys exposed to dioxin (Rier 2001).

Exposure to TCDD (dioxin) and xeno-oestrogens from contaminated fatty foods such as meat and dairy probably reduces fertility – these factors are explored further in Chapter 11. Two dietary mechanisms that may help to counteract these effects are supplementation of cleaned omega-3 fatty acids and vitamin B3 (nicotinamide). MK Johnson of the Medical Research Council reported in 1975 that nicotinamide (vitamin B3) was the only nutrient that would take the organophosphate-pesticides out through the liver. More research is required to investigate the profound effects on human fertility and health, as epigenetic and transgenerational effects encompass several generations. Research in Australia suggests that organic foods cleanse the body, and whilst it is only a small-scale study, results look promising. After eating organic food for one week, pesticide levels were cut by 90 per cent (Oates *et al.* 2014). Thirteen people were given a diet of 80 per cent organic food for seven days, then the diet was changed to seven days on 80 per cent conventional food. Urine samples were taken each week on day seven. The researchers tested for six chemicals, including organophosphates, and dialkyl phosphates (DAPs). The body produces DAPs as it attempts to break down pesticides. In the organic food group, DAP levels were 89 per cent lower than in those eating foods containing pesticides (Oates *et al.* 2014).

### Table 5.2 The dirty dozen (Environmental Working Group 2012)

| Most contaminated (buy organic) | Least contaminated |
|---|---|
| 1. Peaches | 1. Onions |
| 2. Apples | 2. Avocado |

| | |
|---|---|
| 3. Sweet bell peppers | 3. Sweetcorn |
| 4. Celery | 4. Pineapple |
| 5. Nectarines | 5. Mango |
| 6. Strawberries | 6. Asparagus |
| 7. Cherries | 7. Sweet peas |
| 8. Pears | 8. Kiwi fruits |
| 9. Grapes | 9. Bananas |
| 10. Spinach | 10. Cabbage |
| 11. Lettuce | 11. Broccoli |
| 12. Potatoes | 12. Papaya |

## 15. Effects of nutrition (good and bad) on endometriosis

Dietary factors have been the focus of a growing number of endometriosis patient-directed books and websites. A hospital-based Italian case-controlled study on 504 patients observed a statistically significant protective effect of current green vegetable (OR=0.3; CI=0.2–0.5) and fruit (OR=2.0; CI=1.4–2.8) consumption and a significant risk of endometriosis with greater red meat consumption (OR=2.0; CI=1.4–2.8) (Parazzini *et al.* 2004). The research also showed that women who eat meat once a day are up to twice as likely to have endometriosis compared with those who eat less red meat and more fruit and vegetables.

Diets high in saturated animal fat are seen to increase concentrations of serum oestrogen, so eating in moderation is important (Nagata *et al.* 2000). Studies by Goldin *et al.* in 1982 have shown that women with the highest intake of red meat increase their risk of endometriosis by between 80 and 100 per cent, while those with the highest intake of fresh fruit and vegetables lowered their risk of endometriosis by 40 per cent. Reducing consumption of foods high in saturated fats and replacing them with fruit and vegetables such as broccoli, cauliflower and cabbage, which contain indoles (compounds that break oestrogen down), improves oestrogen metabolism (Goldin *et al.* 1982; Gorbach and Goldin 1987). Vegetarian women excrete 2–3 times more oestrogen in their stools and have 50 per cent lower free oestrogen in their blood compared with meat eaters. High-fibre diets may help explain lower pre-menstrual-syndrome symptoms, as excess oestrogen binds to soluble fibre and can then be excreted from the body (Goldin *et al.* 1982).

Randomised controlled trials (RCTs) show that dietary intervention (vitamins, minerals, salts, lactic ferments and fish oils) following endometriosis surgery appears to be an effective alternative to hormone treatment that is associated with similar pelvic pain reduction and quality of life improvement (Sesti *et al.* 2007; Sesti *et al.* 2009). A small trial on patients with dysmenorrhoea by Proctor and Murphy in 2001 showed that fish oils (omega-3 fatty acids) were more effective than placebo for pain relief. Cellular immunity is reduced in women with endometriosis (Ishimura and Masuzaki 1991). The presence of endometriosis increased oxidative stress, and depletion of anti-oxidants may contribute to excessive growth of endometrial cells (Foyouzi *et al.* 2004; Shanti *et al.* 1999). Research also suggests that vitamins B1 and B6 are beneficial (Proctor and Murphy 2001) while the use of magnesium also shows some benefit in pain reduction (Proctor and Murphy 2001).

Oxidative stress has been implicated in the pathogenesis of infertility related to endometriosis. A positive association between advanced endometriosis stage and increased serum levels of hyperperoxides suggesting an increased production of reactive-species in women with endometriosis III/IV. Donabela *et al.* (2010) demonstrated decreased levels of glutathione.

Missmer *et al.* (2007) found that trans-fats (hydrogenated oils) are linked to an increased risk of endometriosis and omega-3 fish oils are linked to a lower risk. 120,000 US nurses (25–42 years of age) not diagnosed with endometriosis were tracked over 12 years. Those who developed endometriosis were eating diets higher in trans-fats (Missmer *et al.* 2007; Missmer *et al.* 2010). In a group of Danish women, a higher intake of omega-3 fatty acids or a higher ratio of omega-3/omega-6 fatty acids was associated with reduced menstrual pain (Deutch 1995). Women should reduce their saturated and trans-fatty-acid intake by half, then oestrogen levels would be 20 per cent lower. This research advised the use of oily fish, nuts, seeds, dark leafy vegetables, cold-pressed extra virgin olive and walnut oils (Parazzini *et al.* 2004). Dietary fibre increases excretion of excess oestrogen from the body; fibres such as lignins in rye and seeds are changed by gut flora to form anti-oestrogen compounds, which protect against cancers (Stock 1995) and probably endometriosis.

Eating moderate saturated fats and cold pressed cis-oils is vital for hormone production and fat-soluble vitamin storage. Soluble fibre binds to oestrogen and inhibits its reabsorption. 'Good quality fibre encourages a hormone known as SHBG... Whilst oestrogen is bound to the SHBG, it cannot exert any biological effect within the body' (Cowan 1981). If fibre intake is low then the oestrogen has a biological effect, triggering endometrial implant growth. Vegetarian, low-fat diets reduced period pain and increased SHBG (Barnards *et al.* 2000).

Eating vegetables from the cruciferous family, rich in B complex vitamins and magnesium, such as cabbage, sprouts, broccoli, cauliflower, kale, turnip, swede, radish, horseradish, mustard and cress, is protective. Brassica vegetables contain three compounds – indoles, dithiolethiones and isothiocyanates. These influence enzymes that rev up the body's degradation system, so that oestrogen is 'metabolised' and ultimately excreted from the body (Cowan 1981).

Other protective factors may be the phytoestrogens from a moderate soy intake and a high natural level of selenium in foods (Spallholz *et al.* 1973). Phytoestrogens are coumestans, isoflavones and lignans. Coumestans are in split-peas, pinto and lima beans and alfalfa; isoflavones are in soy, green beans, chick peas, peanuts and red clover; lignans are in flax/linseed and sesame seeds, oat, nuts and other plant foods. While phytoestrogens are orders of magnitude less potent than natural oestrogen made within the body, nevertheless an excess of phytoestrogens may not be beneficial as they can cause hormonal disruption; there is enormous complexity in phytoestrogen biochemistry. Women's body biochemistry varies, especially where exposed to xeno-oestrogens (pesticides and plasticisers). If liver function is disrupted, oestrogen biotransformation and clearance may be compromised.

Table 5.3 Food sources of oestrogen (Shepperson Mills and Vernon 2002)

**Should be eaten in moderation, not to excess:**

| | | | | |
|---|---|---|---|---|
| Chickpeas | Chasteberry | Cloves | Yams | Nettle |
| Beans | Caffeine | Chamomile | Parsley | Barley |
| Lentils | Carrots | Barley | Pumpkin | Dandelion |
| Rye | Sunflower seeds | Aniseed | Apples | Spices |
| Alfalfa | Pomegranate | Corn | Green beans | Pepper |
| Citrus fruits | Fennel | Papaya | Oats | Turmeric |
| Soy (milk, tofu) | Liquorice | Potatoes | Peas | Almond |
| Flaxseeds | Oregano | Squash | Red Beans | Peanuts |
| Red clover | Cumin | Cucumber | Olives | Wheat |
| Black cohosh | Plums | Beetroot | Clover | Farmed fish |
| Dong quai | Nutmeg | Cherries | Pears | Rice |

## 16. Case studies

There is no single 'correct' intervention programme for a given situation. Real-world specific interpretations and prescriptions differ between practitioners presented with the same case, as they have different experiences and knowledge. Scientific literature and data may be controversial, incomplete and at times contradictory. Decisions should be informed and reflect biochemical imbalances (Nicolle and Woodriff-Beirne 2010). We must treat each patient as a unique individual and look at their particular needs in their case with functional integrated medicine (Grimaldi *et al.* 2003).

The author uses a MYMOP medical audit 'measure yourself medical outcome profile' form from the Medical Research Council (MRC) with each patient at consultations, for example with scores dropping from 3.3 to 0.75 during the course of the programme. MYMOP was devised by Dr Charlotte Paterson of MRC. The research looked at symptoms, activity, medications, supplements and dietary changes (Paterson 1996). The data is collected on the Clinic-Aid database so that research statistics can be analysed (Mills 2011). This can be done individually to watch the progress of each client or for 100–200 clients to assess overall improvements and look for a commonality within the cohort (Shepperson Mills 2011b).

Table 5.4 Results of the Endometriosis and
Fertility Clinic UK (Shepperson Mills 2006)

| MYMOP-collated results: in measurements on 198 women taken over 6 months: |
|---|
| 50 per cent reported reduction in pain scores |
| 34 per cent reported infertility as a problem |
| 52 per cent of the subfertile group fell pregnant |
| 26 per cent of the rest fell pregnant |
| 82 per cent reported adverse reactions from wheat |
| 55 per cent reported adverse reactions from bovine dairy food |

## 17. Case history 1

This lady presented with viral ear infection and endometriosis. Puberty was age ten years, with pains beginning five years later. The GP prescribed Ponstan (mefenamic acid), an NSAID. At 19 years, weight was low and periods ceased until age twenty, when blood loss lasted three weeks, so the GP prescribed the cyclic OCP for three years continuously, but daily spotting occurred. From 24 to 31 years she stopped the OCP and felt fine, but failed to fall pregnant. By 37 years (on continuous OCP) she became unwell, having weeks off work with vertigo, exhaustion, ear infections, constant antibiotics and pains in the right ovary. The GP dismissed this as a grumbling appendix. She haemorrhaged and was rushed to A&E. A scan showed a failed pregnancy. The bowel was stuck by adhesions to the womb and ovaries. An operation removed the adhesions and mild endometriosis. Small implants were lasered from the bowel, bladder, ovaries, cervix and Pouch of Douglas.

She was put on Prostap SR (leuprorelin acetate) for three months, but side-effects were severe so she stopped treatment. IVF was offered but she felt too ill. Six months later scans showed endometriosis implants. Periods lasted six days with brown sludge-like blood, with a 26-day cycle. She experienced sharp-glass cutting pain lasting for twenty-one days. Quality of life was poor. The pain did not resolve after the laparoscopy.

Her husband carried her into the first consultation and the priority was to reduce pain. Digestion was compromised with bloating, constipation and discomfort. Fertility was on hold until health improved, after spending 22 years using the medical route to treat abnormal bleeding, pain and infertility. Limited finances meant concentrating on using fresh foods and a few quality supplements.

### 17.1 Dietary advice

A vegetarian, she ate mainly green beans and lettuce. The main source of protein was from dairy, so goat, sheep and buffalo sources were recommended with more eggs, nuts, seeds and pulses to vary the protein intake and increase cis-fatty-acid intake to reduce inflammation. Proanthocyanidins (berries) and pine bark were used to reduce inflammation (Masquelier 1981).

Dysbiosis was suspected, so cooked green leafy vegetables were recommended for the first two weeks, to help reduce the inflamed gut membrane and increased magnesium intake. Green vegetables contain indoles, which aid oestrogen balance in the body, and vegans have a greater excretion of oestrogen in the stools. Recipes and menu suggestions included two weeks of vegan and two weeks of vegetarian menu plans, to increase variety in her intake of nutrients from foods.

## 17.2 Nutritional supplement protocol

### ··· BOX 5.3 NUTRITIONAL SUPPLEMENTS ························

Recommended for the first 4 weeks (revised monthly):

> Multivitamin-mineral (25mg B complex, low iron), 1 at breakfast
>
> Microcell essential fatty acids (1000mg linseed, 660mg borage oil), 1 at breakfast, 1 at dinner
>
> Magnesium malate (116mg), 1–2 at dinner
>
> Vitamin E (300IU), 1 at breakfast (optional)
>
> Bioacidophilus (20 billion LAB4B complex),1 at breakfast
>
> Vegan digestive enzymes, 1 at dinner.

A multivitamin-mineral with iron was suggested due to the extreme fatigue, pale skin, eyelids and nails, weak nails and itchy legs and as the GP test showed low iron status (Chavarro et al. 2006). The B vitamin content would also assist with energy production, as could the vitamin C and magnesium (Chavarro et al. 2008). The B vitamins, B1, B6 and B12, are involved with pain reduction (Greenwood 1964; Misra et al. 1977). Additionally, low B vitamins (folic acid, vitamin B12) may lead to elevated homocysteine levels which can predispose women to early miscarriage (Bohles et al. 1999).

Eicosanoids are vital hormone-like substances involved in important cellular functions. As a vegetarian, omega-3 fatty acids were used from hemp, linseed and walnut oils. Lignans from flaxseed stimulate production of SHBG (Haggans et al. 1999; Martin *et al.* 1996). This was to balance a higher ratio of omega-3 to omega-6 fatty acids to help reduce menstrual pain (Deutch 1995).

Advice was given to reduce saturated and trans-fatty-acid intake by half – hoping to reduce oestrogen levels and to use nuts, seeds, leafy vegetables and cold pressed extra virgin olive oil. These foods are also rich in minerals. Adequate calcium and magnesium are important preventatives against miscarriage (Molina 2005). Magnesium from vegetables also relaxes smooth muscle and produces ATP (adenosine triphosphate) which produces energy; deficiency is associated with cramps, spasms and convulsions (Bell *et al.* 1975).

Probiotics inhibit the faecal bacterial enzymes, which convert oestrogen to more toxic forms and decrease the reabsorption of excreted, detoxified oestrogen. Soluble fibre (wheat-free gluten-free oats) absorbs degraded oestrogen for excretion. Eating onions, asparagus, pectin from fruits, alginates from seaweed, oat bran, vegetables, nuts, seeds, bananas and maple syrup encourages good gut flora. Herbal teas such as lemon and ginger, sweet peppermint and fennel were recommended to support digestion. Lime-blossom tea was also advised to relax the nervous system.

··· **BOX 5.4 TEST RESULTS** ························································

| Gliadin antibodies (IgG) | Gliadin Antibodies (IgA) |
|---|---|
| Negative: <7 U/ml | Negative: <7 U/ml |
| Equivocal: 7-10 U/ml | Equivocal: 7-10 U/ml |
| Positive: >10 U/ml | Positive: >10 U/ml |

Gluten grains were avoided: wheat, rye, oats, barley, spelt, etc. The gluten-sensitivity blood test came back positive and then a biopsy was done. After eating corn, rice, buckwheat, millet, quinoa, banana, chestnut, arrowroot and tapioca she felt well.

## 17.3 Summary

This lady's energy levels improved. Research shows that many individuals without apparent symptoms who are found to have coeliac disease remark on a new-found vitality and sense of wellbeing when started on a gluten-free diet (Cronin and Shahan 1997). Pain levels were alleviated by normal wheat-free paracetamol. Periods consisted of red blood for five days only, moderate flow, and felt 'fantastic'. Digestion was improved and normal peristalsis returned. 'I have a life now – a good quality of life, I'm not just existing any more. My husband says I am a new woman. I have never felt this good before. Pain is greatly reduced, energy levels are higher, and this is a home full of laughter again.' After six months they fell pregnant and a healthy little boy was born.

## 18. Case history 2

This lady presented with a diagnosis of period pain, polycystic ovaries and fibroids and was being managed by treatment with ibuprofen and tranexamic acid. The GP suggested the OCP but as pregnancy was being attempted she refused, and in the past OCP use had triggered depression. The laparoscopy had been undertaken seven days earlier. Severe stage IV endometriosis had been diagnosed, adhesions in the abdomen had been discovered and both tubes were blocked and both ovaries had endometriomas. The gynaecologist left the endometriosis and adhesions in situ. He suggested the OCP or GnRH analogues as treatment to dry out endometriotic tissue over six months. After the operation, periods worsened and became ten days long with brown-sludge-like blood. Shortly after, she was rushed to A&E with a ruptured ovarian cyst and was sent home with opiate painkillers.

Periods began when she was aged 11 years; they were always heavy with debilitating pain. Bleeds lasted ten days and the blood was dark red with large brown/black clots. Mefenamic acid (NSAID) helped reduce pains, but PMS was seven days of agitation, weeping, breast pain, fatigue and headaches. The GP suggested antidepressants but she refused. She reported that sleep was never refreshing. Teeth-grinding was severe with a tooth guard worn at night, indicating high stress levels. Heels on her feet were cracked, memory was poor and she felt clumsy when pre-menstrual. It was suspected that adrenal stress was manifesting with the teeth-grinding (bruxism) being indicative of low vitamin B5 levels (Pelton *et al.* 1999). She was in a very stressed state, as her brother had just been diagnosed with ulcerative colitis and her father with suspected bowel cancer. Her mother was in remission from breast cancer. With fertility threatened and three sick family members to support, it was all too much. Digestive problems included daily bloating, burning sensations in the abdomen; she reported that peppermint tea helped. She also craved everything sweet, including sugary cakes, biscuits and chocolates. She experienced night sweats and thirst.

A referral to the John Radcliffe Hospital Specialist Endometriosis Centre in Oxford was organised. Fertility would improve only after an operation to remove the endometriosis implants, cysts, adhesions and unblock the fallopian tubes. Before operations all supplements were stopped for five days.

Tests for blood sugar balance ruled out diabetes. Chromium is the mineral involved in insulin production, with excellent glucose-lowering properties and anti-oxidant activity in the liver and kidneys (Lieberman *et al.* 2007). Nutritional intervention such as for subclinical chromium deficiency can be supported if metabolic syndrome develops (Kelly 2000).

Conserving fertility was paramount. Digestion may have been compromised by the NSAIDs used to alleviate the pain, known to trigger bleeding in the gut and deplete folic acid (Pelton *et al.* 1999).

Breakfast included muesli with live yoghurt, lunch was a sandwich, with fish, meat and vegetables for dinner. Diet Coke was drunk daily, containing aspartame, and care must be taken during pre-conception until more research is done to show safety levels (Roberts 1990).

## 18.1 Tests

The GP tested red cell magnesium, iron and vitamin D levels. The red cell magnesium levels were borderline (normal range being 2.08 to 3.00). Research shows a strong link between magnesium deficiency and insulin resistance (Humphries *et al.* 1999). Vitamin D levels were fine. Homocysteine test was fine (Forges 2007). The GP tests showed that haemoglobin was low at 9.8mg. Two hundred mg of ferrous sulphate caused constipation and black stools; this was changed to iron citrate and vitamin C as better tolerated. Research shows that low iron may lead to anovulatory infertility (Chavarro *et al.* 2006). She was eating frozen foods such as pineapple and berries. This compulsive desire to chew ice happens with low iron levels and is known as pagophagia (Parry-Jones 1992; Watts 1999). The use of vitex-agnus-castus (through

Specialist Herbal Supplies – UK-registered medical herbalist advice) helped normalise menstrual function by supporting pituitary function. It corrects luteal phase defects and improves menstrual irregularities, affecting the hypothalamic–pituitary axis (Trickey 1998).

The magnesium, essential fatty acids in the fish oils and the selenium were used to reduce inflammation. Research has shown that women with endometriosis have lower anti-oxidant intakes of vitamin C, vitamin E, selenium and zinc (Hernandes-Guerrero *et al.* 2006). The presence of endometriosis, increased oxidative stress and depletion of anti-oxidants (Foyouzi *et al.* 2004) suggest that this may contribute to excessive growth of endometrial cells.

## 18.2 Dietary advice

A more hunter-gatherer style diet was recommended: cook everything from fresh whenever possible, use oily and white fish three times a week, lean pasture-fed meat (wild game or lamb), fresh fruits and vegetables in season, and berries to help reduce inflammation; avoid oranges and grapefruits. Bovine dairy was reduced, in favour of goat, sheep and buffalo sources. Wheat was excluded from the diet as the GP blood test showed gluten sensitivity and following biopsy coeliac disease was diagnosed. When a first-degree relative is diagnosed it is crucial that all relatives be tested (both brother and father tested positive for coeliac disease). After two months, digestion improved. Slippery elm was recommended to help the gut-membrane, reducing IBS and constipation. Gut flora balance was supported with acidophilus to increase the body's own B vitamin production. The use of B vitamins seems to be crucial for women with endometriosis, and regular use of multivitamin supplements may decrease the risk of ovulatory infertility (Chavarro *et al.* 2008).

Energy improved, sleep became refreshing and deep. No painkillers were being used at this point, but she was taking the homeopathic remedy Mag phos. A Cambridge Nutritional Sciences Food Intolerance Test was performed and showed reactions to wheat, rice, rye, almond, Brazil, cashew, cow's dairy, whole egg, peanuts, soya beans, cocoa beans and yeasts. Menu plans were written and recipes found for corn, millet, buckwheat, quinoa, chestnut, banana, coconut flour, tapioca and arrowroot.

## 18.3 Nutritional supplement protocol

The judicious use of nutritional supplements whilst the diet is being corrected may improve reproductive health. Harvard University and the American Dietetics Association both advise that a multivitamin-mineral should be taken each day (Willett and Stampfer 2006). Basic supplements (see * in Box 5.5) were used for one month, then changes made were reviewed monthly.

··· BOX 5.5 NUTRITIONAL SUPPLEMENTS ··························

*Multivitamin-mineral, 1 per day (low-dose Vitamin A, 25mg B complex, no iron)

*Omega-3 fish oil (1200mg-5:1DHA/EPA), 1 at breakfast, 1 at dinner

Vitamin E (200IU), 1 at lunch

Magnesium taurine (146mg), 1 at breakfast (supports bile production)

*Magnesium malate (116mg), 1 at dinner (supports energy in Kreb cycle)

Magnesium plus pantothenate (400mg), 1 per day

Chromium (110µg), 1 drop per day

*Permatrol (1 billion acidophilus, 700mg glutamine), 1–2 a day

Slippery elm (600mg), 1–2 a day.

Supplements were used according to test results. Fifty-five per cent of all women in their childbearing years reported taking vitamin-mineral supplements (Czeizel *et al.* 1998). Should women at high risk for nutritional inadequacy be given a supplement as part of a pre-conceptional care programme (Keen *et al.* 1994)? More research is required in this area to look at the needs of women in the population where poor nutrition may be a factor in the present UK births, with high levels of low birth weight and premature babies.

## 18.4 Lifestyle advice

Gentle exercise was undertaken, as BMI was 27. Fresh air and natural daylight are supportive of pituitary function, so walks at lunchtime were important. People at work were noticing improvement and commented that she was 'glowing'.

## 18.5 Nutritional therapy

After correcting iron and magnesium levels we used anti-oxidants to support immune system function. The period pains became normal mild aches, tolerable without medication. Supplements were reduced to one B complex, omega-3 fish oil, magnesium and probiotic. Four months after the operation she fell pregnant and later a healthy son was born.

# References

Adamson, G.D., Kennedy, S.H., and Hummelshoj, L. (2010) 'Creating solutions in endometriosis: global collaboration through World Endometriosis Research Foundation.' *Journal of Endometriosis 2*, 13–16.

Allen, C., Hopewell, S., *et al.* (2009) 'Non-steroidal anti-inflammatory drugs for pain: women with endometriosis.' *Cochrane Database of Systematic Reviews 2*, CD004753.

An, P., Rice, T., Gagnon, J., *et al.* (2000) 'Genetic study of sex-hormone-binding-globulin measured before-and-after 20 week endurance-exercise training programme: Heritage-family-study.' *Metabolism 49*, 1014–1020.

Arruda, M.S., Petta, C.A., *et al.* (2003) 'Time elapsed from onset of symptoms of endometriosis in a cohort study of Brazilian women.' *Human Reproduction 18*, 756–759.

Barnards, N.D., Scialli, A.R., *et al.* (2000) 'Diet and sex-hormone-binding-globulin, dysmenorrhea and PMS.' *Obstetrics and Gynaecology 2*, 245–250.

Barnhart, K., Dunsmoor, S., *et al.* (2002) 'Effects of endometriosis: in-vitro-fertilisation.' *Fertility and Sterility 77*, 6, 1148–1155.

Bell, L.T., Branstrator, M., *et al.* (1975) 'Chromosomal abnormalities in maternal and fetal tissues: magnesium and zinc-deficient rats.' *Teratology 12*, 221–226.

Birnbaum, L.S. (1994) 'Endocrine effects of prenatal exposure to PCBs, dioxins, xenobiotics: implications for policy and future research.' *Environmental Health Perspectives 102*, 676–679.

Blaser, M.J., and Falkow, S., (2009) 'The consequences of the disappearing microbiota?' *Nature – Review – Microbiology 7*, 887–894.

Bohles, H., *et al.* (1999) 'Maternal plasma-homocysteine, placenta status, docosahexaenoic-acid concentration in erythrocyte-phospholipids of newborns.' *European Journal of Pediatrics 158*, 243–246.

British National Formulary (2004) '10.1.1. Musculoskeletal and Joint Diseases.' *British Medical Association 478*.

Brown, J., Kives, S., and Akhtar, M. (2012) 'Progestogens and anti-progestogens for pain associated with endometriosis.' *Cochrane Database of Systematic Reviews 3*, CD002122.

Bruner-Tran, K.L., Crispens, M.A., *et al.* (2008) 'Dietary supplements with omega-3-fatty-acids reduces reproductive impact of developmental TCDD in mice.' *Fertility and Sterility 90* (suppl. 1), S-50.

Bruner-Tran, K.L., Yeaman, G.R., *et al.* (2008) 'Dioxin may promote inflammation-related development of endometriosis.' *Fertility and Sterility 89*, 3, 1287–1298.

Chandler, J.G., Corson, S.L., *et al.* (2001) 'Three spectra of laparoscopic entry access injuries.' *Journal of American College of Surgery 192*, 478.

Chavarro, J.E., *et al.* (2008) 'Use of multi vitamins, intake of B vitamins, and risk of ovulatory infertility.' *Fertility and Sterility 89*, 668–676.

Chavarro, J.E., Rich-Edwards, J.W., *et al.* (2006) 'Iron intake and risk of ovulatory infertility.' *Obstetrics and Gynaecology 108*, 1145–1152.

Ciacci, C.C., *et al.* (1996) 'Coeliac disease and pregnancy outcome.' *American Journal Gastroenterology 91*, 4, 718–722.

Clayton, P. (2004) *Health Defence, 2nd Edition.* Accelerated Learning Systems Ltd, 44.

Collin, P., Salmi, J., Halstrom. O., *et al.* (1994) 'Autoimmune thyroid disorders and coeliac disease.' *European Journal Endocrinology 130*, 2, 137–140.

Counsell, C., *et al.* (1994) 'Coexistence of celiac and thyroid disease.' *Gut 35*, 6, 844–846.

Cowan, L.D. (1981) 'Breast-cancer incidence in women with history of progesterone deficiency.' *American Journal of Epidemiology 114*, 209–217.

Cronin, C.C., and Shahan, F. (1997) 'Insulin dependent diabetes-mellitis and coeliac disease.' *Lancet 349*, 1096–1097.

Crosignani, P.G., Luciano, A., *et al.* (2006) 'Subcutaneous depot medroxyprogesterone-acetate versus leuprolide-acetate in treatment of endometriosis-associated pain.' *Human Reproduction 21*, 1, 248–256.

Cuoco, L., Certo, M., *et al.* (1999) 'Prevalance and early diagnosis of coeliac-disease in auto-immune-thyroid disorders.' *Italian Journal of Gastro-Hepatology 31*, 4, 283–287.

Czeizel, A., *et al.* (1998) 'Periconceptional folic-acid containing multi-vitamin-supplementation.' *European Journal of Obstetric-Gynaecological Reproductive-Biology 78*, 2, 151–161.

D'Hooghe, T., and Hummelshoj, L. (2006) 'Multidisciplinary-centres and networks of excellence for endometriosis management research: a proposal.' *Human Reproduction 21*, 11, 2743–2748.

Davis, L., Kennedy, S., *et al.* (2007) 'Modern combined-oral-contraceptives for pain associated with endometriosis.' *Cochrane Database of Systematic Reviews 3*, CD001019.

Dayan, C.M. (2001) 'Interpretation of thyroid funtion tests.' *Lancet 357*, 619–624.

Deutch, B. (1995) 'Menstrual pain in Danish women correlated with low omega-3-polyunsaturated fatty-acid intake.' *European Journal of Clinical Nutrition 49*, 500–516.

De-Vas, M., Devroey, P., *et al.* (2010) 'Primary ovarian insufficiency.' *Lancet 376*, 911–921.

Donabela, F.C., Andrade, A.Z., *et al.* (2010) 'Influence of pituitary-suppression and controlled-ovarian-hyperstimulation (COH) on oxidative-stress markers of infertile patients with endometriosis and controls.' *Fertility and Sterility 94*, 4, S205–S205.

Donabela, F.C., *et al.* (2010) 'Serum markers of oxidative-stress in infertile women with endometriosis and controls.' *Fertility and Sterility 94*, 4, S40.

Drago, S., *et al.* (2006) 'Gliadin, zonulin and gut permeability: effects on coeliac and non-coeliac intestinal-mucosa and intestinal-cell-lines.' *Scandanavian Journal of Gastroenterology 4*, 4, 408–419.

Elizabeth, V., Menshikova, M., *et al.* (2006) 'Effects of exercise on mitochondrial content and function, aging human skeletal muscle.' *Journal of Gerontology Biological Science Medical Science 61*, 6, 534–540.

Environmental Working Group (2012) *The Dirty Dozen.* Available at www.ewg.org, accessed on 19 May 2015.

Fasano, A., *et al.* (2000) 'Zonulin, a newly discovered modulator of intestinal permeability and its expression in coeliac disease.' *Lancet 355*, 9214, 1518–1519.

Fasano A. (2011). 'Zonulin and its Regulation of Intestinal Barier Function: The Biological Door to Inflammation, Autoimmunity, and Cancer.' *Physiology Review 91*, 151–175. Doi:10.1152Physrev00003,2008.

Forges, T. (2007) 'Impact of folate and homocysteine metabolism on human reproductive health.' *Human Reproduction Update 13*, 3, 225–238.

Foyouzi, N., *et al.* (2004) 'Effects of oxidants and anti-oxidants on proliferation of endometrial-stromal-cells.' *Fertility and Sterility 82*, 3, 1019–1022.

Fredericks, C. (1989) *Guide to Women's Nutrition: Dietary Advice for Women of All Ages.* New York, NY: Perigee Books.

Fulcher, K.Y. and White, P.D. (1997) 'Randomised controlled trial of graded exercise in patients with chronic fatigue syndrome.' *British Medical Journal 314*, 1647–1652.

Gambert, S.R. (1991) 'Factors that Control Thyroid Function: Environmental Effects and Physiologic Variables.' In L.E. Braverman and R.D. Utiger (eds) *The Thyroid Gland.* Philadelphia, PA: Lippincott.

Gerhard I., Runnebaum B. (1992) 'The limits of hormone substitution in pollutant exposure and fertility disorders' [in German]. *Zentralble Gynakology 114*, 593–602.

Giudice, L.C. (2010) 'Clinical practice: endometriosis.' *New England Journal Medicine 362*, 25, 2389–2398.

Glinoer, D., Riahi, M., *et al.* (1994) 'Risk of sub-clinical-hypothyroidism in pregnant women with asymptomatic autoimmune-thyroid-disorder.' *Journal Clinical Endocrinology and Metabolism 79*, 197–204.

Goldin, B.R., Adlercreutz, H., *et al.* (1982) 'Oestrogen-excretion patterns and plasma-levels in vegetarian and omnivorous women.' *New England Journal Medicine 307*, 1542–1547.

Gorbach, S.L., and Goldin, B.R. (1987) 'Diet and the excretion and enterohepatic-cycling of estrogens.' *Preventative Medicine 16*, 525–531.

Gorbach, S.L., and Goldin, B.R. (1992) 'Nutrition and gastrointestinal-microflora.' *Nutrition Review 50*, 12, 378–381.

Granges, G., and Littlejohn, G.O. (1993) 'Comparative study of clinical-signs in fibromyalgia-fibrositis-syndrome, healthy and exercising subjects.' *Journal of Rheumatology 20*, 344–351.

Grant, E. (1994) *Sexual Chemistry.* London: Cedar.

Greenwood, J. (1964) 'Optimum vitamin C intake: a factor in the preservation of disc integrity.' *Medical Annals 33*, 274.

Grimaldi, K., Gill-Garrison, R., and Roberts, G. (2003) 'Personalised nutrition: an early win from the human genome project.' *Integrated Medicine 2*, 34–45.

Guo, S.W., *et al.* (2009) 'Reassessing the evidence for the link between dioxin and endometriosis: from molecular biology to clinical epidemiology.' *Molecular Human Reproduction 15*, 10, 609–624.

Guzick, D.S., Huang L.S., *et al.* (2011) 'Randomised trial of leuprolide versus continuous-oral-contraceptives in treatment of endometriosis-associated pelvic-pain.' *Fertility and Sterility 95*, 5, 1568–1573.

Hadfield, R., Mardon, H., *et al.* (1996) 'Delay in the diagnosis of endometriosis: a survey of women from the USA and the UK.' *Human Reproduction 11*, 4, 878–880.

Haggans, C.J., *et al.* (1999) 'Lignans in flaxseed stimulate SHBG.' *Nutrition and Cancer 33*, 188–195.

Halme, J.K (1996) 'Role of peritoneal inflammation in endometriosis associated with infertility. Endometriosis Today: advances in research and practice.' *The Proceedings of the Vth World Congress on Endometriosis.* Yokahama, Japan, October 1996. Parthenon Publishing, 132–135.

Halme, J.K. (1997) 'Role of Peritoneal Inflammation in Endometriosis Associated Infertility.' In X. Minaguchi and O. Sugimoto (eds) *Endometriosis Today: Advances in Research and Practice, Proceedings of the Vth World Congress on Endometriosis, Yokahama, Oct 1996.* New York and London: Parthenon.

Hansen, K., *et al.* (2014) 'Visceral syndrome in endometriosis patients.' *European Journal of Obstetrics and Gynaecology and Reproductive Biology 179,* 198–223.

Harada, T., Momoeda, M., *et al.* (2008) 'Low-dose-oral-contraceptive-pill for dysmenorrhoea associated with endometriosis: placebo-controlled, double-blind-randomized-trial.' *Fertility and Sterility 90,* 5, 1583–1588.

Hernandes-Guerrero, C.A., *et al.* (2006) 'Endometriosis and deficient intake of antioxidant-molecules related to peripheral-oxidative-stress.' *Ginecologic Obstetric Mexico 74,* 20–28.

Humphries, S., *et al.* (1999) 'Magnesium-deficiency and insulin-resistance.' *American Journal of Hypertension 12,* 747–756.

Huntington, A., and Gilmour, J.A. (2005) 'A life shaped by pain: women and endometriosis.' *Journal of Clinical Nursing 14,* 9, 1124–1132.

Ishimura, T., and Masuzaki, H. (1991) 'Peritoneal endometriosis; endometrial-tissue implantation as primary etio-logic mechanism.' *American Journal of Obstetrics and Gynaecology 165,* 210–214.

Johnson, M.K. (1975) 'Delayed neuropathy caused by some organophosphate-esters: Mechanisms and challenges. Critical reviews.' *Toxicology 289,* 313–314.

Jones, P.H. (2006) *Celiac Disease: A Hidden Epidemic.* New York, NY: HarperCollins.

Keen, C.L., and Zidenberg-Cherr, S. (1994) 'Should vitamin-mineral-supplements be recommended for all women with childbearing potential?' *American Journal Clinical Nutrition 59,* 532S–539S.

Kelly, D.E. (2000) 'Overview: what is insulin-resistance?' *Nutrition Review 58,* S2–S3.

Kennedy, S., Bergqvist, A., *et al.* (2005) 'ESHRE guideline for the diagnosis and treatment of endometriosis.' *Human Reproduction 20,* 2698–2704.

Kennedy, S.H., Mardon, H.J., *et al.* (1995) 'Familial endometriosis.' *Journal of Assisted Reproductive Genetics 12,* 32.

Khalili, H., Higuchi, L.M., *et al.* (2013) 'Contraceptives, reproduction factors and risk of inflammatory bowel disease.' *Gut 62,* 8, 1153–1159.

Kohler, G., Faustmann, T.A., *et al.* (2010) 'Dose-ranging study to determine the efficacy and safety of 1, 2 and 4mg doses of dienogest daily for endometriosis.' *International Journal Gynaecology and Obstetrics 108,* 21–25.

Koninckx, P.R., Braet, P., *et al.* (1994) 'Dioxin pollution and endometriosis in Belgium.' *Human Reproduction 9,* 1001–1002.

Koninckx, P.R., DeMoor, P., *et al.* (1980) 'Diagnosis of the lutenized-unruptured-follicle-syndrome by steroid-hormone assays on peritoneal fluid.' *European Journal of Obstetrics and Gynaecology 87,* 929–934.

Laufer, M.R., and Ballweg M.L. (2003) 'Adolescent endometriosis: state of the art forum.' *Journal of Paediatric and Adolescent Gynaecology 16,* 3, Supplement 1.

Laufer, M.R., Gitein, L., *et al.* (1997) 'Prevalence of endometriosis in adolescent girls with chronic-pelvic-pain not responding to conventional therapy.' *Journal of Pediatric and Adolescent Gynaecology 10,* 199–202.

Lee, J.R. (1994) *Natural Progesterone.* Sebastopol, CA: BLL Publishing.

Lessey, D.A. (2011) 'Assessment of endometrial-receptivity.' *Fertility and Sterility 96,* 522–529.

Lieberman, S., and Bruning, N. (2007) *The Real Vitamin & Mineral Book.* New York, NY: Avery.

Lu, R. (2000) 'Affinity purification and patial characterisation of zonulin/zonula-occludens-toxin (ZOT) receptor from human brain.' *Journal of Neurochemistry 74,* 1, 320–326.

Martin, N.E., et al. (1996) 'Phytoestrogens stimulate SHBG.' *Life Sciences 58*, 429–436.

Marziali, M. (2012) 'Gluten-free-diet: new strategy for management of painful endometriosis.' *Minerva Chir. 67*, 96, 499–504.

Masquelier, J. (1981) 'Pycnogenols: recent advances in the therapeutical activity of procyanadins.' *National Production of Medical Agents 1*, 243–256.

Maubon, A., Faury, A., et al. (2010) 'Uterine junctional-zone at magnestic-resonance-imaging: a predictor of In-Vitro Fertilisation implantation failure.' *Journal of Obstetrics and Gynaecological Review 36*, 3, 61108.

Misra, A.L., et al. (1977) 'Differential effects of opiates on incorporation of (14C) thiamine in central nervous systems of rats.' *Experimentia 33*, 372–374.

Missmer, S.A., Chavarro, J.E., et al. (2010) 'Trans-fats linked to increased risk of endometriosis.' *Human Reproduction 10*, 1093.

Missmer, S.A., Willett, W.C., et al. (2007) 'Dietary-fats and the incidence of endometriosis.' *American Journal of Epidemiology 165*, 11, S24.

Molina, H. (2005) 'Complement system during pregnancy.' *Immunol. Res. 32*, 187–192.

Momoeda, M., Harada, T., et al. (2009) 'Long term use of dienogest for treatment of endometriosis.' *Obstetrics and Gynaecological Review 35*, 6, 1069–1076.

Nagata, C., Takatsuka, N., et al. (2000) 'Total monounsaturated-fat intake and serum-oestrogen concentrations in premenopausal Japanese women.' *Nutrition and Cancer 38*, 37–39.

Nayyar, T., Bruner-Tran, K.L., et al. (2007) 'Developmental exposure of mice to TCDD elicits a similar uterine-phenotype in adult animals as observed in women with endometriosis.' *Reproductive Toxicology 23*, 3, 326–336.

Nicolle, L. (2007) 'Nutrigenomics in practice: The use of genetic and allied screening tools on a client with known genetic risks for developing a chronic disease.' *Nutrition Practitioner 8*, 3, 4–12.

Nicolle, L., and Woodriff-Beirne, A. (2010) *Biochemical Imbalances in Disease*. London: Singing Dragon.

Nnoaham, K.E., Hummelshoj, L., et al. (2011) 'Impact of endometriosis on quality of life and work productivity: a multi-centre study across ten countries.' *Fertility and Sterility 96*, 2, 366–373.

Oates, L., et al. (2014) 'Organic Consumption Survey.' *Journal of Environmental Research 132*, 105–111.

Osteen, K.G. and Bruner-Tran, K.L. (2014) 'Dioxin exposure and the invasive pathogenesis of endometriosis.' National Institutes of Health. National Institute of Environmental Sciences. Research Project 5R01ES014942-09. APPLICATION 8899540. [Awaiting publication.]

Pabona, J.M., Simmen, F.A., et al. (2012) 'Kruppel-like-factor-9 and progesterone-receptor co-regulation of decidualising-endometrial stromal-cells: implications for pathogenesis of endometriosis.' *Journal of Clinical Endocrinology and Metabolism 97*, 376–392.

Parazzini, F., Chiaffarino, F., et al. (2004) 'Selected food intake and risk of endometriosis.' *Human Reproduction 19*, 8, 1755–1759.

Parry-Jones, B. (1992) 'Pagophagia: compulsive ice consumption: historical perspectives.' *Psychological Medicine 22*, 3, 561–571.

Paterson, C. (1996) 'Measuring outcomes in primary care: patient generated measure, MYMOP. Compared with the SF-36 health survey.' *British Medical Journal 312*, 1016.

Pelton, R., LaValle, J.B., et al. (1999) *Drug-Induced-Nutrient-Depletion Handbook. Vitamin B5*. Lexi-Comp Clinical Reference Library. New York: Barnes and Noble.

Petraglia, F., de Zegler, D., et al. (2012) 'Inflammation: links between endometriosis and preterm birth.' *Fertility and Sterility 98*, 1, 36–40.

Poppe, K., and Velkeniers, B. (2002) 'Thyroid and infertility.' *Verhandelingen Koninklijke Academie Geneeskunde van Belgium 64*, 6, 389–399.

Potdar, N., Gelbaya, T., and Nardo, L.G. (2012) 'Endometrial injury to overcome recurrent embryo implantation failure: a systematic review and meta-analysis.' *Reproductive Biomedicine Online.* December 25, 6, 561–71.

Proctor, M., and Murphy, P.A. (2001) 'Herbal and dietary-therapies for primary and secondary-dysmenorrhoea.' *Cochrane Database of Systematic Reviews 2*, CD002124.

Rabizadeh, S., and Sears, C. (2008) 'New horizons for the infectious diseases specialist: how gut microflora promote health and disease.' *Current Infectious Disease Report 10*, 2, 92–98.

Rier, S. (2001) 'Serum levels of TCDD and dioxin-like-chemicals in rhesus-monkeys chronically exposed to dioxin: correlation of increased serum PCB-levels with endometriosis.' *Toxiological Sciences 59*, 1, 147–159.

Roberts, H. (1990) *Aspartame.* Philadelphia, PA: Charles Press.

Rock, J.A., and Hurst, B.S. (1990) 'Clinical Significance of Prostanoid-Concentrations in Women with Endometriosis.' In D.R. Chadha and V.C. Buttram (eds) *Current Concepts in Endometriosis.* New York: Alan R. Liss.

Roman, J.D. (2010) 'Adolescent endometriosis in the Wakato region, New Zealand – comparative cohort study with a mean follow up time of 2.6 years.' *Australian and New Zealand Journal of Obstetrics and Gynaecology 50*, 579–583.

Schindler, A.E. (2011) 'Dienogest in long-term-treatment of endometriosis.' *International Journal of Women's Health 3*, 175–184.

Schlaff, W.D., Carson, S.A., *et al.* (2006) 'Subcutaneous injection of depot medroxyprogesterone-acetate compared with leuprolide-acetate in the treatment of endometriosis-associated pain.' *Fertility and Sterility 85*, 2, 314–325.

Sesti, F., Capozzolo, T., *et al.* (2009) 'Recurrence rate of endometriomas after laparoscopic cystectomy: comparative-randomized-trial between post-operative hormonal-suppression treatment or dietary-therapy vs. placebo.' *European Journal of Obstetrics and Reproductive Biology 47*, 1, 72–77.

Sesti, F., Pietropolli, A., *et al.* (2007) 'Hormonal suppression-treatment or dietary-therapy versus placebo in control of painful symptoms after conservative surgery for endometriosis(stage-III-IV). Randomized-comparative-trial.' *Fertility and Sterility 88*, 6, 1541–1547.

Shanahan, F. (1994) 'The Intestinal Immune System.' In Johnson, L.R., Christensen, J., Jackobson, E., Walsh, J.H., Eds. *Physiology of the gastrointestinal tract, 3rd Edition.* New York: Raven Press, 643–684

Shanti, A., *et al.* (1999) 'Auto-antibodies to markers of oxidative-stress are elevated in women with endometriosis.' *Fertility and Sterility 71*, 1115–1118.

Shepperson Mills, D. (2006) 'Nutritional therapy provides an effective method of improving fertility rates and reducing abdominal pain in women with endometriosis. "What is one man's meat is another man's poison" may presumably have a chemical basis. Integrated medicine at the point of diagnosis may enhance treatment of women with compromised fertility and abdominal pain.' *Fertility and Sterility 86*, 2, S270–S271.

Shepperson Mills, D. (2011a) 'A conundrum: wheat/gluten avoidance and its implication with endometriosis patients.' *Fertility and Sterility 96*, 3, S139.

Shepperson Mills, D. (2011b) 'MYMOP2 in action using Clinic-Aid: from clinical practice to research – The Endometriosis and Fertility Clinic.' *Journal of Nutritional Therapy 4*, 28, 1–12.

Shepperson Mills, D., and Vernon, M.W. (2002) *Endometriosis: A Key to Healing and Fertility Through Nutrition.* Thorsons/HarperCollins.

Simoens, S. (2012) 'The burden of endometriosis: costs and quality of life of women with endometriosis, treated in referral centres.' *Human Reproduction 27*, 1292–1299.

Sinaii, N., Cleary, S.D., *et al.* (2002) 'High rates of autoimmune and endocrine disorders, fibromyalgia, chronic fatigue syndrome and atopic diseases among women with endometriosis: a survey analysis.' *Human Reproduction 17*, 10, 2715–2724.

Singh, A., Dantas, Z.N., *et al.* (1995) 'Presence of thyroid-antibodies in early-reproductive-failure: biochemical versus clinical pregnancies.' *Fertility and Sterility 63*, 2, 277–281.

Spallholz, J.E., *et al.* (1973) 'Immunological responses of mice fed diets supplemented with selenite-selenium.' *Proceedings Society Experimental Biological Medicine 143*, 685–689.

Stanner, S., Thompson, R., *et al.* (2009) 'Healthy Ageing: The Skin.' In *Healthy Ageing: The Role of Nutrition and Lifestyle.* London: Wiley-Blackwell.

Stock, S. (1995) 'Nutrition and hormones.' *Nutrition Therapy Today. Society for the Promotion of Nutritional Therapy 3–4*, 1–5.

Stoll, B.A. (2000) 'Adiposity as a risk determinant for postmenopausal breast-cancer.' *International Journal of Obstetric Related Metabolic Disorders 24*, 527–533.

Stratton, P., and Berkley, K.J. (2011) 'Chronic pelvic pain and endometriosis: translational evidence of the relationship and implications.' *Human Reproduction Update 17*, 327–346.

Strowitzki, T., Faustmann, T., *et al.* (2010) 'Dienogest in the treatment of endometriosis-associated pelvic pain: 12 week, randomized-double-blind-placebo-controlled study.' *European Journal of Obstetrics and Gynaecology Reproductive Biology 151*, 2, 193–198.

Strowitzki, T., Marr, J., *et al.* (2010) 'Dienogest: as effective as leuprolide-acetate in treating the painful symptoms of endometriosis: 24 week, randomized-multicentre, open-label trial.' *Human Reproduction 25*, 3, 633–641.

The Doctors Laboratory (2015) 'Tumour-Markers/-Sites.' *Laboratory Guide, January 2015.* Available at www.tdlpathology.com/media/4144/TAP2540_TDL_Labguide2015_NP_V3_WEB.pdf, accessed on 19 May 2015.

Treloar, S., Hadfield, R., *et al.* (2002) 'International Endogene Study Group. The International Endogene Study: a collection of families for genetic research in endometriosis.' *Fertility and Sterility 78*, 4, 679–685.

Trickey, R. (1998) *Women, Hormones & The Menstrual Cycle.* London: Allen Unwin.

Tummon, I.S. (1987) 'Occult ovulatory-dysfunction in women with minimal endometriosis or unexplained infertility.' *Fertility and Sterility 50*, 716.

Tworoger, S.S., Missmer, S.A., *et al.* (2007) 'Physical activity and inactivity in relation to sex-hormones, prolactin and insulin-like-growth-factor concentrations in premenopausal women: exercise and premenstrual-hormones.' *Cancer Causes Control 18*, 743–752.

Vercellini, P., Crosignani, P., *et al.* (2011) 'Waiting for Godot: commonplace approach to medical treatment of endometriosis.' *Human Reproduction 26*, 1, 3–13.

Vercellini, P., Pietropauolo, G., *et al.* (2006) 'Reproductive performance in infertile women with rectovaginal-endometriosis: is surgery worthwhile?' *American Journal of Obstetrics and Gynaecology 195*, 5, 1303–1310.

Watts, D. (1999) *Trace Elements and other Essential Nutrients.* Addison, TX: Trace Elements. Available at www.traceelements.com/EducationalResources/BookStore.aspx, accessed on 19 May 2015.

Weetman, A.P. (1997) 'Hypothyroidism: screening and subclinical disease.' *British Medical Journal 314*, 1175–1178.

Willett, W.C., and Stampfer, M.J. (2006) 'Rebuilding the food pyramid.' *Scientific American Reports 16*, 4, 3.

Wykes, C.B., Clark, T.J., *et al.* (2004) 'Accuracy of laparoscopy in the diagnosis of endometriosis: a systematic quantitative review.' *British Journal of Obstetrics and Gynaecology 111*, 11, 1204–1212.

Ylikorkala, O. (1984) 'Peritoneal-fluid prostaglandin in endometriosis, tubal disorders and unexplained infertility.' *Obstetrics and Gynaecology 63*, 616–620.

# Chapter 6

# Male Factor Infertility

*Clare Casson BA (Hons), MA, MSc, Dip. BCNH, Dip. ION, mBANT, CNHC, Registered Nutritional Therapist practising at a private fertility clinic in London, associate lecturer at BCNH, the UK College of Nutrition and Health*

## 1. Prevalence of male infertility

It is estimated that 1 in 20 men of reproductive age is infertile (McLachlan and O'Bryan 2010). In Europe, 1 in 5 men have a sperm count below the WHO (World Health Organisation) lower reference level (Olea *et al.* 2010). In the USA, 9.4 per cent of men aged 15–44 and 12 per cent of men aged 25–44 self-report some form of infertility or subfertility (Chandra and Copen 2013). In the UK, 30 per cent of infertility cases are attributable to a male factor and 40 per cent involve both male and female factors (NICE 2013). Similarly, in the USA one-third of cases is attributable to a male factor and two-thirds to a combination of male and female factors (Office on Women's Health 2012). However, estimates of the prevalence of male factor infertility vary and data is patchy. A WHO multicentre study some years ago found that a male factor is solely responsible in about 20 per cent of infertile couples (WHO 1987). It is estimated to be a contributory factor, alongside female factors, in 30 per cent to 50 per cent of cases (Jarow *et al.* 2002; WHO 1987).

## 2. Anatomy and physiology of sperm production

Some readers will already be familiar with male reproductive anatomy and physiology. For those who are not, this brief overview of sperm production and its hormonal control will aid understanding of the various causes and risk factors for male infertility and the rationale for male fertility investigations and treatment.

### 2.1 The testes

The testes contain the seminiferous tubules where sperm are produced; Leydig cells, which produce the hormones that control the process; and Sertoli cells, which are tightly joined to form the blood–testis barrier. This effectively seals off the tubules from the rest of the body, protecting the developing sperm from extraneous substances, and preventing their exposure to the immune system. The significance of this will be discussed in the section on anti-sperm antibodies. The Sertoli cells also nourish the developing sperm.

The seminiferous tubules are lined with germ cells (spermatogonia). Type A spermatogonia self-replicate to maintain the supply of germ cells. Type B spermatogonia self-replicate to give rise to sperm. This process is illustrated in Figure 6.1. The tubules contain sperm at different stages of development, with the more mature spermatocytes located closer to the lumen of the tubule.

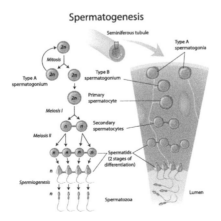

Figure 6.1 The stages of spermatogenesis, which takes place in the seminiferous tubules

## 2.2 Spermatogenesis

The process of sperm production is known as spermatogenesis, described by Hirsch (2015) as follows. It is a highly complex process of cell division involving mitosis, in which cells duplicate themselves, and meiosis, during which chromosomes are 'shuffled' to ensure genetic variation between sperm. In the later stages of development, genetic material becomes highly condensed; the enzyme-filled acrosome cap is formed; finally the tail (flagellum) structures develop, and the energy-producing mitochondria fuse to form a spiral round the midpiece. Any remaining unnecessary cell contents are removed and absorbed by the Sertoli cells. This means that sperm lack the structures responsible for DNA repair and are hence highly vulnerable to DNA damage. The resulting spermatozoa are mature, but are immotile. In the final stage, managed by the Sertoli cells, the spermatozoa are released into the lumen of the seminiferous tubule. They are carried by peristalsis (the contraction of the tubular walls) in the testicular fluid, secreted by the Sertoli cells, to the epididymis. There they become motile and hence capable of fertilising an ovum. Groups of germ cells pass through spermatogenesis and develop together as a 'generation' of sperm.

The whole process of spermatogenesis takes 86 days – almost 3 months: the development of germ cells into mature spermatazoa takes 74 days; another 12 days is required for transport of the spermatozoa through the epididymis and their maturation into motile, fertile sperm (Hirsch 2015), so male pre-conceptual care should ideally begin at least three months before attempting to conceive naturally or before fertility treatment begins. However, recent data from studies in which developing sperm were labelled with 2H2O (heavy water) show that the length of spermatogenesis is variable, even within individuals, averaging just 64 days, and could be as low as 42 days (Agarwal and Esteves 2011). It follows that it may still be worth starting a programme of male pre-conceptual care within six weeks of trying to conceive. Spermatogenesis continues throughout life, from puberty to old age.

## 2.3 Hormonal control of spermatogenesis

Spermatogenesis is initiated at puberty and from then on is controlled by the hypothalamic–pituitary–gonadal (HPG) axis: the interaction of the hypothalamus, pituitary gland and Leydig cells in the testes. Gonadotrophin-releasing hormone (GnRH) is released by the hypothalamus in short pulses, every 70 to 90 minutes. This triggers the release of luteinising hormone (LH) by the pituitary gland, which in turn stimulates the Leydig cells in the testes to produce testosterone. The production of testosterone is controlled by a negative feedback mechanism: rising testosterone suppresses production of LH (University of Ottawa 2013). As well as secreting testosterone, the Leydig cells also secrete other hormones, transmitters and growth factors which stimulate cell growth, proliferation and differentiation, such as IGF1 (Insulin-like Growth Factor 1), TGFβ (Transforming Growth Factor Beta) and NGF (Nerve Growth Factor). These have various functions which are not well understood but include regulating blood flow within the testes; maintaining the Sertoli cells; controlling cellular functions and developmental processes of germ cells; and controlling the peristaltic movements of the seminiferous tubules which transport spermatozoa (Hirsch 2015).

GnRH (gonadotrophin-releasing hormone) also stimulates the pituitary gland to release FSH (follicle-stimulating hormone). This stimulates production of androgen-binding protein by the Sertoli cells, which enables testosterone to be concentrated in the Sertoli cells to levels high enough to trigger and maintain spermatogenesis (Hirsch 2015). The activity of the Sertoli cells is controlled via a negative feedback mechanism involving the production of inhibin, which suppresses production of FSH by the pituitary (Hirsch 2015). This is illustrated in Figure 6.2.

Clearly, any disruption in the delicate balance and feedback mechanisms involved in the HPG axis could potentially have a significant impact on male fertility. Hormonal causes of male infertility are explored later in this chapter.

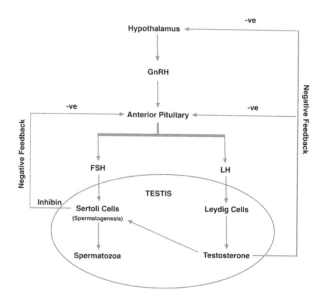

Figure 6.2 The HPG axis (hypothalamic–pituitary–gonadal axis) in men

*LH and FSH stimulate testosterone secretion by the Leydig cells and spermatogenesis by the Sertoli cells. Rising levels of testosterone and the release of inhibin by Sertoli cells inhibits the release of GnRH, FSH and LH via a negative feedback mechanism.*

## 3. Main issues with sperm

Male fertility is defined in terms of sperm and semen quality and quantity – typically semen volume and pH; sperm number, concentration, motility, morphology and vitality (NICE 2013). Other parameters such as semen viscosity, the quality of sperm DNA, and the presence of leucocytes or anti-sperm antibodies are also relevant (Raheem, Ralph and Minhas 2012). Semen parameters, while important, are of limited diagnostic value, however, since some infertile men have normal parameters and some men with abnormal parameters are fertile (Irvine 1998). Nevertheless, the WHO (2010) values for normal parameters are based on over 4000 men in 14 countries with proven fertility, whose partners were known to conceive by them in the previous 12 months. These are the parameters commonly used in semen analysis tests and are detailed in the section on male fertility investigations. The common issues with sperm relate to the quantity and quality of sperm produced, and include the following.

## 3.1 Semen volume

- Hypospermia or hypozoospermia – low semen volume

- Aspermia – absence of semen (not to be confused with azoospermia)

- Hyperzoospermia – high semen volume; related to low sperm concentration because the sperm are diluted by an excessive volume of semen (Cooke, Tyler and Driscoll 1995).

## 3.2 Sperm count

- Oligozoospermia – low sperm concentration

- Azoospermia – no measurable sperm count

- Cryptozoospermia – very low sperm count; may easily be mistaken for azoospermia.

## 3.3 Sperm morphology

- Sperm morphology refers to the observable structural form of head, midpiece and flagellum ('tail') of the sperm. A very high percentage of abnormal forms, in many permutations and combinations, may be present without affecting infertility so long as there is a good sperm count and concentration. Figure 6.3 shows various abnormal forms.

- Teratozoospermia or teratospermia refers to a degree of abnormality likely to affect fertility.

- Globozoospermia refers specifically to a condition where the acrosome is absent or there is a small acrosome, giving the sperm heads a rounded appearance.

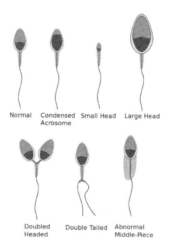

Figure 6.3 Different types of abnormal sperm
forms found in teratozoospermia

*"Abnormalsperm" by Xenzo at English Wikipedia Licensed under CC BY-SA 3.0
found at http://creativecommons.org/licenses/by-sa/3.0/ via Wikimedia Commons
http://commons.wikimedia.org/wiki/File:Abnormalsperm.svg#mediaviewer/
File:Abnormalsperm.svg. Full terms of the Creative Commons license can be
found at: http://creativecommons.org/licenses/by-sa/3.0/legalcode*

### 3.4 Sperm motility

Motility refers to the ability of sperm to swim. Athenozoospermia or astenozoospermia refers to reduced motility. This may be immotility, or non-progressive motility, where the tail beats but the head does not move forward, or moves in small circles.

### 3.5 OAT syndrome

Oligozoospermia, asthenozoospermia and teratozoospermia may occur together as oligo-astheno-teratozoospermia (OAT) syndrome. In this case there is an increased incidence of genetic abnormalities and obstruction of the male genital tract (EAU 2014).

### 3.6 Sperm vitality

Sperm vitality measures the number of sperm that are dead or alive. Necrozoospermia refers to a high proportion of immotile, non-viable sperm.

## 3.7 Viscosity

Semen is composed of fluids secreted by the prostate and seminal vesicles. Their dysfunction can lead to imbalanced composition of proteins in the semen which affects coagulation and liquefaction and hence the viscosity of seminal fluid. Increased viscosity can impair motility and can lead to decreased sperm count due to a 'blocking' effect on sperm progression in the seminal tubules (Du Plessis, Gokul and Agarwal 2013).

## 3.8 Agglutination

Agglutination refers to motile spermatozoa sticking to each other. It can affect motility and concentration, and may be caused by sperm antibodies, but there are other causes, and antibodies may not cause agglutination (WHO 2010).

## 3.9 Anti-sperm antibodies

Anti-sperm antibodies are produced when the body's immune system mistakes a man's sperm as foreign to the body and therefore potentially invading pathogens. They are released into semen and bind to sperm. This can cause agglutination and also interfere with the acrosome reaction and zona binding during fertilisation. Not all anti-sperm antibodies actually affect sperm function. A sperm-mucus penetration test is carried out to determine whether or not they do (Bohring and Krause 2003; WHO 2010).

## 3.10 Altered semen pH

The pH of semen reflects the balance between the pH values of the different accessory gland secretions, mainly the secretions of the seminal vesicles (alkaline) and prostatic secretions (acidic) and is an indicator of their function.

## 3.11 Altered zinc, fructose and glucosidase

The levels of zinc, fructose and neutral glucosidase are biochemical tests for prostate and seminal vesicle function. Poor quality semen may be linked to testicular dysfunction or post-testicular damage in the epididymis or ejaculate due to abnormal glandular secretions (WHO 2010).

## 3.12 Presence of non-sperm cells – leukocytes and 'peroxidase-positive leukocytes'

Leukocytes are white blood cells. Leukocytospermia or pyospermia means there is an excessive number of leukocytes (WHO 2010). Their presence, especially when active (peroxidase positive), combined with a small ejaculate volume may point to infection of the prostate or seminal vesicles. This can lead to obstruction or oxidative damage to sperm (EAU 2014) leading to poor motility and DNA integrity (WHO 2010).

## 3.13 Presence of high levels of reactive oxygen species

ROS (reactive oxygen species), also known as free radicals (FRs), are highly reactive molecules. They have functional roles in sperm (as in other cells and tissues) but in excess they cause a state of 'oxidative stress' in the body. This leads to cellular damage (including to sperm), pathological processes and dysfunction. Oxidative stress is discussed in more detail later in this chapter. Around 40 to 80 per cent of infertile patients have high levels of seminal ROS (Venkatesh *et al.* 2009).

## 3.14 DNA fragmentation

Conventional semen analysis is limited in that it does not discriminate between the sperm of fertile and infertile men and is not clinically predictive; hence sperm morphology, motility and concentration reference values are no more than a guide to reproductive potential (Guzick *et al.* 2001). Conventional parameters take no account of any damage to sperm DNA ('DNA fragmentation'), although the extent of DNA fragmentation correlates negatively with standard sperm parameters (Irvine *et al.* 2000).

Sperm lack the cellular structures necessary to repair DNA (Venkatesh *et al.* 2009) and even though the oocyte (egg) may be able to carry out sperm DNA repair after fertilisation, more extensive damage may introduce mutations associated with poor fertilisation capacity, deficient embryo development and repeated miscarriage

(Bungum *et al.* 2007; Meseguer *et al.* 2008; Seli *et al.* 2004; Zini *et al.* 2008). DNA fragmentation has been linked to impaired fertilisation, disrupted pre-implantation embryo development, miscarriage and birth defects in the offspring (Lewis *et al.* 2013).

It is estimated that a significant proportion of men whose infertility is hitherto 'unexplained' have a cause attributed after sperm DNA testing (Bungum *et al.* 2007). Simon *et al.* (2013) found that in 80 per cent of 239 couples with unexplained or idiopathic infertility, the male partner had high sperm DNA damage. A DNA fragmentation rate of under 15 per cent sperm was seen in the sperm of fertile men, but at 25 per cent plus, it significantly reduced the chance of pregnancy, even with some forms of fertility treatment (Simon *et al.* 2013). A growing number of studies report sperm DNA damage to be useful as a diagnostic tool for male infertility and as a predictor of treatment success (Lewis *et al.* 2013).

## 4. Declining male fertility

A number of studies and meta-analyses suggest that sperm parameters have been falling over the last 20 to 50 years (Carlsen *et al.* 1992; Swan, Elkin and Fenster 1997). However, many of the studies have been criticised for poor methodology, in particular unrepresentativeness and selection bias (Fisch 2008). The authors of one of the largest ever studies, carried out recently in France, argue that their methodology largely overcomes these problems and that although they were unable to control for socioeconomic status, this would make their estimates of sperm parameters higher, if anything, than in the general population (Rolland *et al.* 2013). They concluded that there has been a continuous decrease in semen concentration in French men between 1989 and 2005, of about 1.9 per cent per year, and a decrease in morphologically normal sperm, consistent with findings in other recent studies carried out across the world. Nevertheless, whether or not there has actually been a global decline in male fertility continues to be debated. One hypothesis for the postulated decline is the impact of environmental toxins such as pesticides, phthalates, dioxins and PCBs (polychlorinated biphenyls), which have been shown to damage sperm DNA and negatively affect the function of Sertoli or Leydig cells via oestrogenic action (Mortimer *et al.* 2013; Sengupta and Banerjee 2013). This is explored further in Chapter 11.

## 5. Male fertility investigations

Assessment of male fertility begins with a detailed medical history and physical examination. Semen analysis is also carried out as standard, and other possible tests include tests for infections, sperm DNA testing, other genetic tests and hormonal tests.

### 5.1 Standard semen analysis

Standard semen analysis is usually carried out using WHO (World Health Organisation) reference values (WHO 2010), with a repeat test for abnormal results.

---

··· BOX 6.1 SEMEN ANALYSIS ·········································

- ▶ Semen volume: 1.5 ml or more

- ▶ pH: 7.2 or more

- ▶ Sperm concentration: 15 million spermatozoa per ml or more

- ▶ Total sperm number: 39 million spermatozoa per ejaculate or more

- ▶ Total motility (percentage of progressive motility and non-progressive motility): 40 per cent or more

- ▶ Motile: 32 per cent or more with progressive motility

- ▶ Vitality: 58 per cent or more live spermatozoa

- ▶ Sperm morphology (percentage of normal forms): 4 per cent or more.

---

Some studies have shown that IVF outcomes (using 'classic' techniques) are improved if a lower limit of >14 per cent normal forms (at least 15%) is applied (Svalander *et al.* 1996), so this has been adopted by many IVF clinics. However, findings are not consistent (Ghirelli-Filho *et al.* 2012) and outcomes of IVF using intra cytoplasmic sperm injection (ICSI) do not appear to be any less successful when a lower limit of >4 per cent normal forms is applied, probably because the embryologist will always try to choose the best sperm (French *et al.* 2010; Svalander *et al.* 1996).

## 5.2 Specialist tests

Specialist semen analysis such as leukocyte counts, anti-sperm antibody tests and sperm viability testing is not required for the diagnosis of male infertility but may be useful to identify a specific male factor contributing to unexplained male infertility or to inform the selection of assistive reproductive techniques (ART) (American Urological Association 2010).

··· BOX 6.2 SPECIALIST TESTS IDENTIFIED BY WHO (2010) ·

▶ Peroxidase-positive leukocytes. This refers to the presence of activated leukocytes in the ejaculate. Their number may reflect the severity of an inflammatory condition or degree of oxidative attack.

▶ MAR test (mixed agglutination reaction) or immunobead (IB) test for the presence of anti-sperm antibodies. If positive, a sperm-mucus penetration test is carried out to determine whether the antibodies interfere with sperm function.

▶ Seminal zinc, fructose and neutral glucosidase, which are indicators of functioning of the prostate and seminal vesicles.

▶ Presence of non-sperm cells which may indicate damage to the testicles or efferent ducts.

▶ Viscosity and agglutination – which can be linked respectively to prostate and seminal vesicle function, or sperm autoimmunity.

▶ Seminal pH: low pH (acidic semen) with low volume and low sperm numbers may indicate an ejaculatory duct obstruction or congenital bilateral absence of the vas deferens (CBAVD).

## 5.3 DNA fragmentation testing

Conventional semen analysis is limited in that it does not discriminate between the sperm of fertile and infertile men and is not clinically predictive, hence sperm morphology, motility and concentration reference values are no more than a guide to reproductive potential (Guzick *et al.* 2001). Conventional parameters take no account of any damage to sperm DNA, although the extent of DNA fragmentation correlates negatively with standard sperm parameters (Irvine *et al.* 2000). Common methods for investigating DNA fragmentation include the sperm chromatin structure assay (SCSA), the TdT (terminal deoxynucleotidyl transferase)-mediated dUDP nick-end labelling (TUNEL) and Comet assays, and the sperm chromatin dispersion test (SCD) also known as the Halo test (Lewis *et al.* 2013). The major limitation of all these assays is that the sperm tested cannot be used for clinical purposes, for example for IVF (Wright, Milne and Leeson 2014).

A number of proxy tests for sperm DNA damage and sperm-selection procedures have been developed. These do not measure DNA damage directly but correlate with it and assist embryologists in selecting sperm with low levels of DNA damage. These include birefringence, intracytoplasmic morphologically selected sperm injection (IMSI) and hyaluronic acid-selection of spermatozoa for ICSI; however, there is currently little research to evaluate their success (Lewis *et al.* 2013).

DNA fragmentation testing remains largely experimental: there is a limited evidence base both for the benefits of testing and for therapies to correct an abnormal test result (Bungum 2012).

## 5.4 Genetic testing

Genetic tests can help to identify any genetic causes for idiopathic (unexplained) male infertility (Jungwirth *et al.* 2014) although only a limited set of tests has yet been validated (McLachlan and O'Bryan 2010). NICE (2013b), EAU guidelines (Jungwirth *et al.* 2014) and AUA guidelines (AUA 2010) all recommend genetic testing in cases of severe non-obstructive azoospermia, severe oligozoospermia or OAT syndrome, as the presence of genetic abnormalities may inform decisions around the use of donor sperm where abnormalities are heritable. Genetic testing is also recommended in men with conditions linked to common chromosomal disorders such as congenital bilateral or unilateral absence of the vas deferens (CAVD), which is associated with mutations in the cystic fibrosis transmembrane regulator (CFTR) gene which causes cystic fibrosis (Jungwirth *et al.* 2014); in recurrent miscarriage (Jungwirth *et al.* 2014) which may be caused by chromosome defects (Dada *et al.* 2011); and in men undergoing IVF, especially ICSI, to prevent the transmission of genetic defects which may underlie these problems (Dada *et al.* 2011).

## 5.5 ROS test (reactive oxygen species)

In semen, ROS are produced both by sperm themselves and by leucocytes (white blood cells involved in the immune system) so high levels may be linked to infection and further tests may be indicated (WHO 2010). Anti-oxidant therapy can be used to counteract oxidative stress. It may be useful to carry out a ROS test, which measures the levels of ROS in semen, in order to determine whether anti-oxidant supplementation is indicated: physiological concentrations of ROS are essential for normal sperm function and excessive or unnecessary anti-oxidant supplementation may lead to 'reductive stress' (O'Flaherty, de Lamirande and Gagnon 2005). Food therapy and supplementation are considered in further detail in Chapter 10.

## 5.6 Hormone testing

Hormonal investigations may be carried out to help determine the underlying causes of abnormal semen parameters, or if there is impaired sexual function, or other clinical findings which may indicate a particular endocrinopathy (AUA 2010). These usually include determining levels of FSH, LH, testosterone and sex hormone-binding globulin (SHBG).

## 5.7 Microbiological assessment

Microbiological assessment can help to eliminate causes linked to 'silent' or evident urinary tract infections (UTIs), male accessory gland infections (MAGI) and sexually transmitted diseases (STDs).

Microbiological assessment is also recommended where peroxidase-positive leukocytes are present as this may point to infection of the prostate or seminal vesicles, or an STI such as *Neisseria gonorrhoeae* or, commonly, *Chlamydia trachomatis* (Jungwirth *et al.* 2014).

## 5.8 Other assessments

Ultrasonography (US) may be used in cases of azoospermia or oligospermia with low semen volume to detect any obstruction or other relevant lesions such as varicocele, testicular tumours, prostatic cysts or stenosis (narrowing) of the ejaculatory ducts (AUA 2010). Testicular biopsy may be carried out to help diagnosis in the case of azoospermia or extreme OAT when FSH levels and testicular volume are normal (Jungwirth *et al.* 2014).

## 6. Causes and risk factors

Male infertility is often characterised as being due to either primary or secondary hypogonadism. Hypogonadism means low testicular function characterised by a deficiency in testosterone (Kumar *et al.* 2010). Primary hypogonadism may be characterised by hormonal disturbances but usually has another underlying cause rather than hormonal dysfunction (McClure 2005). Secondary hypogonadism occurs where the endocrine (hormonal) system, the HPG axis, which regulates the chain of hormonal events that enable sperm production is dysfunctional. There are a wide range of underlying causes and risk factors including physical causes such as tubal blockages, undescended testicles and testicular trauma; genetic factors; and environmental factors such as nutrition, lifestyle and toxic exposure which may affect testicular function or its hormonal control (Jungwirth *et al.* 2012). In addition, two per cent of infertile men have sexual dysfunction which impairs ejaculation (Raheem *et al.* 2012).

About one-third of cases of male infertility are due to a physical cause (Edey and Sidhu 2008). Obstructive causes, where there is normal sperm production but there is a blockage in the genital tract, occur in 60 per cent of cases; non-obstructive causes, where there is a problem with sperm production by the testes, occur in 38 per cent of cases (Raheem *et al.* 2012). Non-obstructive causes may be hormonal, genetic or linked to nutrition, lifestyle and environmental factors. These are all explored in greater depth throughout this book.

In a significant proportion of cases there is no identifiable cause of a man's infertility. This is known as idiopathic infertility. One study of 1549 men found there was an identifiable cause of abnormal semen parameters in only 66 per cent of cases (Pierik *et al.* 2000).

Unexplained infertility, where the semen analysis is normal and female infertility factors have been ruled out, accounts for up to 45 per cent of cases but the extent to which individual patients are fully investigated varies widely (Moghissi and Wallach 1983). For example, there may be high levels of DNA fragmentation even if standard semen parameters appear normal, but this is not routinely assessed.

## 6.1 Obstructive infertility

Obstructive azoospermia or severe oligozoospermia, where sperm production is normal but there is a blockage in the genital tract, occurs in 60 per cent of cases (Raheem *et al.* 2012). The blockage may be in the testes, usually as a result of scar tissue linked to trauma and inflammation (Jungwirth *et al.* 2012); the epididymis, often due to inflammation linked to infection (Jequier 1985); the seminal ducts, including CBAVD, which occurs in most men with cystic fibrosis and 85 per cent of men with a defect in the gene linked to cystic fibrosis (Oates and Amos 1994); or the ejaculatory ducts, where obstruction can be congenital, due to cysts in the prostate, or inflammation and scarring following urethral prostatitis or pelvic surgery (Jungwirth *et al.* 2012).

Previous surgery is a significant cause: orchidopexy (to release undescended testicles), vasectomy reversal, prostate, bladder, scrotal, inguinal and other pelvic surgery can all cause injury to the epididymis, vas deferens or spermatic vessels. This may result in the formation of scar tissue and hence obstruction which may not be noticed until the patient presents with fertility issues (Summerton *et al.* 2012).

Functional – as opposed to mechanical – obstruction can occur due to neuropathy, such as diabetic neuropathy which can affect the functioning of seminal vesicles (La Vignera *et al.* 2011).

## 6.2 Non-obstructive causes

Cryptorchidism (undescended testicles) occurs when the testes fail to descend from the abdominal cavity into the scrotum towards the end of pregnancy. It occurs in about one per cent to four per cent of babies born at term (Kolon, Patel and Huff 2004), and up to 21 per cent in those born prematurely (Urology Care Foundation 2013). If the testes have not descended after three months, hormonal or surgical treatment (orchidopexy) is required. Ten per cent of infertile men have a history of cryptorchidism and orchidopexy (Grasso, Buonaguidi and Lania 1991). Cryptorchidism is associated with azoospermia and lower fertility rates than in men with normally descended testicles, particularly in untreated bilateral cryptorchidism where the incidence is 98 per cent (Chung and Brock 2011).

The impact on fertility may be due to overheating of the testes inside the body which can damage the germ cells (Docimo, Silver and Cromie 2000). There may also be underlying genetic abnormalities affecting testicular function since men who undergo orchidopexy have an increased risk of testicular cancer (Raheem *et al.* 2012). If cryptorchidism is untreated, fibrosis develops leading to damage and dysfunction (Chung and Brock 2011).

The cause of cryptorchidism usually isn't known, although, especially in pre-term boys, there may be hormonal dysfunction of the HPG axis which does not develop until the latter stages of pregnancy (Chung and Brock 2011). One risk factor is exposure of male foetuses to excess oestrogen in the uterus resulting in a reduced androgen–oestrogen ratio, affecting descent of the testes (Chung and Brock 2011). This may be linked to maternal obesity, but not all studies have found an association between maternal obesity and increased risk of cryptorchidism (Adams *et al.* 2011).

## 6.3 Varicocele

A varicocele is an abnormal swelling in a vein within the pampiniform plexus, a network of veins found in the spermatic cord which runs through the abdomen down to the testicle. The pampiniform plexus acts as a heat exchanger to cool blood and maintain the optimal temperature for sperm production (Einer-Jensen and Hunter 2005). There are no valves in the veins of the pampiniform plexus, so varicoceles can be caused by retrograde blood flow or the pooling of blood. Risk factors include low BMI (body mass index) (Nielsen *et al.* 2006), family history indicating a possible genetic factor (Raman, Walmsley and Goldstein 2005) and intense physical activity over several years (Di *et al.* 2001).

A varicocele is found in up to 40 per cent of infertile patients (Weidner, Pilatz and Altinkilic 2010) and is associated with lowered testosterone, smaller testicles (Said *et al.* 1992) and impaired sperm parameters (Kantarzi *et al.* 2007).

Possible mechanisms for reduced sperm production include disruption in the heat-exchange mechanism, increasing the temperature in the testicles; increased intra-testicular pressure and hypoxia due to constriction of blood flow; reflux of toxic metabolites from the adrenal glands; and hormonal abnormalities (Kantarzi *et al.* 2007). Oxidative stress may also be involved, leading to damage to sperm membranes, impaired morphology and motility (Miyaoka and Esteves 2012), and also sperm DNA damage: varicocele are associated with high levels of sperm DNA fragmentation, even when other sperm parameters are normal (Smith *et al.* 2006).

The link between varicocele and infertility remains controversial as about two-thirds of men with varicocele remain fertile and those who don't may not see any improvement in fertility after surgical treatment (varicocelectomy) (Miyaoka and Esteves 2012).

## 6.4 Torsion, hernia and other testicular trauma

Testicular torsion occurs when the spermatic cord is twisted, cutting off the blood supply to the testes. Up to 1.2 per cent of infertile men have a history of torsion, and up to 40–70 per cent of men with a history of torsion have abnormal semen (Singh *et al.* 2012). One or both testes may have to be removed during treatment but where they are left intact, in vitro studies suggest sperm production is adversely affected due to the release of free radicals causing oxidative stress during both infarction (when the blood supply is cut off) and reperfusion (return of the blood flow). This leads to oxidation of membrane lipids, sperm DNA damage and cell death in the testes (Minutoli *et al.* 2009; Turner, Bang and Lysiak 2004). Impairment of hormonal functions of the testes has also been reported (Romeo *et al.* 2010). Animal studies suggest that testicular torsion may also be linked to the development of anti-sperm antibodies if the blood–testes barrier is breached during the injury itself or corrective surgery (Merimsky, Orni-Wasserlauf and Yust 1984).

A hernia occurs when tissue protrudes through a defect in its encapsulating walls, such as an inguinal hernia which occurs in the groin. As with torsion, this can interrupt blood flow to the testes either directly or during corrective surgery, causing damage to their functioning, and surgery may lead to breach of the blood–testes barrier, triggering the production of anti-sperm antibodies. Scar tissue may also form, leading to obstructive oligozoospermia or azoospermia (Dy, Rust and Ellsworth 2012). The incidence of obstruction of the vas deferens may be as high as 26.7 per cent in subfertile patients who underwent inguinal hernia repair in childhood (Chen *et al.* 2014).

## 6.5 Mumps orchitis

The incidence of mumps orchitis in males contracting mumps after puberty is as high as 40 per cent (Davis *et al.* 2010). The virus attacks the testicular glands, leading to inflammation which directly damages sperm production. Leydig cell function may also be damaged leading to hormonal disturbances, but this usually resolves after the acute phase (Davis *et al.* 2010). Where only one testicle is affected, the effect on sperm parameters is usually short-lived (Berhrman, Kliegman and Jenson 2004), but where both testicles are affected then 30–87 per cent of patients experience infertility (Casella *et al.* 1997). Overall, subfertility results in about 13 per cent of patients (Davis *et al.* 2010). It has been suggested that there may be a causal link between mumps orchitis and anti-sperm antibodies, but one small study found that the incidence and level of serum anti-sperm antibodies in 21 patients who had or had previously had mumps orchitis was low (Kalaydjiev, Dimitrova and Tsvetkova 2001).

## 6.6 Hormonal imbalances

Endocrine (hormonal) causes of male infertility are well recognised, but account for less than three per cent of cases (Sigman and Jarow 1997). The most common endocrine cause is a disorder of the hypothalamus or pituitary gland in the brain (Anawalt 2013), which together control all the hormonal systems in the body, but this only accounts for 0.5 per cent or less of male infertility cases (Skakkebaek, Giwercman and de Kretser 1994).

The underlying cause of a hormonal imbalance may be genetic (e.g. Klinefelter's syndrome), physical (e.g. cryptorchidism), or acquired, for example subsequent to orchitis, testicular torsion, testicular tumour, systemic illness, or cytotoxic therapy such as radio- or chemotherapy (Jungwirth *et al.* 2014). Systemic disorders such as chronic illnesses, nutritional deficiencies and obesity have also been identified as causes (Friedman and Dull 2012). Alternatively, the hormonal control system itself – HPG axis – may be dysfunctional.

Other hormonal disturbances such as thyroid and adrenal dysfunction can influence fertility.

## BOX 6.3 DYSFUNCTION OF THE HPG AXIS – OVERVIEW OF DIFFERENT ··· PROBLEMS (STANFORD UNIVERSITY 2014) ··················

▶ The hypothalamus does not release enough GnRH to stimulate testosterone synthesis and sperm production.

▶ The pituitary does not produce enough LH and FSH to stimulate the testes and testosterone/sperm production.

▶ The Leydig cells in the testes may not produce testosterone in response to LH stimulation.

▶ A man may produce or be exposed to other hormones or endocrine-disrupting substances, which interfere with the sex-hormone balance. (These are discussed in Chapter 7.)

The most common cause of hypothalamic–pituitary dysfunction is a pituitary tumour or other brain tumour (Skakkebaek *et al.* 1994). Tumours can cause hyperprolactinaemia, present in around 11 per cent of oligospermic men. Hyperprolactinaemia inhibits the secretion of GnRH and in turn FSH, LH and testosterone, and hence lowers sperm production, motility and quality (Singh *et al.* 2011).

Other common causes include congenital factors such as Kallmann's syndrome, which occurs in 1 in 10,000 men and is associated with GnRH deficiency, often leading to undescended testicles and delay or failure of puberty (Skakkebaek *et al.* 1994). In androgen resistance syndromes, cells become unresponsive to testosterone, leading to raised testosterone production and elevated LH due to lack of feedback regulation by androgen receptors in the hypothalamus and pituitary (McClure 2005). Other congenital syndromes such as Prader-Willi syndrome, Laurence-Moon-Bardet-Biedle syndrome, Lowe's syndrome and Möbius' syndrome (McClure 2005) are also associated with HPG dysfunction.

Other hormonal problems include oestrogen excess, which suppresses gonadotrophin secretion in the pituitary. It may be due to tumours in the adrenal cortex, Sertoli cells, interstitial cells in the testes or cirrhosis of the liver (responsible for biotransformation and excretion of excess oestrogen) (McClure 2005). Another factor may be obesity, due to increased aromatisation of testosterone to oestradiol in adipose tissue (Schindler, Ebert and Friedrich 1972). Exogenous oestrogen exposure may also disrupt male reproductive hormone function. A recent report for the World Health Organisation (Bergman *et al.* 2013) reviews an extensive body of epidemiological and animal studies linking exposure to environmental oestrogens such as PCBs, dioxins, phthalates and pesticides to declining sperm counts and other problems associated with male infertility such as cryptorchidism.

Leptin resistance – common in obesity – may also play a role: a small number of human studies of leptin-deficient men, supported by strong evidence from animal studies, indicate that leptin is essential for male fertility via stimulation of GnRH, which in turn stimulates FSH and LH secretion from the pituitary (Teerds, de Rooij and Keijer 2011).

Primary adrenal insufficiency, also known as Addison's disease, occurs when the adrenal glands fail to produce adequate amount of hormones despite a normal stimulation by ACTH (adrenocorticotrophic hormone). It may underlie hypothyroidism (discussed below) and lead to oligospermia (Kowal, Turco and Nangia 2006). Cushing's disease, where the adrenal glands are overactive, is associated with low LH and low testosterone leading to hypergonadism (Jequier 2000).

Hypothyroidism and hyperthyroidism affect levels of SHGB (sex hormone-binding globulin) and sex steroids, disrupting normal spermatogenesis, with hyperthyroidism linked to abnormal sperm motility, and hypothyroidism to abnormal morphology (Krassas, Poppe and Glinoer 2010).

Diabetes mellitus (commonly known as diabetes) can be divided into Type 1 (T1DM) and Type 2 (T2DM). T1DM is an autoimmune condition caused by dysfunction of the immune system, with a strong genetic component. T2DM is a metabolic disorder which involves a degree of genetic susceptibility but is also significantly linked to lifestyle factors such as obesity and inactivity. Men with T1DM may have decreased serum testosterone due to impaired Leydig cell function (Amaral, Oliveira and Ramalho-Santos 2009) and animal studies provide some good evidence that low insulin affects serum levels of FSH, LH and prolactin, leading to reduced sperm output and fertility (Agabaje *et al.* 2007). However, Sexton and Jarrow (1997) argue that research findings are conflicting and T1DM is unlikely to impair reproductive function without the presence of other factors such as oxidative stress due to high levels of glucose causing damage to developing sperm. Oxidative stress and its impact are discussed elsewhere in this chapter. T2DM in men is also associated with low testosterone and low LH or FSH, possibly due to increased conversion of testosterone to oestrogen in adipose tissue leading to suppression of GnRH and impairment of sperm production; or in cases where T2DM is not associated with obesity, impaired insulin signalling (a feature of T2DM) at the hypothalamic level may impair function of the HPG axis (Dandona *et al.* 2009).

Taken either as prescribed medications or otherwise obtained, anabolic androgenic steroids may cause subfertility by disrupting normal hormonal output. They suppress endogenous testosterone production usually resulting in azoospermia. This may be reversible over a 3–6-month period but normal pituitary function does not always return (Kobayashi, Nagao and Nakajima 2012).

Commonly available medical therapies for hypogonadotrophism-related infertility include gonadotrophin replacement therapy, aromatase inhibitors, and selective oestrogen receptor modulators (SERMs, e.g. clomiphene) but may take months or even years to take maximal effect, so assisted reproduction should also be considered (Anawalt 2013).

## 6.7 Genetic causes

The normal human genetic complement is 23 pairs of chromosomes. The genes located on a particular pair of chromosomes, known as the sex chromosomes, determine sex. Females have two X chromosomes so are 'XX'; males have one X chromosome and one Y chromosome so are 'XY'. A significant proportion of male infertility is likely to result from abnormalities of Y chromosome genes involved in the regulation of spermatogenesis (NICE 2013b). A study of 1263 infertile couples by Kjessler (1972) found the overall incidence of chromosomal abnormalities to be 6.2 per cent; where the sperm count was less than 10m the incidence was 11 per cent and in those with azoospermia it was 21 per cent.

Chromosome abnormalities can be numerical or structural, for example inversions or translocations of genes, and may be on the X or Y sex chromosome, or may occur on other chromosomes (Jungwirth *et al.* 2014) in which case they are known as autosomal abnormalities.

··· BOX 6.4 Y CHROMOSOME DEFECTS ···························

The azoospermic factor (AZF) is a common microdeletion (defect) which occurs on the Y chromosome and is associated with oligozoospermia and azoospermia (McClure 2005). Some Y chromosome deletions may lead to abnormalities in offspring born by ICSI (McLachlan and O'Bryan 2010) so men with severe oligozoospermia or azoospermia should be offered genetic testing prior to undergoing assisted reproduction.

(NICE 2013b)

··· BOX 6.5 X CHROMOSOME DEFECTS ···························

Abnormalities can also occur on the X chromosome. The most common is Klinefelter's syndrome, characterised by an extra X chromosome in the male, which leads to hormonal disturbances, small testicles and sclerosis of the seminiferous tubules. It accounts for 3 per cent of male infertility and is found in 5 to 10 per cent of men with oligospermia and azoospermia (Wattendorf and Muenke 2005). ICSI may be an option for some patients as techniques using testicular microdissection have been successful in identifying viable sperm for IVF with resulting pregnancies.

(Tournaye et al. 1996)

·····································································

Androgen insensitivity syndrome can also be due to a mutation in the AR gene, located on the long arm of the X chromosome, which may result in androgen insensitivity, infertility and varying degrees of feminisation of the external genitalia (Jungwirth et al. 2014).

About 10 per cent of Caucasians have a mutation of the methylenetetrahydrofolate reductase (MTHFR) gene, called the MTHFR C677T polymorphism, on both genes in the relevant pair (a homozygous mutation) (Botto and Yang 2000). The lowest occurrence is in West Africans (Forges et al. 2007). Polymorphisms of the MTHFR gene reduce functioning of the enzyme 5,10-MTHFR which converts 5,10-methyleneTHF (inactive folate) into 5-methylTHF (active folate or folic acid). This disrupts an important metabolic process, the homocysteine-methionine cycle, leading to the build-up of homocysteine called hyperhomocysteinaemia (Harmon et al. 1996).

Elevated homocysteine impairs another important metabolic process, methylation, involved in gene expression and DNA repair. It also triggers an inflammatory response and reduces the availability of nitric oxide, leading to oxidative stress, impairment of blood flow to the testes, and the activation of apoptosis (cell 'suicide'), all of which may be linked to impairment of sperm production or function and hence male (and female) infertility (Forges et al. 2007). However, findings of research into the links between the presence of the MTHFR C677T polymorphism and male infertility risk (azoospermia and oligozoospermia) are inconsistent. This may be due to the clinical effects of polymorphisms being masked by higher intakes of B6, B12 and folate (the key vitamins involved in the homocysteine-methionine cycle and methylation) in some populations compared with others (Singh et al. 2005). Lack of active folate (folic acid) also leads to an increased risk of neural tube defects such as spina bifida. Another MTHFR polymorphism, MTHFR A1298C, does not seem to be associated with hyperhomocysteinaemia or a greater risk of male infertility (Park *et al.* 2005; van der Put *et al.* 1998).

Cystic fibrosis (CF) is the most common genetic disease of Caucasians and four per cent are carriers (Jungwirth *et al.* 2014). The condition is due to mutations involving the CTFR gene (CF transmembrane conductance regulator). This is involved in formation of the ejaculatory duct, seminal vesicle, vas deferens and epididymis. CFTR gene mutations are associated with CBAVD and were found in approximately 2 per cent of men with obstructive azoospermia attending a clinic in Edinburgh, Scotland (Donat *et al.* 1997). During diagnosis, CBAVD is easy to miss, so careful examination is recommended, especially in men with low semen volume (Jungwirth *et al.* 2014).

Other more common autosomal disorders include: Noonan syndrome (male Turner syndrome) which affects 1 in 1000 to 1 in 2500 children (van der Burgt 2007), 75 per cent of whom are born with cryptorchidism that may affect fertility (Sharland *et al.* 1992); primary ciliary dyskinesia (PCD)/Kartagener's syndrome, with an incidence of 1 in 3000 to 1 in 20,000 (Hempel and Buchholz 2009), associated with the impairment or inability of sperm flagella (tails) to beat, resulting in immotility, although not all men with PCD have immotile sperm (Munro *et al.* 1994); and Kallman's syndrome, which affects 1 in 8000 men and causes hypogonadism, delayed sexual maturation and maldescended testicles amongst other symptoms (Hempel and Buchholz 2009).

Other autosomal abnormalities associated with male fertility include: Prader-Willi syndrome, Bardet-Biedle syndrome, cerebellar ataxia, dominant polycystic kidney disease and 5-α reductase deficiency (Jungwirth *et al.* 2014). It is likely that many others are yet to be discovered, and it is possible that many or most cases of idiopathic male infertility are caused by as yet unknown genetic mutations or polymorphisms (Nuti and Krausz 2008).

## 6.8 Infections

Infection is a recognised factor which may impair male infertility via organ damage due to the organism itself or via inflammation which may damage cells, contribute to oxidative stress and consequent sperm damage, or block ducts (Ochsendorf 2010). The main infections of relevance are the urogenital infections: urethritis, usually associated with sexually transmitted chlamydia and gonococcal infections (Schiefer 1998); prostatitis; epididymitis; and orchitis (infections of the testes), usually chronic and attributable to viral infection including mumps, Coxsackie virus types, Epstein–Barr, influenza and HIV (Rusa et al. 2012). There are some indications that herpes simplex virus (HSV) and human papilloma virus (HPV) may also negatively affect sperm parameters (Ochsendorf 2010).

The most significant impact may be from silent (asymptomatic) infections. Silent infections of the testes are commonly found in infertile men when testicular biopsy is performed (Schuppe et al. 2010). Similarly, according to the US Centers for Disease Control and Prevention (CDC 2014), most people with chlamydia have no symptoms. Prostate infections can also be silent and may have a negative impact on sperm density, motility and morphology due to the effects of oxidative stress when sperm are exposed to inflammatory prostatic fluid following ejaculation, but research results are inconsistent (Potts and Pasqualotto 2003; Diemer et al. 2003). The role of silent infections as a primary or contributing factor in male infertility is probably significantly underestimated (Schuppe et al. 2010). A case study showing how silent infections were implicated in the couple's infertility is included in Chapter 9. Infection may also give rise to anti-sperm antibodies which bind to sperm (Schuppe and Meinhardt 2005).

## 6.9 Anti-sperm antibodies

Antigens are proteins on cell membranes. The immune system uses them to recognise the body's own cells so that it does not attack them. Normally, sperm is made and stored within a sealed system in the testes, bound by the blood–testis barrier. This means that new antigens expressed on the membranes of developing spermatocytes and spermatids are unknown in the rest of the body and hence mature sperm appear 'foreign' to the immune system. If they do somehow come into contact with the rest of the body (for example as a result of surgery such as a biopsy or vasectomy, following an infection or injury to the testes, or even through gastrointestinal exposure), immunocompetent white blood cells, which form part of the immune system, will mistake the sperm for invading organisms and start to form anti-sperm antibodies to deal with the 'threat' they pose. The injury may heal, but the body continues to produce the antibodies. These are released into semen. At the point of ejaculation, when semen and sperm mix, the antibodies bind to the sperm. This can cause agglutination and also interfere with the acrosome reaction and zona binding during fertilisation. Not all anti-sperm antibodies actually affect sperm function. A sperm-mucus penetration test is carried out to determine whether or not they do (Bohring and Krause 2003; WHO 2010).

Treatments for anti-sperm antibodies include immunosuppressive corticosteroids or cyclosporine; assisted reproductive techniques (ART) such as ICSI; and laboratory techniques such as sperm washing, immunomagnetic sperm separation and proteolytic enzyme treatment (Naz 2004).

## 6.10 Oxidative stress

ROS are highly reactive molecules that have functional roles in sperm (as in other cells and tissues) but in excess can cause oxidative damage to cellular lipids, protein and DNA, initiating pathological processes. Most cells are protected by enzymatic anti-oxidant systems (superoxide dismutase, glutathione peroxidase and catalase) or non-enzymatic systems such as ascorbic acid (vitamin D) or alpha-tocopherol (vitamin E). Sperm are particularly vulnerable to damage by ROS because mature sperm lack cytoplasm, which is the main source of anti-oxidants, although some anti-oxidant enzymes are present. They also lack a nucleus and hence are unable to repair their own DNA. This is compensated for by anti-oxidant enzyme systems and other enzymes in semen (Venkatesh *et al.* 2009). These neutralise and balance ROS, but these defences may be overwhelmed, leading to excessive ROS build-up and a state of oxidative stress, sperm damage and consequent impairment of sperm function (WHO 2010). Around 40 to 80 per cent of infertile patients have high levels of seminal ROS (Venkatesh *et al.* 2009).

It is thought that excessive ROS may be generated primarily as a by-product of defective metabolism in the sperm's mitochondria (responsible for cellular energy production); infection and the presence of leucocytes in the genital tract (white blood cells involved in the immune system); exposure to xenobiotics (foreign chemicals) such as environmental pollutants; and by defective sperm themselves, in particular those with excess residual cytoplasm (Aitken and de Iuliis 2007; Koppers *et al.* 2008). Wright *et al.* (2014) also identify age, smoking, obesity, mobile phone radiation, heat and exposure to toxic metals as factors associated with oxidative stress and negative impacts on sperm. A low intake of anti-oxidant nutrients may also be a factor. These nutritional and environmental factors are explored in more detail in Chapters 10 and 11.

## 6.11 DNA fragmentation

DNA fragmentation is damage to sperm DNA. It is widely hypothesised that the main cause is oxidative stress (Aitken and de Iuliis 2010). This is supported by the research, including a study of 101 infertile men, which found that an increase in seminal ROS levels by 25 per cent was associated with a 10 per cent increase in sperm DNA fragmentation (Mahfouz *et al.* 2010). Subsequent studies have found similar results (Aktan *et al.* 2013; Atig *et al.* 2013; Khosravi *et al.* 2012). Another study comparing sperm DNA from a cohort of 50 assisted conception patients with that of a group of donors concluded that DNA fragmentation arises from a process involving oxidative stress, leading to the oxidation of DNA bases, DNA fragmentation and cell death (Aitken *et al.* 2010).

DNA fragmentation has been linked to impaired fertilisation, disrupted pre-implantation embryo development, miscarriage and birth defects in the offspring (Lewis *et al.* 2013). It is estimated that a significant proportion of men whose infertility is hitherto 'unexplained' have a cause attributed after sperm DNA testing (Bungum *et al.* 2007). Simon *et al.* (2013) found that in 80 per cent of 239 couples with unexplained or idiopathic infertility, the male partner had high levels of sperm DNA damage. At 25 per cent or more it significantly reduced the chance of pregnancy, even with some forms of fertility treatment (Simon *et al.* 2013). A growing number of studies report sperm DNA damage to be useful as a diagnostic tool for male infertility and as a predictor of treatment success (Lewis *et al.* 2013).

Following fertilisation, the oocyte (egg) may be able to carry out some sperm DNA repair but more extensive damage may introduce mutations associated with poor fertilisation capacity, deficient embryo development and repeated miscarriage (Bungum *et al.* 2007; Meseguer *et al.* 2008; Seli *et al.* 2004; Virro, Larson-Cook and Evenson 2004; Zini *et al.* 2008).

## 6.12 Mitochondrial function

Mitochondria are the energy 'power houses' of cells. They are responsible for producing energy in the form of ATP (adenosine triphosphate) via the electron-transport chain. Mitochondria have their own DNA which encodes for the polypeptides involved in the electron-transport chain. Sperm motility depends on the production of energy by mitochondria in a densely packed group forming a chain round the base of the flagellum (Nakada *et al.* 2006). Defects in the arrangement of mitochondria can affect the motility (Venkatesh *et al.* 2009). Low motility is found in sufferers of mitochondrial diseases caused by mitochondrial DNA mutations, and mitochondrial DNA mutations have been found in semen samples of men with fertility problems, suggesting that the accumulation of DNA mutations contributes to sperm dysfunction and infertility (Nakada *et al.* 2006).

As a by-product of their respiratory/energy-producing function, mitochondria produce ROS, which are needed at low levels by sperm for physiological functions including sperm capacitation and the acrosome reaction (Venkatesh *et al.* 2009). However, if the anti-oxidant defence systems are insufficient, and generation of ROS overwhelms them, this can lead to oxidative stress, resulting in damage to the mitochondrial membranes and mitochondrial DNA and hence reduced energy production and sperm function (Venkatesh *et al.* 2009). Animal studies have found that depletion of the mitochondrial anti-oxidant, mitochondrial glutathione peroxidase, by lack of selenium, can cause male infertility, owing to impaired sperm quality and structural abnormalities in the midpiece (Schneider *et al.* 2009).

## 6.13 Cancer treatment

Chemotherapy damages the DNA in stem cells in the testes and hence spermatogenesis. The effects of chemotherapy on male fertility depend on the particular therapy, and may be temporary or permanent. Even if temporary, recovery of spermatogenesis may take many years (Lee *et al.* 2006). Radiotherapy directly to the testes damages the highly sensitive germinal epithelium, resulting in temporary or permanent azoospermia, depending on the dose. Higher doses can also affect production of testosterone by Leydig cells. Recovery of spermatogenesis may take years, and for higher doses there is a risk of permanent infertility. Combined with chemotherapy, total body radiotherapy will cause sterility (Royal College of Physicians 2007).

Sperm and embryo cryopreservation (freezing and banking) are the standard methods of preserving fertility, but are less effective once treatment has started as the sperm DNA may already have been damaged (Loren *et al.* 2013). Azoospermic men may sometimes be producing limited sperm within the testes, and testicular sperm retrieval for ICSI – in which sperm are removed directly from the testes via aspiration or microdissection of the seminiferous tubules – may be offered but this should be considered an experimental procedure (Loren *et al.* 2013).

## 6.14 Effects of other medications

Medications can also affect sperm production by damaging the germ cells, their supporting cells, or by disruption of the HPG axis (McClure 2005). They may also cause erectile dysfunction or ejaculatory problems (Brezina, Yunus and Zhao 2012) or reduce libido (Nudell, Monoski and Lipshulz 2002). The most commonly prescribed medication which affects male fertility is cimetidine, used to reduce stomach acid production in relation to stomach ulcers and acid reflux/GERD (gastroesophageal reflux disease), which also reduces sperm density and causes gynaecomastia. A study of 300 men concluded that it does not reduce circulating androgen levels but is an androgen antagonist, affecting peripheral androgen action (Carlson, Ippoliti and Swerdloff 1981). A wide range of other medications have been linked to male fertility including SSRIs (selective serotonin reuptake inhibitors) used for depression; calcium channel blockers used for hypertension; alpha adrenergic blockers used to treat lower urinary tract syndrome associated with benign prostatic hyperplasia (BPH); anti-epilepsy medications; colchicine and allopurinol used to treat gout; methotrexate used for rheumatoid arthritis, psoriatic arthritis and psoriasis; sulfasalazine used for inflammatory bowel disease or IBS; and anti-retrovirals used to treat HIV (Brezina *et al.* 2012; Ehrenfeld *et al.* 1986; French and Koren 2003; Nudell *et al.* 2002; Toovey *et al.* 1981). Data evaluating the effects of most medications on semen is lacking, and where it exists is often inconclusive (Brezina *et al.* 2012).

Another significant effect of medication is the impact of diethylstilbestrol (DES), a synthetic oestrogen, on the male offspring of mothers who took it to prevent miscarriage and other pregnancy complications in the USA from 1938 to 1971. The sons of women who took DES during pregnancy are three times more likely than unexposed men to have epididymal cysts, undescended testes, small testes or other genital structural abnormalities, and also sperm and semen abnormalities, although overall they do not seem to have an increased risk of infertility as a result (Schrager and Potter 2004).

## 6.15 Other illnesses

Coeliac disease is an autoimmune condition that primarily effects the small intestine, triggered by exposure to dietary gluten. Common symptoms include chronic diarrhoea, malabsorption and consequent weight loss, but there is increasing recognition that it may be a 'silent' condition, with few, if any, digestive symptoms (Freeman 2010). Studies from the UK show that 20 per cent of married coeliacs experienced infertility, associated with androgen resistance, poor sperm morphology and reduced motility, which may improve following removal of gluten from the diet (Farthing *et al.* 1982). Common nutrient deficiencies due to malabsorption in coeliac disease include folic acid, vitamin B12, iron, and vitamin D (Malterre 2009), all of which are important for fertility. Coeliac disease is also an inflammatory condition and this may play a role, given that inflammation can contribute to oxidative stress (Sakar *et al.* 2011). The impact of oxidative stress on male fertility is discussed elsewhere in this chapter. The impact of coeliac disease on both male and female fertility is explored in more depth in Chapter 7.

The hormonal impact of type 1 and type 2 diabetes mellitus on male infertility is discussed elsewhere in this chapter. As with coeliac disease, another important dimension of both type 1 diabetes (T1DM) and type 2 diabetes (T2DM) is oxidative stress. A study involving 18 men with T1DM found they had greater oxidative stress and lower sperm parameters than healthy controls, probably contributing to their infertility (Vignera *et al.* 2009). In addition, 50 per cent of men with T1DM experience sexual dysfunction, such as erectile problems, due to oxidative damage to blood vessels (Amaral *et al.* 2009). A small study comparing semen parameters of 25 men with T2DM and 25 men without found lower values for semen parameters in the diabetic group, concluding that T2DM negatively affects male fertility potential (Singh *et al.* 2014). Increased oxidative stress in the diabetic group is one possible explanation: a small study of 40 men found that increased lipid peroxidation in T2DM men with poor glycaemic control was associated with low sperm quality (La Vignera *et al.* 2012). There may also be other contributing factors: a study of 857 Qatari men found that male infertility is significantly associated with T2DM. However, they also found that age, smoking and obesity were the significant major contributors for infertility in diabetic men (Bener *et al.* 2009).

A combination of hormonal imbalances, toxic accumulation and nutritional deficiencies involved in renal failure contribute to erectile problems and decreased libido as well as decreased spermatogenesis (Handelsman 1985).

Cirrhosis of the liver is associated with testicular atrophy, impotence and gynaecomastia due to altered metabolic clearance of hormones. The condition is usually due to alcohol abuse which also directly reduces testosterone synthesis in the testes (Nitsche *et al.* 2014).

## 6.16 Erectile and ejaculatory problems

Peyronie's disease is a connective tissues disorder which begins as an inflammatory condition, leading progressively to the formation of fibrous scar tissue under the skin of the penis leading it to bend, especially during erection (Jungwirth *et al.* 2014). This may make sexual intercourse difficult and painful. It may be congenital or triggered by damage to the penis. The incidence is hard to determine due to patient embarrassment but is estimated at up to 23 per cent of men between the ages of 40 and 70 in varying degrees of severity (Urology Care Foundation 2014).

Erectile dysfunction is the persistent inability to attain and maintain an erection sufficient to permit satisfactory sexual performance. Estimates of the prevalence vary widely but are probably in the region of 20 per cent to 50 per cent and correlate positively with age, due to an increased incidence in older men of lower urinary tract symptoms (LUTS)/benign prostatic hyperplasia (BPH) and cardiovascular disease, all of which affect erectile function (Jungwirth *et al.* 2014).

Retrograde ejaculation, which may appear as anejaculation (no ejaculation), occurs when the seminal fluid flows backwards into the bladder instead of forwards during orgasm, due to the failure of the bladder neck to close. The main symptoms are little or no semen released during orgasm or cloudy urine after orgasm. Causes include paralysis, multiple sclerosis and diabetes, which may all involve damage to the nerves to the bladder; surgery, which may damage the nerves to the bladder; anti-hypertensive medications; and some mood-altering drugs. Drug treatments, where applicable, include pseudoephedrine or imipramine (Vorvick, Liou and Zieve 2012).

## 6.17 Age

Until relatively recently it was thought that all men remained fertile into old age. However, the impact of age on male fertility is now being recognised. Even after adjusting for the age of the female partner, conception during a 12-month period was found to be 30 per cent less likely for men over age 40 years compared with men under 30 years (Stephen and Chandra 1998). A decline in HPG function and testosterone output, which can impact all semen parameters as well as sexual function, begins around age 40 (Harris *et al.* 2011). Rapid progression and total motility of sperm may start to decline as early as 35 years old (Siddighi *et al.* 2007). Semen volume and sperm morphology may also decline with advancing age (Plastira *et al.* 2007). The rate of DNA fragmentation (associated with infertility and increased risk of miscarriage) is twice that in men aged 45 plus compared with men less than 30 years old (Moskovtsev, Willis and

Mullen 2006). Age-related male factor infertility is likely to be increasingly significant given the trend towards older fatherhood as well as older motherhood (Harris *et al.* 2011).

## References

Adams, S.V., Hastert, T.A., Huang, Yi., and Starr, J.R. (2011) 'No association between maternal pre-pregnancy obesity and risk of hypospadias or cryptorchidism in male newborns.' *Birth Defects Research Part A: Clinical and Molecular Teratology 91*, 4, 241–248.

Agabaje, I.M., Rogers, D.A., McVicar, C.M., McClure, N., *et al.* (2007) 'Insulin dependant diabetes mellitus: implications for male reproductive function.' *Human Reproduction 22*, 7, 1871–1877.

Agarwal, A., and Esteves, S.C. (2011) 'Novel concepts in male infertility.' *International Brazilian Journal of Urology 37*, 1, 5–15.

Aitken, R.J., and De Iuliis, G.N. (2007) 'Origins and consequences of DNA damage in male germ cells.' *Reproductive Biomedicine Online 14*, 727–733. Available at www.rbmojournal.com/article/S1472-6483(10)60676-1/pdf, accessed on 19 May 2015.

Aitken, R.J., and De Iuliis, G.N. (2010) 'On the possible origins of DNA damage in human spermatozoa.' *Molecular Human Reproduction 16*, 3–13

Aitken, R.J., De Iuliis, G.N., Finnie, J.M., Hedges, A., and McLachlan, R.I. (2010) 'Analysis of the relationships between oxidative stress, DNA damage and sperm vitality in a patient population: development of diagnostic criteria.' *Human Reproduction 25*, 2415–2426.

Aktan, G., Dogru-Abbasoglu, S., Kucukgergin, C., Kadioglu, A., Ozdemirler-Erata, G., and Kocak-Toker, N. (2013) 'Mystery of idiopathic male infertility: is oxidative stress an actual risk?' *Fertility and Sterility 99*, 1211–1215.

Amaral, S., Oliveira, P.J., and Ramalho-Santos, J. (2009) 'Diabetes and the impairment of reproductive function: possible role of mitochondria and reactive oxygen species.' *Current Diabetes Reviews 4*, 1, 46–54.

American Urological Association (AUA) (2010) *The Optimal Evaluation of the Infertile Male: AUA Best Practice Statement.* Maryland: American Urological Association Education and Research Inc.

Anawalt, B.D. (2013) 'Approach to male infertility and induction of spermatogenesis.' *Journal of Clinical Endocrinology and Metabolism.* Online. Available at http://press.endocrine.org/doi/abs/10.1210/jc.2012-2400, accessed on 19 May 2015.

Atig, F., Kerkeni, A., Saad, A., and Ajina, M. (2013) 'Effects of reduced seminal enzymatic antioxidants on sperm DNA fragmentation and semen quality of Tunisian infertile men.' *Journal of Assistive Reproduction and Genetics.* e-publication ahead of print. Available at http://link.springer.com/article/10.1007%2Fs10815-013-9936-x, accessed on 19 May 2015.

Bener A., Al-Ansari, A.A., Zirie, M., and Al-Hamaq, A.O. (2009) 'Is male fertility associated with type 2 diabetes mellitus?' *International Urology and Nephrology 41*, 4, 777–784.

Bergman, A., Heindel, J.J., Jobling, S., Kidd, K.A., and Zoeller, R.T. (eds) (2013) *State of the Science of Endocrine Disrupting Chemicals – 2012.* United Nations Environment Programme and the World Health Organisation. Available at www.who.int/ceh/publications/endocrine/en, accessed on 19 May 2015.

Berhrman, R.E., Kliegman, R.M., and Jenson, H.B. (eds) (2004) *Nelson Textbook of Pediatrics* (17th edition). Philadelphia, PA: Saunders.

Bohring, C., and Krause, W. (2003) 'Immune infertility: towards a better understanding of sperm (auto)-immunity.' *Human Reproduction 18*, 5, 915–924.

Botto, L.D., and Yang, Q. (2000) '5,10-methylenetetrahydrofolate reductase gene variants and congenital anomalies: a HuGE Review.' *American Journal of Epidemiology 151*, 862–877.

Brezina, P.R., Yunus, F.N., and Zhao, Y. (2012) 'Effects of pharmaceutical medications on male fertility.' *Journal of Reproduction and Infertility 13*, 1, 3–11.

Bungum, M. (2012) 'Role of Sperm DNA Integrity in Fertility.' In L.V. Pereira (ed.) *Embryology – Updates and Highlights on Classic Topics.* Rijeka: InTech Europe. Available at http://cdn.intechopen.com/pdfs-wm/34557.pdf, accessed on 19 May 2015.

Bungum, M., Humaidan, P., Axmon, A., Spano, M., *et al.* (2007) 'Sperm DNA integrity assessment in prediction of assisted reproduction technology outcome.' *Human Reproduction 22*, 174–179.

Carlsen, E., Giwercman, A., Keiding, N., and Skakkebaek, N.E. (1992) 'Evidence for decreasing quality of semen during past 50 years.' *British Medical Journal 16854*, 609–613.

Carlson, H.E., Ippoliti, A.F., and Swerdloff, R.S. (1981) 'Endocrine effects of an acute and chronic cimetidine administrations.' *Digestive Diseases and Sciences 26*, 5, 428–432.

Casella, R., Leibundgut, B., Lehmann, K., and Gasser, T.C. (1997) 'Mumps orchitis: report of a mini-epidemic.' *Journal of Urology 7*, 158, 2158–2161.

CDC (Centers for Disease Control and Prevention) (2014) *Chlamydia – CDC Factsheet.* Available at www.cdc.gov/std/chlamydia/stdfact-chlamydia.htm, accessed on 19 May 2015.

Chandra, A., and Copen, C.E. (2013) *Infertility and Impaired Fecundity in the United States, 1982–2010: Data From the National Survey of Family Growth.* National Center for Health Statistics Reports Number 67. Hyattsville, MD: National Center for Health Statistics.

Chen, X.F., Wang, H.X., Liu, Y.D., Sun, K., *et al.* (2014) 'Clinical features and therapeutic strategies of obstructive azoospermia in patients treated by bilateral inguinal hernia repair in childhood.' *Asian Journal of Andrology 16*, 745–748.

Chung, E., and Brock, G.B. (2011) 'Cryptorchidism and its impact on male fertility: a state of art review of current literature.' *Canadian Urological Association Journal 5*, 3, 210–214.

Cooke, S., Tyler, J.P.P., and Driscoll, G.L. (1995) 'Hyperspermia: the forgotten condition?' *Human Reproduction 10*, 2, 367–368.

Dada, R., Thilagavathi, J., Venkatesh, S., Esteves, S.C., and Agarwal, A. (2011) 'Genetic testing in male infertility.' *The Open Reproductive Science Journal 3*, 42–56.

Dandona, P., Dhindsa, S., Chandel, A., and Topiwala, S. (2009) 'Low testosterone in men with type 2 diabetes – a growing public health concern.' *Diabetes Voice 54*, 2, 27–29.

Davis, N.F., McGuide, B.B., Mahon, J.A., Smyth, A.E., O'Malley, K.J., and Fitzpatrick, J.M. (2010) 'The increasing incidence of mumps orchitis: a comprehensive review.' *BJU International 105*, 8, 1060–1065.

Di, L., Gentile, V., Pigozzi, F., Parisi, A., Giannetti, D., and Romanelli, F. (2001) 'Physical activity as a possible aggravating factor for athletes with varicocele: impact on the semen profile.' *Human Reproduction 16*, 6, 1180–1184.

Diemer, T., Huwe, P., Ludwig, M., Hauck, E.W., and Weidner, W. (2003) 'Urogenital infection and sperm motility.' *Andrologia 35*, 283–287.

Docimo, S.G., Silver, R.I., and Cromie, W. (2000) 'The undescended testicle: diagnosis and management.' *American Family Physician 61*, 9, 2037–2044.

Donat, R., McNeill, A.S., Fitzpatrick, D.R., and Hargreave, T.B. (1997) 'The incidence of cystic fibrosis gene mutations in patients with congenital bilateral absence of the vas deferens in Scotland.' *British Journal of Urology 79*, 1, 74–77.

Du Plessis, S.S., Gokul, S., and Agarwal, A. (2013) 'Semen hyperviscosity: causes, consequences, and cures.' *Frontiers in Bioscience (Elite Edition) 1*, 5, 224–231.

Dy, G.W., Rust, M., and Ellsworth, P. (2012) 'Detection and management of pediatric conditions that may affect male fertility.' *Urology Nursing 32*, 5, 237–248.

EAU (European Association of Urology) (2014) *Pocket Guidelines 2014 Edition.* Arnhem: EAU Guidelines Office. Available at www.uroweb.org/guidelines/online-guidelines/?no_cache=1, accessed on 19 May 2015.

Edey, A.J., and Sidhu, P.S. (2008) 'Male infertility: role of imaging in the diagnosis and management.' *Imaging 20*, 139–146.

Ehrenfeld, M., Levy, M., Margalioth, E.J., and Eliakim, M. (1986) 'The effects of long-term colchicine therapy on male fertility in patients with familial Mediterranean fever.' *Andrologia 18*, 4, 420–426.

Einer-Jensen, N., and Hunter, R.H.F. (2005) 'Counter-current transfer in reproductive biology.' *Reproduction 129*, 9–18.

Farthing, M.J., Edwards, C.R., Rees, L.H., and Dawson, A.M. (1982) 'Male gonadal function in coeliac disease: 1. Sexual dysfunction, infertility, and semen quality.' *Gut 23*, 608–614.

Fisch, H. (2008) 'Declining worldwide sperm counts: disproving a myth.' *Urology Clinics of North America 55*, 137–146.

Forges, T., Monnier-Barbarino, P., Alberto, J.M., Gueant-Rodriguez, R.M., Daval, J.M., and Gueant, J.L. (2007) 'Impact of folate and homocysteine metabolism on human reproductive health.' *Human Reproduction Update 13*, 3, 225–238.

Freeman, H.J. (2010) 'Reproductive changes associated with celiac disease.' *World Journal of Gastroenterology 16*, 46, 5810–5814.

French, A.E., and Koren, G. (2003) 'Effect of methotrexate on male fertility.' *Canadian Family Physician 49*, 577–578.

French, D.B., Sabanegh, E.S., Goldfarb, J., and Desai, N. (2010) 'Does severe teratozoospermia affect blastocyst formation, life birth rate, and other clinical outcome parameters in ICSI cycles?' *Fertility and Sterility 93*, 4, 1097–1103.

Friedman, S.K., and Dull, R.B. (2012) 'Male infertility: an overview of the causes and treatments.' *US Pharmacist 37*, 6, 39–43. Available at www.uspharmacist.com/content/c/35115/#sthash.z3zHCsk7.dpuf, accessed on 19 May 2015.

Ghirelli-Filho, M., Mizrahi, F.E., Pompeo, A.C.L., and Glina, S. (2012) 'Influence of strict sperm morphology on the results of classic *in vitro* fertilization.' *International Brazilian Journal of Urology 38*, 4, 519–528.

Grasso, M., Buonaguidi, A., and Lania, C. (1991) 'Postpubertal cryptorchidism: review and evaluation of fertility.' *European Urology 20*, 126–128.

Guzick, D.S., Overstreet, J.W., Factor-Litvak, P., Brazil, C.K., *et al.* (2001) 'Sperm morphology, motility, and concentration in fertile and infertile men.' *New England Journal of Medicine 345*, 1388–1393.

Handelsman, D.J. (1985) 'Hypothalamic-pituitary ponadal dysfunction in renal failure, dialysis and renal transplantation.' *Endocrine Reviews 6*, 151–182.

Harmon, D.L., Woodside, J.V., Yarnell, J.W.G., McMaster, D., *et al.* (1996) 'The common "thermolabile" variant of methylene tetrahydrofolate reductase is a major determinant of mild hyperhomocysteinaemia.' *QJM – An International Journal of Medicine 89*, 571–577.

Harris, I.D., Fronczak, C., Roth, L., and Meacham, R.B. (2011) 'Fertility and the aging male.' *Reviews in Urology 13*, 4, 184–190.

Hempel, M., and Buchholz, T.J. (2009) 'Rare syndromes associated with infertility.' *Reproduktionsmed Endokrinol 6*, 1, 24–26.

Hirsch, I. H. (2015) 'Male Reproductive Endocrinology.' In Merck & Co. Inc. Merck Manual Professional Version. Available online at http://www.merckmanuals.com/professional/genitourinary-disorders/male-reproductive-endocrinology-and-related-disorders/male-reproductive-endocrinology, accessed on 16 July 2015. New Jersey: Merck, Sharp and Dohme Corp.

Irvine, D.S. (1998) 'Epidemiology and aetiology of male infertility.' *Human Reproduction 13 Suppl.*, 1, 33–44.

Irvine, D.S., Twigg, J.P., Gordon, E.L., Fulton, N., Milne, P.A., and Aitken, R.J. (2000) 'DNA integrity in human spermatozoa: relationships with semen quality.' *Journal of Andrology 21*, 33–44.

Jarow J.P., Sharlip I.D., Belker A.M., Lipshultz L.I., *et al.* (2002) 'Best practice policies for male infertility.' *Journal of Urology 167*, 5, 2138–2144.

Jequier, A.M. (1985) 'Obstructive azoospermia: a study of 102 patients.' *Clinical Reproductive Fertility 3*, 21–36.

Jequier, A.M. (2000) *Male Infertility: A Guide for the Clinician.* Oxford: Blackwell.

Jungwirth, A., Diemer, T., Dohle, G.R., Giwercman, A., *et al.* (2014) *Pocket Guidelines 2014 Edition: Guidelines for the Investigation and Treatment of Male Infertility.* Arnham: EAU (European Association of Urology), Guidelines Office. Available at www.uroweb.org/guidelines/online-guidelines/?no_cache=1, accessed on 19 May 2015.

Jungwirth, A., Giwercman, A., Tournaye, H., Diemer, T., *et al.* (2012) 'European Association of Urology Guidelines on Male Infertility: The 2012 Update.' *European Urology 62*, 324–332.

Kalaydjiev, S., Dimitrova, P., and Tsvetkova, D. (2001) 'Serum sperm antibodies unrelated to mumps orchitis.' *Andrologia 33*, 69–70.

Kantarzi, P.D., Goulis, C.D. Goulis G.D., and Patadimas, I. (2007) 'Male infertility and varicocele: myths and reality.' *Hippokratia 11*, 3, 99–104.

Khosravi, F., Valojerdi, M.R., Amanlou, M., Karimian, L., and Abolhassani, F. (2012) 'Relationship of seminal reactive nitrogen and oxygen species and total antioxidant aapacity with sperm DNA fragmentation in infertile couples with normal and abnormal sperm parameters.' *Andrologia 46*, 17–23.

Kjessler, B. (1972) 'Facteurs génétiques dans la subfertilité male humaine.' In *Fecondité et Stérilité du Male.* Acquisitions récentes. Paris: Masson.

Kobayashi, H., Nagao, N., and Nakajima, K. (2012) 'Review article: Focus issue on male infertility.' *Advances in Urology.* Article ID 823582. Available at www.hindawi.com/journals/au/2012/823582, accessed on 19 May 2015.

Kolon, F.T., Patel, P.R., and Huff, S.D. (2004) 'Cryptorchidism: diagnosis, treatment and long-term prognosis.' *Urologic Clinics of North America 31*, 469–480.

Koppers, A.J., De Iuliis, G.N., Finnie, J.M., McLaughlin, E.A., and Aitken, R.J. (2008) 'Significance of mitochondrial reactive oxygen species in the generation of oxidative stress in spermatozoa.' *Journal of Clinical Endocrinology and Metabolism 93*, 3199–3207.

Kowal, B.F., Turco, J., and Nangia, A.K. (2006) 'Addison's disease presenting as male infertility.' *Fertility and Sterility 85*, 4, 1059.

Krassas, G.E., Poppe, K., and Glinoer, D. (2010) 'Thyroid function and human reproductive health.' *Endocrine Reviews 31*, 702–755.

Kumar, P., Kumar, N., Singh Thakur, D., and Patidar, A. (2010) 'Male hypogonadism: symptoms and treatment.' *Journal of Advanced Pharmaceutical Technology and Research 1*, 3, 297–301.

La Vignera, S., Condorelli, R.A., Vicari, E., D'Agata, R., and Calogero, A.E. (2011) 'Seminal vesicles and diabetic neuropathy: ultrasound evaluation in patients with couple infertility and different levels of glycaemic control.' *Asian Journal of Andrology 13*, 872–876.

La Vignera, S., Condorelli, R.A., Vicari, E., D'Agata, R., Salemi, M., and Calogero, A.E. (2012) 'High levels of lipid peroxidation in semen of diabetic patients.' *Andrologia* *44, Suppl. 1*, 565–570.

Lee, S.J., Schover, L.R., Partridge, A.H., Patrizio, P., *et al.* (2006) 'American Society of Clinical oncology recommendations on fertility preservation in cancer patients.' *Journal of Clinical Oncology 24*, 2917–2931.

Lewis, S.E., Aitken, R.J., Conner, S.J., Iuliis, G.D., *et al.* (2013) 'The impact of sperm DNA damage in assisted conception and beyond: recent advances in diagnosis and treatment.' *Reproductive BioMedicine Online 27*, 325–337. Available at www.rbmojournal.com/ article/S1472-6483(13)00363-5/fulltext, accessed on 19 May 2015.

Loren, A.W., Mangu, P.B., Beck, L.N., Brennan, L., *et al.* (2013) 'Fertility preservation for patients with cancer: American Society of clinical oncology clinical practice guideline update.' *Journal of Clinical Oncology 31*, 19, 2500–2510.

Mahfouz, R., Sharma, R., Thiyagarajan, E., Kale, V., *et al.* (2010) 'Semen characteristics and sperm DNA fragmentation in infertile men with low and high levels of seminal reactive oxygen species.' *Fertility and Sterility 94*, 6, 2141–2146.

Malterre, T. (2009) 'Digestive and nutritional considerations in celiac disease: could supplementation help?' *Alternative Medicine Review 14*, 3, 247–257.

McClure, R.D. (2005) 'Endocrinology of Male Infertility.' In P.E. Patton and D.E. Battaglia (eds) *Office Andrology*. New Jersey: Humana Press.

McLachlan, R.I., and O'Bryan, M.K. (2010) 'State of the art for genetic testing of infertile men' *Journal of Clinical Embryology and Metabolism 95*, 3. Available at http://press. endocrine.org/doi/abs/10.1210/jc.2009-1925?url_ver=Z39.88-2003&rfr_ id=ori:rid:crossref.org&rfr_dat=cr_pub%3dpubmed, accessed on 19 May 2015.

Merimsky, E., Orni-Wasserlauf, R., and Yust, I. (1984). 'Assessment of immunological mechanism in infertility of the rat after experimental testicular torsion.' *Urological Research 12*, 3, 179–182.

Meseguer, M., Martínez-Conejero, J.A., O'Connor, J.E., Pellicer, A., Remohi, J., and Garrido, N. (2008) 'The significance of sperm DNA oxidation in embryo development and reproductive outcome in an oocyte donation program: a new model to study a male infertility prognostic factor.' *Fertility and Sterility 89*, 1191–1199.

Minutoli, L., Antonuccio, P., Polito, F., Bitto, A., *et al.* (2009). 'Mitogenactivated protein kinase 3/mitogenactivated protein kinase 1 activates apoptosis during testicular ischemia-reperfusion injury in a nuclear factor-kappaB-independent manner.' *European Journal of Pharmacology 14*, 27–35.

Miyaoka, R., and Esteves, S.C. (2012) 'A critical appraisal on the role of varicocele in male infertility.' *Advances in Urology*. Article ID 59749. Available at www.hindawi.com/ journals/au/2012/597495, accessed on 19 May 2015.

Moghissi, K.S., and Wallach, E.E. (1983) 'Unexplained infertility.' *Fertility and Sterility 39*, 5–21.

Mortimer, D., Barratt, C.L.R., Björndahl, L., de Jager, C., Jequler, A.M., and Muller, C.H. (2013) 'What should it take to describe a substance as "sperm safe"?' *Human Reproduction Update 19, Suppl. 1*, i1–i45.

Moskovtsev, S.I., Willis, J., and Mullen, J.B. (2006) 'Age-related decline in sperm deoxyribonucleic acid integrity in patients evaluated for male infertility.' *Fertility and Sterility 85*, 496–499.

Munro, N.C., Currie, D.C., Lindsay, K.S., Ryder, T.A., *et al.* (1994) 'Fertility in men with primary ciliary dyskinesia presenting with respiratory infection.' *Thorax 49*, 684–687.

Nakada, K., Sato, A., Yoshida, K., Morita, H., Tanaka, H., and Inoue, S.-I. (2006) 'Mitochondrial-related male infertility.' *PNAS 103*, 41, 15148–15153.

National Institute for Health and Care Excellence (NICE) (2013a) *Investigation of Fertility Problems and Management Strategies.* Available at http://pathways.nice.org.uk/pathways/fertility#path=view%3A/pathways/fertility/investigation-of-fertility-problems-and-management-strategies.xml&content=view-node%3Anodes-semen-analysis, accessed on 19 May 2015.

National Institute for Health and Clinical Excellence (NICE) (2013b) *Fertility: Assessment and Treatment for People with Fertility Problems.* NICE Clinical Guideline 156 issued February 2013. Available at www.nice.org.uk/CG156, accessed on 19 May 2015.

Naz, R.K. (2004) 'Modalities for treatment of antisperm antibody mediated infertility: novel perspectives.' *American Journal of Reproductive Immunology 51*, 5, 390–397.

Nielsen, M.E., Zderic, S., Freedland, S.J., and Jarow, J.P. (2006) 'Insight on pathogenesis of varicoceles: relationship of varicocele and body mass index.' *Urology 86*, 2, 392–396.

Nitsche, R., Coelho, J.C.U., de Freitas, A.C.T., Zeni Neto, C., and Martins, E. (2014) 'Testosterone changes in patients with liver cirrhosis before and after orthotopic liver transplant and its correlation with meld.' *Arquivos de Gastroenterologica 51*, 1, 59–63.

Nudell, D.M., Monoski, M.M., and Lipshulz, L.I. (2002) 'Common medications and drugs: how they affect male fertility.' *Urology Clinics of North America 29*, 4, 965–973.

Nuti, F., and Krausz, C. (2008) 'Gene polymorphisms/mutations relevant to abnormal spermatogenesis.' *Reproductive Biomedicine Online 16*, 4, 504–513.

O'Flaherty, C., de Lamirande, E., and Gagnon, C. (2005) 'Reactive oxygen species and protein kinases modulate the level of phospho-MEK-like proteins during human sperm capacitation.' *Biology of Reproduction 73*, 94–105.

Oates, R.D., and Amos, J.A. (1994) 'The genetic basis of congenital bilateral absence of the *vas deferens* and cystic fibrosis.' *Journal of Andrology 15*, 1–8.

Ochsendorf, F.R. (2010) 'What Are the Consequences of Sexually Transmitted Infections on Male Reproduction.' In B. Robert and P. Chan (eds) *Handbook of Andrology* (2nd edition). American Society of Andrology. Lawrence, KS: Allen Press. Available at www.andrologysociety.com/docs/handbook-2nd/Handbook-of-Andrology-Second-Edition-English.aspx, accessed on 19 May 2015.

Office on Women's Health (2012) *Infertility Factsheet.* Washington: Office on Women's Health. Available at www.womenshealth.gov/publications/our-publications/fact-sheet/infertility.html, accessed on 19 May 2015.

Olea, N., Sharp, R., Jegou, B., Toppari, J., Skakkebaek, N.E., and Schlatt, S. (2010) *Male Reproductive Health: Its Impacts in Relation to General Wellbeing and Low European Fertility Rates.* Science Policy Briefing 40. Strasbourg: European Science Foundation.

Park, J.H., Lee, H.C., Jeong, Y.M., Chung, T.G., *et al.* (2005) 'MTHFR C677T polymorphism associates with unexplained infertile male factors.' *Journal of Assisted Reproduction and Genetics 22*, 361–368.

Pierik F.H., Van Ginneken A.M, Dohle, G.R., Vreeburg, J.T.,and Veber, R.F (2000) 'The advantages of standardized evaluation of male infertility.' *International Journal of Andrology 23*, 340–346.

Plastira, K., Msaouel, P., Angelopoulou, R., Zanioti, K., *et al.* (2007) 'The effects of age on DNA fragmentation, chromatin packaging and conventional semen parameters in spermatozoa of oligoasthenoteratozoospermic patients.' *Journal of Assisted Reproduction and Genetics 24*, 437–443.

Potts, J.M., and Pasqualotto, F.F. (2003) 'Seminal oxidative stress in patients with chronic prostatitis.' *Andrologia 35*, 5, 304–308.

Raheem, A.A., Ralph, D., and Minhas, S. (2012) 'Male infertility.' *Journal of Clinical Urology 5*, 5, 254–268.

Raman, J.D., Walmsley, K., and Goldstein, M. (2005) 'Inheritance of varicoceles.' *Urology 65*, 6, 1186–1189.

Rolland, M., Le Moal, J., Wagner, V., Royere, D., and De Mouzon, J. (2013) 'Decline in semen concentration and morphology in a sample of 26,609 men close to general population between 1989 and 2005 in France.' *Human Reproduction 28*, 2, 462–470.

Romeo, C., Impellizzeri, P., Arrigo, T., Antonuccio, P., *et al.* (2010). 'Late hormonal function after testicular torsion.' *Journal of Pediatric Surgery 45*, 2, 411–413.

Royal College of Physicians (RCP), The Royal College of Radiologists, Royal College of Obstetricians and Gynaecologists (2007) *The Effects of Cancer Treatment on Reproductive Functions: Guidance on Management. Report of a Working Party*. London: RCP.

Rusa, A., Pilatz, A., Wagenlehner, F., Linn, T., *et al.* (2012) 'Influence of urogenital infections and inflammation on semen quality and male fertility.' *World Journal of Urology 30*, 1, 23–30.

Said, S.A., Aribarg, A., Virutamsen, P., Chutivongse, S., *et al.* (1992) 'The influence of varicocele on parameters of fertility in a large group of men presenting to infertility clinics.' *Fertility and Sterility 57*, 6, 1289–1293.

Sakar, O., Bahrainwala, J., Chandrasekaran, S., Kothari, S., Mathur, P.P., and Agarwal, A. (2011) 'Impact of inflammation on male fertility.' *Frontiers in Bioscience (Elite Edition)* 3, 247–257.

Schiefer, H.G. (1998) 'Microbiology of male urethroadnexitis: diagnostic procedures and criteria for aetiologic classifcation.' *Andrologia 30, Suppl. 1*, 7–13.

Schindler, A.E., Ebert, A., and Friedrich, E. (1972) 'Conversion of androstenedione to estrone by human tissue.' *Journal of Clinical Endocrinology and Metabolism 35*, 627–630.

Schneider, M., Forster, H., Boersma, A., Seller, A., *et al.* (2009) 'Mitochondrial glutathione peroxidase 4 disruption causes male infertility.' *FASEB Journal 9*, 3233–3242.

Schrager, S., and Potter, B.E. (2004) 'Diethylstilbestrol exposure.' *American Family Physician 69*, 10, 2395–2400.

Schuppe, H.C., and Meinhardt, A. (2005) 'Immune privilege and inflammation of the testis.' *Chemical Immunology and Allergy 88*, 1–14.

Schuppe, H.C., Pilatz, A., Hossain, H. Meinhardt, A., Bergmann, M., and Haidl, G. (2010) 'Orchitis and male infertility. *Der Urologe Ausg A 49*, 629–635.

Seli, E., Gardner, D.K., Schoolcraft, W.B., Moffatt, O., and Sakkas, D. (2004) 'Extent of nuclear DNA damage in ejaculated spermatozoa impacts on blastocyst development after *in vitro* fertilization.' *Fertility and Sterility 82*, 378–383.

Sengupta, P., and Banerjee, R. (2013) 'Environmental toxins: alarming impacts of pesticides on male fertility.' *Human and Experimental Toxicology.* e-publication ahead of print. Available at http://het.sagepub.com/content/early/2013/12/13/0960327113515504.abstract?maxtoshow=&HITS=10&hits=10&RESULTFORMAT=&fulltext=male+fertility+environmental+toxins&andorexactfulltext=and&searchid=1&FIRSTINDEX=0&resourcetype=HWCIT, accessed on 19 May 2015.

Sexton, W.J., and Jarrow, J.P. (1997) 'Effect of diabetes mellitus upon male reproductive function.' *Urology 149*, 508–513.

Sharland M., Burch M., McKenna W.M., and Patton M.A. (1992) 'A clinical study of Noonan syndrome'. *Archives of Diseases in Childhood 67*, 178–83.

Siddighi, S., Chan, C.A., Patton, W.C., Jacobson, J.D., and Chan, P.J. (2007) 'Male age and sperm necrosis in assisted reproductive technologies.' *Urologia Internationalis 9*, 231–234.

Sigman, M., and Jarow, J.P. (1997) 'Endocrine evaluation of infertile men.' *Urology 50*, 5, 659–664.

Simon, L., Proutski, I., Stevenson, M., Jennings, D., *et al.* (2013) 'Sperm DNA damage has a negative association with live-birth rates after IVF.' *Reproductive BioMedicine Online 26*, 1, 68–78. Available at www.rbmojournal.com/article/S1472-6483(12)00590-1/pdf, accessed on 19 May 2015.

Singh, A.K., Tomar, S., Chaudhari, A.R., Singh, R., and Verma, N. (2014) 'Type 2 diabetes mellitus affects male fertility potential.' *Indian Journal of Physiology and Pharmacology* 58, 4, 403–406.

Singh, K., Singh, S.K., Sah, R., Singh, I., and Raman, R. (2005) 'Mutation C677T in the methylenetetrahydrofolate reductase gene is associated with male infertility in an Indian population.' *International Journal of Andrology 28*, 115–119.

Singh, P., Singh, M., Cugati, G., and Singh, A.K. (2011) 'Hyperprolactinemia: an often missed cause of male infertility.' *Journal of Human Reproductive Science 4*, 2, 102–103. Available at www.ncbi.nlm.nih.gov/pmc/articles/PMC3205532, accessed on 19 May 2015.

Singh, R., Hamada, A.J., Bukavina, L., and Agarwal, A. (2012) 'Physical deformities relevant to male infertility.' *Nature Reviews in Urology 9*, 156-174. Available at www.nature.com/nrurol/journal/v9/n3/full/nrurol.2012.11.html, accessed on 19 May 2015.

Skakkebaek, N.E., Giwercman, A., and de Kretser, D. (1994) 'Pathogenesis and management of male infertility.' *Lancet 343*, 8911, 1473.

Smith, R., Kaune, H., Parodi, D., Madariaga, M., *et al.* (2006) 'Increased sperm DNA damage in patients with varicocele: relationship with seminal oxidative stress.' *Human Reproduction 21*, 4, 986–993.

Stanford University (2014) *What Causes Male Infertility?* Stanford University Online. Available at http://web.stanford.edu/class/siw198q/websites/reprotech/New%20 Ways%20of%20Making%20Babies/causemal.htm, accessed on 19 May 2015.

Stephen, E.H., and Chandra, A. (1998) 'Updated projections of infertility in the United States: 1995–2025.' *Fertility and Sterility 70*, 30–34.

Summerton, D.J., Kitrey, N.D., Lumen, N., Serafentinidis, E., and Djakovic, N. (2012) 'EAU Guidelines on Iatrogenic Trauma.' *European Urology 62*, 628–639.

Svalander, P., Jakobsson, A.-H., Forsberg, A-S., Bengtsson, A.-C., and Wilkland, M. (1996). 'The outcome of intracytoplasmic sperm injection is unrelated to "strict criteria" sperm morphology.' *Human Reproduction 11*, 5, 1019–1022.

Swan, S.H., Elkin, E.P., and Fenster, L. (1997) 'Have sperm densities declined? A reanalysis of global trend data.' *Environmental Health Perspectives 11*, 1228–1232.

Teerds, K.J., de Rooij, D.G., and Keijer J. (2011) 'Functional relationship between obesity and male reproduction: from humans to animal models.' *Human Reproduction Update 17*, 667–683.

Toovey, S., Hudson, E., Hendry, W.F., and Levi, A.J. (1981) 'Sulphalazine and male infertility: reversibility and possible mechanism.' *Gut 22*, 6, 445–451.

Tournaye, H., Staessen, C., Liebaers, I., Van Assche, E., *et al.* (1996) 'Testicular sperm recovery in nine 47, XXY Klinefelter patients.' *Human Reproduction 11*, 1644–1649.

Turner, T.T., Bang, H.J., and Lysiak, J.L. (2004). 'The molecular pathology of experimental testicular torsion suggests adjunct therapy to surgical repair.' *Journal of Urology 172*, 2572–2578.

University of Ottawa (2013) *Spermatogenesis.* Ottawa: University of Ottawa R. Samuel McLaughlin Centre for Population Health Risk Assessment. Available at www.emcom.ca/primer/sperma.shtml, accessed on

Urology Care Foundation (2013) *Undescended Testis (Cryptorchidism).* Urology Care Foundation. The Official Foundation of the American Urological Association. Available at www.urologyhealth.org/urologic-conditions/cryptorchidism, accessed on 19 May 2015.

Urology Care Foundation (2014) *Peyronies.* Urology Care Foundation: The Official Foundation of the American Urological Association. Available at www.urologyhealth.org/urologic-conditions/peyronies-disease, accessed on 19 May 2015.

Van der Burgt, I. (2007) 'Noonan syndrome.' *Orphanet Journal of Rare Diseases 2*, 4. Available at www.ojrd.com/content/2/1/4, accessed on 19 May 2015.

Van der Put, N.M., Gabreels, F., Stevens, E.M., Smeitink, J.A., *et al.* (1998) 'A second common mutation in the methylenetetrahydrofolate reductase gene: an additional risk factor for neural-tube defects?' *American Journal of Human Genetics 62*, 1044–1051.

Venkatesh, S., Deecaraman, R., Shamsi, M.B., and Dada, R. (2009) 'Role of reactive oxygen species in the pathogenesis of mitochondrial DNA (mtDNA) mutations in male infertility.' *Indian Journal of Medical Research 129*, 127–137.

Vignera, S.L., Vicari, E., Calogero, A.E., Condorelli, R., and Lanzafame, F. (2009) 'Diabetes, oxidative stress and its impact on male fertility.' *Journal of Andrological Sciences 16*, 42–46.

Virro, M.R., Larson-Cook, K.L., and Evenson, D.P. (2004) 'Sperm chromatin structure assay (SCSA) parameters are related to fertilization, blastocyst development, and ongoing pregnancy in *in vitro* fertilization and intracytoplasmic sperm injection cycles.' *Fertility and Sterility 81*, 1289–1295.

Vorvick, L.J., Liou, L.S., and Zieve, D. (2012) *Retrograde Ejaculation.* MedlinePlus. National Institutes of Health. Available at www.nlm.nih.gov/medlineplus/ency/article/001282.htm, accessed on 19 May 2015.

Wattendorf, D.J. and Muenke, M. (2005) 'Klinefelter Syndrome.' *American Family Physician 72*, 11, 2259–2262

Weidner, W., Pilatz, A., and Altinkilic, B. (2010) 'Varicocele: an update.' *Andrology 49*, 163–165.

World Health Organisation (WHO) (1987) 'Towards more objectivity in diagnosis and management of male infertility.' *International Journal of Andrology 7, Suppl.,* 1–53.

World Health Organisation (WHO) (2009) 'Revised Glossary on ART Terminology.' *Human Reproduction 24*, 11, 2683–2687.

World Health Organisation (WHO) (2010) *Laboratory Manual for the Examination and Processing of Human Semen* (5th edition). Geneva: World Health Organisation.

Wright, C., Milne, S., and Leeson, H. (2014) 'Sperm DNA damage caused by oxidative stress: modifiable clinical, lifestyle and nutritional factors.' *Male Infertility Reproductive BioMedicine Online 28*, 6, 684–703. Available at www.rbmojournal.com/article/S1472-6483(14)00118-7/fulltext, accessed on 19 May 2015.

Zini, A., Boman, J.M., Belzile, E., and Ciampi, A. (2008) 'Sperm DNA damage is associated with an increased risk of pregnancy loss after IVF and ICSI: systematic review and meta-analysis.' *Human Reproduction 23*, 2663–2668.

# Chapter 7

# Coeliac Disease and Infertility Disorder

*Dr Mohammad Rostami-Nejad, Coeliac Disease Department, Gastroenterology and Liver Diseases Research Center, Shahid Beheshti University of Medical Sciences, Tehran, Iran; Gastroenterology Department, Worcestershire, Royal Hospital Worcester, UK, and Kamran Rostami, Gastroenterology Unit, Alexandra Hospital, Redditch, Worcestershire, UK*

## 1. Undiagnosed coeliac disease and fertility

Infertility is defined as the biological inability of a woman or man to achieve pregnancy after at least one year of trying. Women who are able to get pregnant but then have repeat miscarriages are also considered to be infertile (Gnoth *et al.* 2005; Quaas and Dokras 2008). On the other hand, undiagnosed or untreated coeliac disease can lead to a host of seemingly unrelated problems, including osteoporosis, depression and anaemia (Bradley and Rosen 2004). Now medical researchers, along with some observant obstetrician-gynaecologists, are realising that undiagnosed coeliac disease may be a major cause of otherwise unexplained infertility in both men and women (Rostami *et al.* 2001). Although it is commonly believed that infertility is heavily related to female factors, according to a range of studies in different countries this condition is associated with untreated coeliac disease, and only about one-third of cases of infertility actually stem from the woman (Collin *et al.* 2002). Men with untreated disease may also face fertility issues (Gnoth *et al.* 2005). About one-third of cases originate with the male partner and the remaining cases are a combination of unknown factors or a mix of male and female complications (Gnoth *et al.* 2005). Although these problems were not always recognised as being related to coeliac disease by doctors and other health professionals, this situation is now beginning to change (Jackson *et al.* 2008). Italian researchers have noted that male coeliac disease patients have a greater risk of infertility and other reproductive issues, as well as a greater incidence of androgen (male hormone) deficiency (Stazi and Mantovani 2004).

It is not clear why more people with undiagnosed or untreated coeliac disease suffer from infertility. It is possible that malnutrition resulting from malabsorption of nutrients from food may be to blame, or there may be some as-of-yet undiscovered reason (Pope and Sheiner 2009).

'Gluten intolerance' is the term used when we refer to the entire category of gluten issues including coeliac disease, non-coeliac gluten sensitivity and wheat allergy, and in many cases it is difficult to differentiate between these. Whilst the treatment plan for all of them is to follow a gluten-free diet initially, this could change with the advent of potential medications for coeliac disease.

Coeliac disease is an inherited autoimmune disorder which most often causes intestinal tissue damage, but 'non-coeliac gluten sensitivity' causes the body to mount a stress response (often gluten-intolerance symptoms) different from the immunological response that occurs in those who have coeliac disease.

Many gluten-intolerant women afflicted with fertility problems do not present with the 'classic' digestive complaints associated with coeliac disease but are more apt to suffer from fatigue and anaemia. Often they have no digestive complaints whatsoever. Studies have showed that fertility problems could very well indicate early autoimmune changes, a serious hallmark of gluten intolerance (Rostami *et al.* 2001; Collin *et al.* 2002; Jackson *et al.* 2008) (Figure 7.1).

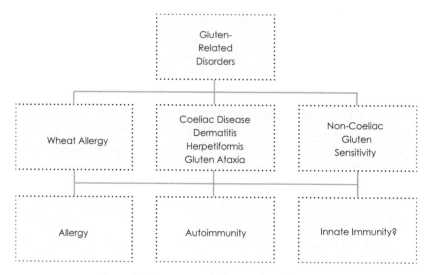

Figure 7.1 Spectrum of gluten-related disorders

## 2. Epidemiology

Over the last 10 years, several studies have examined the link between coeliac disease and infertility and found that women suffering from unexplained infertility may have clinically silent coeliac disease (Ferguson, Holmes and Cooke 1982; Collin *et al.* 1996; Sher and Mayberry 1996; Meloni *et al.* 1999). Hundreds of women from different parts of the world suffering from infertility were found to be afflicted with coeliac disease (Table 7.1) (Ferguson *et al.* 1982; Rostami *et al.* 2001; Collin *et al.* 2002; Shamaly *et al.* 2004; Khoshbaten *et al.* 2011).

### Table 7.1 Rate of infertility in affected women with coeliac disease

| Country | Percentage |
|---------|------------|
| Finland | 2.7 |
| Italy | 3.03 |
| Iran | 1.5 |
| Israel | 2.65 |

The testing methods utilised were strictly those for coeliac disease, including for endomysial antibodies (EMA), anti-tissue transglutaminase (tTG) antibodies and a positive small bowel biopsy (Rostami Nejad *et al.* 2009). If clinicians had included testing such as for deamidated gliadin and anti-gliadin antibodies, they would have identified those women suffering from gluten sensitivity as well (Rostami *et al.* 1999). According to the National Center for Health Statistics, roughly 12 per cent of women in the United States had difficulty getting pregnant or carrying a baby to term in 2002 (Chandra, Copen and Hervey 2013). One study conducted by physicians at Thomas Jefferson University Hospital in Philadelphia found that the rate of recurrent spontaneous abortion (RSA) and infertility in coeliac disease patients is at least four times higher than in the general population (Chandra *et al.* 2013). The authors suggested that patients who experience unexplained infertility or RSA should be screened for coeliac disease. Another study from the Department of Medicine at Tampere University Hospital and Medical School at the University of Tampere, Finland, found that the rate of coeliac disease among women reporting infertility was 4.1 per cent (Collin *et al.* 1996). Although the exact reason for the increased risk remains unknown, the researchers suggested that female coeliac patients who are not adhering to a gluten-free diet have a shortened reproductive period and early menopause. Males with coeliac disease have shown gonadal dysfunction, which could also contribute to fertility complications.

The link between coeliac disease and infertility is currently being evaluated by researchers at Molinette Hospital in Turin, Italy (Sheiner, Peleg and Levy 2006; Zugna *et al.* 2011). Early reports from their research suggest that the prevalence of coeliac disease among women with unexplained infertility is 2.5 per cent to 3.5 per cent higher than in the control population. They suggest that coeliac disease represents a risk for abortion, low-birthweight babies and short breast-feeding periods, all of which can be corrected with a gluten-free diet. In the recent study by Khoshbaten *et al.* in Iran (2011), 100 Iranian couples with unexplained infertility and 200 couples not reporting reproductive problems as controls were investigated for coeliac disease. Positive results of tTGA were detected in 13 infertile patients (6.5%) and coeliac disease was confirmed by biopsy in three (1.5%) of the unexplained infertile patients. The result of this study indicated a higher seroprevalence of coeliac disease in infertile cases in comparison with those with normal fertility.

## 3. Risk factors

There are various factors that increase risk of infertility in women compared with men, as presented in Table 7.2. As this table shows, environmental factors such as smoking and alcohol consumption are risk factors of infertility in men, and habits such as diet and athletic activity are risk factors of infertility in women (www.celiaccentral.org).

### Table 7.2 Factors that increase risk of infertility in men and women

| Risk factor in men | Risk factor in women |
|---|---|
| Chemotherapy and radiation treatment for cancer | Age |
| Drugs | Diet |
| Toxins in the environment such as lead and pesticides | Athletic activity |
| Alcohol consumption | Stress |
| Smoking | Overweight or underweight |
| Coeliac disease | Smoking |
| Abnormality in sperm activity | Alcohol consumption |
| | Sexually transmitted diseases (STDs) |
| | Health problems that cause hormonal changes |
| | Coeliac disease |
| | Hormonal dysfunction |

## 4. Complications of having coeliac disease

Women with coeliac disease are reported to start having periods later and stop menstruating earlier than average (Khoshbaten *et al.* 2011; Rostami Nejad *et al.* 2011). They also suffer more often from secondary amenorrhoea, a condition in which menses start but then stop (Rostami Nejad *et al.* 2011). Together, these menstrual disorders lead to fewer ovulations, which results in less of a chance to get pregnant. Hormonal factors and poor nutrition are thought to play a role in causing these problems. Meanwhile, pregnancy complications such as threatened miscarriage, pregnancy-related hypertension, severe anaemia and intrauterine growth retardation occurred four times more often in women with coeliac disease (Norouzinia *et al.* 2011).

However, there are many causes of infertility, miscarriages and small babies besides unrecognised coeliac disease, and some studies have failed to show that the risks of these problems are actually increased by untreated coeliac disease (Tiboni *et al.* 2006). In any case, early pregnancy loss is frequent in many other autoimmune diseases (e.g. systemic lupus erythematosus (SLE), primary biliary cirrhosis and thyroiditis) (Farthing *et al.* 1982; Molteni, Bardella and Bianchi 1990). In addition, several studies have found that coeliac women who do achieve fertilisation often have higher chances of miscarriages and intrauterine growth (Farthing *et al.* 1982; Kurppa *et al.* 2009). Another study showed that women with coeliac disease had normal fertility, but their fertility had decreased in the two years preceding CD diagnosis (Farthing *et al.* 1982). Previous studies have suggested that women with undiagnosed coeliac disease have a nine-fold relative risk of multiple abortions and low-birthweight babies compared with women with treated coeliac disease (Farthing *et al.* 1982). For men, problems can include abnormal sperm such as lower sperm numbers, altered shape and reduced function. Men with untreated coeliac disease may also have lower testosterone levels (Chandra *et al.* 2013).

Twenty per cent of coeliacs who are married are infertile, and semen analysis reveals abnormalities in sperm shape as well as motility in affected men (Zugna *et al.* 2011). But there is good news in the fact that removal of gluten from the diet improved sperm morphology (Freeman 2010). Similarly, hormonal imbalances found in male coeliacs also normalised on a gluten-free diet (Tersigni *et al.* 2014). Of course, for both men and women, how often a couple have intercourse affects fertility. If someone feels unwell from untreated coeliac disease or gluten intolerance, infrequent sexual activity may be contributing to the problem. Sexual relations occurred less often when one partner had active coeliac disease compared with couples in which the partner's coeliac disease was being treated (National Institute of Diabetes and Digestive and Kidney Diseases 2015; see also BabyMed 2015).

In another Italian study, nearly 20 per cent of the coeliac women had amenorrhoea, or missed menstrual periods, while only 2.2 per cent of the control subjects suffered from amenorrhoea (Freeman 2010). In yet another study, four cases of coeliac disease were found in a group of 99 women with unexplained infertility; none of the coeliac women had extensive malabsorption, but two suffered from iron deficiency anaemia (Tersigni *et al.* 2014). Another study looked at the rate of children born to patients with coeliac disease compared with children born to control subjects. The authors found that women with coeliac disease had significantly fewer children prior to diagnosis – 1.9 children, on average, compared with 2.5 children in controls (Khashan *et al.* 2010). Obviously these are averages! After the women were diagnosed with coeliac disease, the difference began to even out. The researchers concluded that coeliac disease caused the difference in fertility prior to diagnosis, while the gluten-free diet corrected it following diagnosis. Once a woman with active coeliac disease does conceive, other problems that can arise during the pregnancy include miscarriages and smaller babies because of pre-term delivery or delayed growth in the uterus. These conditions are reported to be more common in women with untreated coeliac disease, though miscarriages have many causes and occur in up to a quarter of all pregnancies. Nonetheless, we recommend that if a woman has repeated miscarriages or is unable to conceive, consideration should be given to screening her for coeliac disease by antibody testing and, if negative, gluten intolerance testing should be considered.

## 5. Gluten intolerance

One key factor in reproductive and fertility issues is gluten intolerance. This is rather well known in the literature, but until it becomes standard to evaluate for coeliac and gluten sensitivity in those suffering from infertility, delayed menstruation, poor outcomes of pregnancy, and the like, then it definitely bears repeating that these problems have a strong gluten association. While it is quite well established that coeliacs suffer from infertility, an increased incidence of stillbirths, and perinatal (around the time of birth) deaths, the good news is that once they receive a diagnosis of coeliac disease and begin a gluten-free diet, some markers of infertility (e.g. miscarriage rates) may be corrected.

## 5.1 Diagnosis

Many researchers and clinicians now recommend that patients with unexplained infertility should be screened for coeliac disease, especially if they have any of the classic coeliac disease symptoms or risk factors (Khoshbaten *et al.* 2011; Norouzinia *et al.* 2011).

However, many of the women diagnosed in these infertility studies had subtle symptoms of coeliac disease or even so-called 'subclinical' coeliac disease, in which they had no apparent symptoms. Therefore, one should not rely on their symptoms to determine their risk for the condition. Screening of any infertile men and women with unknown origin, in the first step serologically then confirmed by biopsy, is recommended in all clinical practice; and if negative look at gluten intolerance, especially if there are autoimmune issues (Figure 7.2).

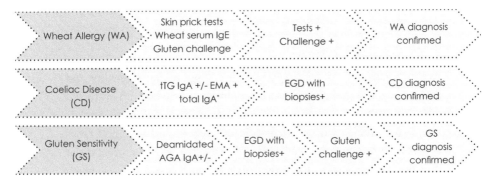

Figure 7.2 Algorithm for the differential
diagnosis of gluten-related disorders
*tTG: tissue transglutaminase; EMA: endomysial antibodies*

### ··· BOX 7.1 GLUTEN IN DIET AND A GLUTEN-FREE DIET ·····

Tolerable gluten thresholds in gluten-free products have long been debated, together with issues of cross-contamination of gluten-free cereals during the milling process. It is well established that a totally gluten-free diet is virtually impossible owing to the presence of traces of gluten. It is estimated that daily consumption of gluten from contaminated gluten-free foods is in the range of 5 to 50 mg.

Permitted levels of gluten in gluten-free foods vary in different areas of the globe. The Codex Alimentarius (World Health Organisation & UN Food and Agriculture Organisation Commission) recommends that 200 parts per million (ppm) of gluten is permitted in foods considered to be free of gluten. An intake of gluten below 10 mg/day is generally considered safe for most coeliac patients and not thought likely to cause histological abnormalities.

Moreover, several recent studies have demonstrated that oats (which contain gluten) can be tolerated by many coeliac patients. The prolamine gliadin in wheat constitutes 40 per cent of the cereal; the percentages are similar for rye and barley. However, in oats, avenins constitute only 15 per cent of the cereal.

(Bold and Rostami 2011)

## 6. Concluding remarks

According to our clinical experience we suggest that infertility and smaller or pre-term babies are more common in women with untreated coeliac disease than in those without. We are sure that some readers could share their own experiences in this regard and the good news is that with proper treatment with a gluten-free diet and correction of nutritional deficiencies, the prognosis for future pregnancies is much improved.

The rate of caesarean delivery increased amongst coeliac parents, according to Decker *et al.* (2010). Should all birth centres screen their mothers for coeliac disease and gluten sensitivity? Pregnant women certainly get screened for other diseases that are far less common. Considering the outcome of pregnancy with a diagnosed coeliac vs. an undiagnosed one, it may very well prove to be an excellent change in protocol.

Imagine if every young woman with a delayed onset of her menstrual cycle or amenorrhoea (no menstrual cycle) was tested for gluten intolerance. How much healthier and happier (remember that balanced hormones help to dictate balanced mood) could such women be? Imagine if women suffering from miscarriages could improve their outcome of a full term healthy baby by removing gluten from their diet. Now that is a recipe for happiness!

## References

BabyMed (2015) *Does Coeliac Disease Cause Infertility?* Available at www.babymed.com/fertility-news/does-celiac-disease-cause-infertility, accessed on 17 September 2015.

Bold, J., and Rostami, K. (2011) 'Gluten tolerance; potential challenges in treatment strategies.' *Gastroenterology and Hepatology From Bed to Bench 4*, 2, 53–57.

Bradley, R., and Rosen, M. (2004) 'Subfertility and gastrointestinal disease: "unexplained" is often undiagnosed.' *Obstetrical & Gynaecological Survey 59*, 108–117.

Chandra, A., Copen, C., and Hervey, E. (2013) 'Infertility and impaired fecundity in the United States, 1982–2010: Data from the National Survey of Family Growth.' *National Health Statistics Reports 67*, 14, 1–18.

Collin, P., Kaukinen, K., Valimaki, M., and Salmi, J. (2002) 'Endocrinological disorders and celiac disease.' *Endocrine Reviews 23*, 464–483.

Collin, P., Vilska, S., Heinonen, P., Hällström, O., and Pikkarainen, P. (1996) 'Infertility and coeliac disease.' *Gut 39*, 3, 382–384.

Decker E, Engelmann G, Findeisen A, Gerner P, Laass M, Ney D, Posovszky C, Hoy L, Hornef MW. (2010) 'Cesarean delivery is associated with celiac disease but not inflammatory bowel disease in children'. *Pediatrics. 2010 Jun*;125(6):e1433–40.

Farthing, M., Edwards, C., Rees, L., and Dawson, A. (1982) 'Male gonadal function in coeliac disease: 1. Sexual dysfunction, infertility and semen quality.' *Gut 23*, 608–614.

Ferguson, R., Holmes, G., and Cooke, W. (1982) 'Coeliac disease, fertility, and pregnancy.' *Scandinavian Journal of Gastroenterology 17*, 65–68.

Freeman, H. (2010) 'Reproductive changes associated with celiac disease.' *World Journal of Gastroenterology 16*, 46, 5810–5814.

Gnoth, C., Godehardt, E., Frank-Herrmann, P., Friol, K., Tigges, J., and Freundl, G. (2005) 'Definition and prevalence of subfertility and infertility.' *Human Reproduction 20*, 5, 1144–1147.

Jackson, J., Rosen, M., McLean, T., Moro, J., Croughan, M., and Cedars, M. (2008) 'Prevalence of celiac disease in a cohort of women with unexplained infertility.' *Fertility and Sterility 89*, 1002–1004.

Khashan, A., Henriksen, T., Mortensen, P., McNamee, R., *et al.* (2010) 'The impact of maternal celiac disease on birthweight and preterm birth: a Danish population-based cohort study.' *Human Reproduction 25*, 2, 528–534.

Khoshbaten, M., Rostami Nejad, M., Farzady, L., Sharifi, N., Hashemi, S., and Rostami, K. (2011) 'Fertility disorder associated with celiac disease in males and females: fact or fiction?' *Journal of Obstetrics and Gynaecology Research 37*,10, 1308–1312.

Kurppa, K., Collin, P., Viljamaa, M., Haimila, K., *et al.* (2009) 'Diagnosing mild enteropathy celiac disease: a randomized, controlled clinical study.' *Gastroenterology 136*, 816–823.

Meloni, G., Dessole, S., Vargiu, N., Tomasi, P., and Musumeci, S. (1999) 'The prevalence of coeliac disease in infertility.' *Human Reproduction 14*, 2759–2761.

Molteni, N., Bardella, M., and Bianchi, P. (1990) 'Obstetric and gynecological problems in women with untreated celiac disease.' *Journal of Clinical Gastroenterology 12*, 37–39.

National Institute of Diabetes and Digestive and Kidney Diseases (2015) *Celiac Disease.* Available at www.niddk.nih.gov/health-information/health-topics/digestive-diseases/celiac-disease/Pages/facts.aspx, accessed on 20 May 2015.

Norouzinia, M., Rostami, K., Amini, M., Lahmi, F., *et al.* (2011) 'Coeliac disease: prevalence and outcome in pregnancy.' *HealthMED 5*, 6, 1537–1541.

Pope, R., and Sheiner, E. (2009) 'Celiac disease during pregnancy: to screen or not to screen?' *Archives of Gynaecology and Obstetrics 279*, 1, 1–3.

Quaas, A., and Dokras, A. (2008) 'Diagnosis and treatment of unexplained infertility.' *Reviews in Obstetrics & Gynaecology 1*, 2, 69–76.

Rostami Nejad, M., Rostami, K., Cheraghipour, K., Nazemalhosseini Mojarad, E., *et al.* (2011) 'Celiac disease increases the risk of toxoplasma gondii infection in a large cohort of Iranian pregnant women.' *American Journal of Gastroenterology 106*, 548–549.

Rostami Nejad, M., Rostami, K., Pourhoseingholi, M., Nazemalhosseini Mojarad, E., *et al.* (2009) 'A typical presentation is dominant and typical for coeliac disease.' *Journal of Gastrointestinal and Liver Diseases 18*, 3, 285–291.

Rostami, K., Kerckhaert, J., Tiemessen, R., Meijer, J., and Mulder, C. (1999) 'The relationship between anti-endomysium antibodies and villous atrophy in coeliac disease using both monkey and human substrate.' *European Journal of Gastroenterology & Hepatology 11*, 439–442.

Rostami, K., Steegers, E., Wong, W., Braat, D., and Steegers-Theunissen, R. (2001) 'Coeliac disease and reproductive disorders: a neglected association.' *European Journal of Obstetrics & Gynaecology and Reproductive Biology 96*, 146–149.

Shamaly, H., Mahameed, A., Sharony, A., and Shamir, R. (2004) 'Infertility and celiac disease: do we need more than one serological marker?' *Acta Obstetricia et Gynecologica Scandinavica 83*, 12, 1184–1188.

Sheiner, E., Peleg, R., and Levy, A. (2006) 'Pregnancy outcome of patients with known celiac disease.' *European Journal of Obstetrics & Gynaecology and Reproductive Biology 129*, 1, 41–45.

Sher, K., and Mayberry, J. (1996) 'Female fertility, obstetric and gynaecological history in coeliac disease: a case control study.' *Acta Paediatrica Supplement 412*, 76–77.

Stazi, A., and Mantovani, A. (2004) 'Celiac disease and its endocrine and nutritional implications on male reproduction.' *Minerva Medica 95*, 3, 243–354.

Tersigni, C., Castellani, R., de Waure, C., Fattorossi, A., *et al.* (2014). 'Celiac disease and reproductive disorders: meta-analysis of epidemiologic associations and potential pathogenic mechanisms.' *Human Reproduction Update 20*, 4, 582–593.

Tiboni, G., de Vita, M., Faricelli, R., Giampietro, F., and Liberati, M. (2006) 'Serological testing for celiac disease in women undergoing assisted reproduction techniques.' *Human Reproduction 21*, 376–379.

Zugna, D., Richiardi, L., Akre, O., Stephansson, O., and Ludvigsson, J. (2011) 'Celiac disease is not a risk factor for infertility in men.' *Fertility and Sterility 95*, 5, 1709–1713, e1–e3.

# Chapter 8

# Unexplained Infertility and Reproductive Immunology (RI)

*Louise Carder BA (Hons), BSc,
Pg. Dip. Nutritional Therapist*

## 1. Introduction

Far from being a single entity, unexplained infertility is an umbrella term that covers many factors, including genetic, lifestyle, nutritional, environmental and of course medical issues. Unexplained infertility, also known as idiopathic infertility, currently has over 2500 entries on the PubMed search facility, each seeking to offer insight into its cause. For the patient, however, it is a very singular thing: the inability to initially achieve and/or then maintain a pregnancy to a successful outcome. The spectrum is a wide one therefore, from being unable to initially achieve even a very early stage pregnancy, with failure coming at implantation stage or even earlier, to recurrent pregnancy loss prior to twenty weeks. Early pregnancy loss is characterised as a loss of pregnancy before twenty weeks gestation or with a foetal weight of less than 500g (Petrozza 2014). Recurrent pregnancy loss has proved harder to define, but epidemiological studies tend to define it as three recurrent losses prior to 20 weeks, which affects 1–2 per cent of women (Stephenson 1996).

This chapter uses a Functional Medicine framework considering genetics as an antecedent, and then lifestyle and environment as triggers and mediators for unexplained infertility. The chapter also focuses on reproductive immunology (RI), as this can occur as a result of one or all of these factors. RI has helped create many families over the past 30 years, but there is still a lack of consensus as to what elements of the immune system have the most impact. What we do know is that in a healthy pregnancy the immune system response adapts to support the growing foetus, but in some cases it is the immune system response that becomes a problem; how exactly this happens is still open to debate. However, by considering RI we are able, as Dr Alan Beer, a pioneer in the field, stated, to examine a new factor to 'explain the unexplained' (Beer, Kantecki and Reed 2006).

## 2. Genetics

Taking genetics first, the following three factors should be given primary consideration based on current research: genes relating to tissue type compatibility; thrombophilia; and inflammatory issues. Whilst studies are still ongoing, and not all fertility doctors test for these genes, if a patient has a problem with even just one of these factors then the studies listed below show that this could be problematic. It also seems that if a patient has a problem with more than one of these genetic areas then this could be even more problematic. It should be noted, however, that genetic single nuclear polymorphisms (SNPs) only confer a predisposition to symptoms or conditions related to the particular polymorphism in question. Since a given polymorphism will often result in the reduced expression of a gene, and the resultant enzyme produced by it, there is a wide range of nutritional and lifestyle factors that can in turn influence gene expression. It should also be noted that homozygosity (two copies of a gene) and heterozygosity (one copy of a gene) might also affect genetic expression.

### 2.1 Tissue type compatibility

In humans the major histocompatibility complex (MHC) is known as human leukocyte antigen (HLA). HLA antigens act as identifying proteins on cell surfaces and contribute to immune signalling allowing the system to communicate a 'self' or 'non-self' message. The most common HLA antigens considered in RI are DQ alpha antigens. The reason for this is that the mother's immune system is also responding to the paternal HLA proteins so their HLA compatibility becomes important. If both parents have one copy of the DQ 0501 genotype then there is a 25 per cent chance that the baby will have this genotype too (Beer *et al.* 2006). The experience of Dr Beer was that 10–15 per cent of his patients had DQ 0501 histocompatibility and that this match was associated with immune flares, sub-chorionic haemorrhages, haematomas, miscarriages, placental abruption, restricted growth and premature delivery (Beer *et al.* 2006).

Dr Kwak-Kim, an obstetric gynaecologist and leading RI researcher, also found that where there is HLA DQ compatibility and recurrent loss of pregnancy, lower levels of anti-paternal cytotoxic antibodies (APCA), anti-idiotypic antibodies (Ab2) and mixed lymphocyte reaction blocking antibodies (MLR-Bf) are commonly found (Kwak-Kim, Kim and Gilman-Sachs 2000). HLA DQ alpha antigens bind to HLA G molecules, which are responsible for mediating the immune response to a pregnancy.

Onno *et al.* (1994) found HLA G molecules prior to implantation, which added to our understanding of how important this is for protecting a trophoblast from aggressive immune responses such as stimulating T2 immune dominance, turning off natural killer (NK) cell receptors (Munz *et al.* 1997), and encouraging the production of T reg cells (Kwak-Kim *et al.* 2000). Where a low level of HLA DQ alpha antigen is found then the reverse occurs, which has the effect of lowering 'tolerance' to an embryo. According to Dr Beer, NK cells are not 'switched off' and can increase (Beer *et al.* 2006).

Recurrent miscarriage has been linked in studies to high levels of CD56+ (Clifford, Flanagan and Regan 1999) and CD57+ NK cells (Vassiliadou and Bulmer 1996) in particular. Interestingly, secondary infertility (where infertility occurs after a first live birth) is also linked to HLA compatibility via the rise in NK cell activity, which has been shown to increase with each histocompatible pregnancy, with studies such as Ho *et al.* (1990) showing this to have a link with recurrent miscarriage. HLA-compatible or -incompatible combinations may therefore affect implantation and success of a pregnancy, but adding in the complex nature of the interactions between uterine natural killer (NK) cells and MHC class molecules highlights the challenges faced in this area and how many factors are required for what Ashley Moffett-King (2002) terms 'reproductive fitness'.

## 2.2 Thrombophilic genes

Women who are pregnant have been found to have as much as a four- to five-fold increase in risk of thromboembolism compared with non-pregnant women (James, Konkle and Bauer 2013). The risk of thromboembolic conditions that may affect a pregnancy is increased in those with a genetic predisposition, with Lipe and Ornstein finding that during pregnancy (and four to six weeks postnatal) clotting risk is increased in such women, with risk also being higher for early- and late-term miscarriages (Lipe and Ornstein 2011). Blood clots can affect maternal health due to the risk of embolism or a stroke, and can affect a growing foetus by restricting placental blood flow. Normal pregnancy modulates coagulation factors thereby increasing thrombogenic potential in women with inherited thrombophilia. Whilst factors such as plasminogen activator inhibitor (PAI-1) type 1 and 2 and levels of other fibrinolytic inhibitors such as thrombin activatable fibrinolytic inhibitor (TAFI) are important to monitor during pregnancy, the genetic polymorphisms relating to inherited thrombophilia listed in Table 8.1 are particularly important to test for prior to conception.

## Table 8.1 Inherited thrombophilia

**Factor V Leiden**
Factor V Leiden polymorphism triggers a condition called Activated Protein C (APC) resistance. APC is required in the blood to help stop clot growth, so APC resistance would mean that there is a reduced ability to mediate clot growth. Ornstein and Cushman (2003) found that Factor V Leiden increases risk of a thrombolytic event such as deep vein thrombosis (DVT) by a factor of seven, while Martinelli et al. (2000) found that Factor V Leiden and prothrombin mutations can triple the risk of late-pregnancy foetal loss.

### Protein C and Protein S deficiencies

Protein C acts as an anticoagulant by combining with Protein S on blood platelet surfaces. Where there is a deficiency of either protein, coagulation risk increases. The deficiency occurs due to inheritance of an abnormal Protein S gene. According to Benedetto et al. (2010) the risk of a thrombotic event where there is a Protein C deficiency is estimated at one in 113 women, compared with one in 42 for antithrombin deficiency type 2, and one in three for antithrombin deficiency type 1. The second and third trimesters are of particular note regarding Protein C deficiency as resistance increases at this time, thus elevating risk (Walker et al. 1997). Protein S deficiency has also been shown to predispose to foetal loss and venous thromboembolic events (VTE) (Ten Kate and Van der Meer 2008). Two systematic review papers have both found that Protein S deficient patients had the highest risk of unexplained stillbirth after 20 weeks, and taking all thrombophilias into consideration had the strongest association with late pregnancy loss (Alfirevic, Roberts and Martlew 2002: Robertson et al. 2006).

### Prothrombin G20120A

Poort et al. (1996) found that a polymorphism with this gene results in elevated prothrombin levels, which has been shown to increase the risk of venous thrombosis. Where lupus anticoagulants were also taken into consideration, Robertson et al. (2006) found that risk of loss beyond 24 weeks for those heterozygous for the G20120A polymorphism was significantly increased and heterozygosity was also noted to be associated with higher risk of later pregnancy loss than early loss.

### Antithrombin deficiency

This polymorphism is found in the SERPINC1 gene. Antithrombin (AT), as a natural anticoagulant, mediates the thrombin protein's blood-clotting activity, which increases the risk of developing blood clots. As with other inherited thrombophilias, AT deficiency is associated with increased risk of clot development and elevated risk of miscarriage or stillbirth (James et al. 2013). James et al. also found that pregnant women with AT deficiency are classified as being vulnerable to VTE, especially during childbirth, due to anticoagulation therapy being withheld due to risk of bleeding complications (James et al. 2013).

## 2.3 Methylenetetrahydrofolate reductase (MTHFR)

A growing area of genetic interest surrounds the MTHFR gene polymorphisms, namely C677T and A1298C. Whilst probably not presenting as serious a thrombophilic risk as the gene variants already detailed, research on this gene is still in its infancy and RI research has focused on investigation relating to hyperhomocysteinaemia. Studies have shown that there are two direct ways that a MTHFR polymorphism may be implicated in infertility. First, as the MTHFR enzyme is involved in amino acid metabolism it influences levels of homocysteine. High homocysteine is independently considered a risk factor for miscarriages due to the increased risk of blood clots (Murphy 2007). Second, the MTHFR enzyme can also impact on folate levels, and other B vitamins more generally. Riboflavin (B2), for example, is a cofactor for MTHFR and the C677T variant has been linked to higher homocysteine levels in those with this variant, where there is also a riboflavin deficiency (Jacques *et al.* 2002). Low vitamin B status has been shown to have an impact on the risk of miscarriage (Townsley 2013) but also the development of the foetus, with neural tube defects being common where there is a B vitamin deficiency (Pickell *et al.* 2009).

More generally, MTHFR is linked with methylation capacity; any polymorphisms may therefore affect methylation. MTHFR is not the sole determinant of methylation status but it is of critical importance. Yin *et al.* (2012) highlighted the importance of embryonic methylation capacity, linking it with abnormal embryonic development that can lead to early pregnancy loss. The study found that abnormal DNA methyltransferase function resulted in lowered implantation rates, increased foetal absorption and poor foetal and placental development (Yin *et al.* 2012). This study is just one of many that indicate the importance of methylation capacity not just in the mother or father, but also the independent methylation capacity of a growing foetus. Whilst maternal polymorphism status is probably considered more important, some studies show that paternal polymorphism status should not be overlooked. Amongst other factors, including hyperhomocysteinaemia, a paternal C677T polymorphism has also been identified as a risk factor for pregnancy loss (Govindaiah *et al.* 2009).

Type of polymorphism can also impact in a specific way; for example, Kim *et al.* (2011) have linked homozygosity for A1298C to miscarriage risk with foetal aneuploidy by 293 per cent. Thrombophilia, whether inherited or acquired (such as via antiphospholipid syndrome or hyperhomocysteinaemia for example), is a major concern for the mother in pregnancy with increased risk for VTE cited at 200 per 100,000 deliveries (Heit *et al.* 2005), but there are also associations for pre-eclampsia, placental abruption, intrauterine growth delay and foetal loss (Battinelli, Marshall and Connors 2013).

## 2.4 Inflammatory genetic predisposition such as TNF alpha

Increasing research since 2000 has shown that certain genes can impact on inflammation levels in the body. Tumour necrosis factor alpha (TNFα) is a pro-inflammatory cytokine, which plays a role in inflammation in the body. Genetic polymorphisms are associated with increased levels of inflammation, especially in those who are homozygous. Studies, such as those by Lee *et al.* (2013) and Zammiti *et al.* (2009), have associated TNFα polymorphisms with miscarriage/ recurrent miscarriage. However, there is limited reporting clearly associating both gene polymorphism and circulating serum levels of TNFα. It is also clear that a balance of TNFα is required, as some studies, such as Boudjenah *et al.* (2014), link a TNFα 308 GA/ AA polymorphism with increased implantation success. This point highlights that some genes act as 'resilience' genes conferring a positive effect on health. Research on inflammatory consequences in early pregnancy is still in its infancy, but it does seem likely that excess TNFα can cause problems, especially when there is an additional thrombophilic risk.

## 2.5 Conclusion – genetics

Whilst the individual genes focused on above have studies supporting their implication in infertility, it seems that increasing numbers of studies are agreeing that multiple gene polymorphisms are in fact a higher risk factor than any one single gene mutation, especially, for example, when clotting genes are also considered along with MTHFR genes (Coulam *et al.* 2006). Two examples cited in the study by Coulam *et al.* (2006) show that homozygous mutations were found in 59 per cent of women with recurrent miscarriage compared with 10 per cent of controls; and that more than three polymorphisms (from the 10 studied) were identified in 68 per cent of women with recurrent miscarriage and only 21 per cent of controls. Where Factor V Leiden and a Protein C deficiency are seen, then thrombolytic risk has also been shown to increase (Mustafa *et al.* 1998).

Studies such as these show that genetic factors, even where there is still a lack of consensus regarding their overall impact, should not be ignored; and whilst they may not be the sole cause of infertility or miscarriage, they probably increase risk. Testing for these genes is of paramount importance so that appropriate individual risk assessment can take place.

Widening the lens a little, studies have also shown that recurrent implantation failure after fertility treatment can be linked with a Th1 response, rather than the pregnancy protective Th2 response (Ng *et al.* 2002). So, whilst genetic predisposition may play a role in unexplained infertility, the way that the body actually expresses a Th1 or Th2 immune response can be equally as impactful.

## 3. Lifestyle and nutrition

Genes provide a foundation for health, and lifestyle and nutrition can impact greatly on the expression of genes, especially where polymorphisms are present. Lifestyle and nutrition are two key areas that are modifiable, and can potentially improve fertility. A 2007 review article by Homan, Davies and Norman (2007) is just one of many that have concluded that lifestyle modification can optimise fertility, with factors such as age, smoking, weight, diet (including caffeine and alcohol consumption), exercise, psychological stress, and exposure to environmental pollutants being key.

Age is important, as studies show that women tend to see a decline in fertility after the age of 35 (Baird *et al.* 2005). Balen and Rutherford (2007) cite age as being a couple's primary determining fertility factor, with women under 25 seeing conception rates of 60 per cent at six months and 85 per cent at twelve months; women over 35 see figures of less than half this. They also cite societal changes as being important with the average age of first-time mothers in Western countries now being around 29.5 compared with 20 years ago when the average age was 25; this is important as age also increases risk during pregnancy (Balen and Rutherford 2007). Not only do clear clinical symptoms become evident with age, such as reduced quantity and quality of oocytes (Angell 1994), miscarriage or foetal abnormalities (Nasseri and Grifo 1998), but also as spontaneous pregnancy rates decline then success with fertility treatments also decline as a woman ages (Chuang *et al.* 2003).

But clearly, as women do achieve and maintain pregnancies beyond the age of 35 there are many more factors to consider. Whether one or other of the couple smokes can impact on fertility rates, with male smoking affecting sperm production, motility and morphology; and in women, smoking may affect luteal phase hormones and the follicular microenvironment (Younglai, Holloway and Foster 2005) (see Chapter 6 for further male factor information). Regardless of gender, smoking has been shown generally to have a detrimental effect on in-vitro fertilisation (IVF) outcome (Klonoff-Cohen *et al.* 2001) and smoking marijuana can also cause abnormal reproductive function, as can use of other recreational drugs (Sharma *et al.* 2013).

Obesity has been clearly identified as a risk factor for infertility; in particular, studies have shown association with miscarriage (Metwally *et al.* 2008) and stillbirth (Chu *et al.* 2007). High BMI has also been shown to have a negative impact on fertility treatment outcomes (Fedorcsak *et al.* 2004). Some studies have reported that success rates can be halved compared with women with a normal BMI (e.g. Wang, Davies and Norman 2000). However, it has been shown that women do not understand these risks as much as they do the cardio-metabolic risks and cancer risk (Cardozo *et al.* 2012). With 64.1 per cent of women in the USA being found to be overweight or obese in a 2010 study, this is a rising problem in the western world (Flegal *et al.* 2010). An Australian lifestyle modification study by Clark *et al.* (1998) took 87 obese women and gave them access to a weekly lifestyle programme for six months where they were given education about diet, exercise and psychological support. There was a pregnancy rate of 77.6 per cent; however, those who did not achieve a pregnancy smoked, maintained a high BMI or attended less than two-thirds of the sessions. When considering unexplained infertility, studies such as that by Clark *et al.* (1998) add to understanding about how lifestyle modifications can sometimes make that all-important difference.

## 3.1 Nutrient deficiencies

B vitamins have been well documented as being linked with fertility. Taking a multivitamin supplement at least three times a week has been shown to reduce the risk of some types of ovulatory infertility, with B vitamins and primarily folic acid mediating this association (Chavarro *et al.* 2008). Most studies seem to focus on ovulatory infertility when it comes to diet. Another study by Chavarro *et al.* showed a higher monounsaturated to trans-fat ratio, high fat rather than low-fat dairy, vegetable rather than animal protein, lowered glycaemic load and higher iron and multivitamin intake being linked to lower infertility rates (Chavarro *et al.* 2007). Nutrient deficiencies may also be found in women with eating disorders, and studies have also shown that women with eating disorders can have a higher risk of fertility issues (Freizinger *et al.* 2010). With caffeine and alcohol consumption also being modifiable factors, it is worth noting that both consistently show in studies that at high levels they too have a detrimental effect on fertility (Hakim, Gray and Zacur 1998; Rasch 2003). For further information about nutritional factors and fertility see Chapters 10 and 11.

Lastly, with regard to diet, in general food sensitivities are relatively under-studied, especially concerning resulting immune reactions and their relationship with fertility. However, coeliac disease has a well-studied link to fertility problems with up to 50 per cent of women experiencing untreated coeliac disease undergoing miscarriage or another unfavourable outcome to a pregnancy (Martinelli *et al.* 2000). One study specifically stated: 'Screening for coeliac disease should be part of the diagnostic work-up of infertile women, particularly when no apparent cause can be ascertained after standard evaluation' (Meloni *et al.* 1999). Martinelli *et al.* echoed this call in 2000 when their study recorded that one in 70 women is affected by coeliac disease, thus making it more common than many of the conditions that pregnant women are routinely screened for. The point is also made that coeliac disease can become refractory with a gluten-free diet, such a diet thereby ameliorating some of the disease risks. Consideration also has to be given here to the link with coeliac disease and intestinal permeability, with a gluten-free diet also perhaps mediating both intestinal permeability and the immune system (Visser *et al.* 2009). For further information about the link with gluten and fertility see Chapter 7.

## 3.2 Stress

Stress is the final modifiable lifestyle factor being considered in this chapter due to its clear links with autoimmunity and infertility. It should also be noted that infertility itself can be incredibly stressful so a negative feedback loop can occur related to testing, treatments, unsuccessful pregnancies and costs associated with fertility treatments (Anderson, Niesenblat and Norman 2010). It is not clear exactly how different types of stress impact on different aspects of fertility, but overall decreased stress levels have also been correlated with fertility improvements (Sharma *et al.* 2013). One way that lowered stress may link with fertility improvements is via changes in the microbiome, and we are seeing studies linking stress with microbiome bacterial changes (Carpenter 2012). Common gut bacteria strains are also found in semen, and Weng *et al.* (2014) suggest that the bacterial make-up of semen can influence male infertility via quality of semen. In the study, *Prevotella* was the predominant bacteria genus found in the lower quality semen, whereas *Lactobacillus* was the predominant bacteria genus in 80.6 per cent of normal semen samples (Weng *et al.* 2014).

## 3.3 Environment

Another factor that needs to be considered regarding unexplained infertility is the environment. Whilst not as easily modifiable as some of the factors in the previous section, awareness is important so that appropriate tests can be undertaken and avoidance or limitation of exposure can be initiated if required. Exposure to plastics such as bisphenol A (BPA) has been associated with recurrent miscarriage (Sugiura-Ogasawara *et al.* 2005). BPA is found in many places, from plastics to till receipts. Pesticides, dioxins, phthalates and solvents have also been linked to fertility problems. Organochlorine compounds have been shown to shorten menstrual cycles in women thereby affecting fertility (Windham *et al.* 2005), and women who lived near farms where pesticides were sprayed showed a 40 to 120 per cent increase in risk of miscarriage, primarily due to birth defects (Bell *et al.* 2001).

Regular exposure to pesticides even before pregnancy has led to studies linking a 300 per cent greater risk of birth defects and even stillbirth (Romero, Barnett and Midtling 1989). Using pesticides at home, especially during the first two months of pregnancy (where there is a particularly vulnerable window between weeks three to eight), has been shown to increase risk of stillbirth by 2.4 times the norm and stillbirth due to congenital defects by 70 per cent (Pastore, Hertz-Picciotto and Beaumont 1997). Women who experience endometriosis, fibroids, miscarriage and persistent infertility have also been shown to have raised dioxin levels in their blood (Gerhard *et al.* 1999). This is explored more fully in Chapters 5 and 11. Occupational as well as household exposure to chemicals, heavy metals and pollution should therefore be considered in cases of unexplained infertility.

## 4. Medical

Most medical causes of infertility are found relatively early on in investigations, such as hydrosalpinx, endometriosis (see Chapters 4 and 5), fibroids, polyps or polycystic ovaries, via laparoscopy or ultrasound. Pelvic inflammatory disease and tubal blockages in particular need prompt diagnosis so that treatment can be initiated to minimise effects on fertility. Infections of the male genito-urinary tract, for example, may account for 15 per cent of male infertility cases, with chlamydia and gonorrhoea being the most common infections affecting both male and female fertility (Pellati *et al.* 2008) (see Chapter 6 for further male factors and Chapters 4 and 5 for female factors). Candida, herpes and cervical dysplasia should be tested for as part of a comprehensive STD panel as they can also have an impact on fertility.

Thyroid conditions are also implicated in infertility (Poppe *et al.* 2002), but consideration needs to be given beyond the thyroid function itself and the hormonal effect on fertility to assess wider antibody levels. Around one in three women who experience miscarriage test positive for thyroid antibodies (Dendrinos *et al.* 2000), and it is the field of RI, which also covers thyroid antibodies, that will be the focus of the remainder of this chapter.

## 4.1 Reproductive immunology

The American Society for Reproductive Immunology was founded in 1981 and from around this time RI has been a developing area of science, which grew from research clearly showing that abnormal autoimmune function could result in reproductive failure, even in patients that were clinically asymptomatic. Gleicher and El-Roeiy (1988) were amongst the first to define reproductive autoimmune failure syndrome (RAFS) as a diagnostic entity. Their evidence suggested that RAFS correlated with 'the woman's need for increased self-tolerance in face of antigenic exposure to the maternal haplotype of the foetus during normal pregnancy' (Gleicher and El-Roeiy 1988). What this means for the patient is, first, that women with abnormal autoimmune activity are at higher risk of reproductive failure; second, that the autoimmune response can vary; and third, that failure may occur at any stage depending on the immune response that is triggered.

When thinking about the type of experience this may result in, we need to consider single or repeated miscarriage, IVF failure, implantation failure, chemical pregnancy and stillbirth. Dr Beer categorised five reproductive immunological factors with, in his clinical experience, category one being the least and category five being the most severe (Beer *et al.* 2006):

1. Tissue type compatibility

2. Blood clotting defects

3. Immunity to pregnancy

4. Antibodies to sperm

5. High NK cells.

Each of the categories can be interlinked, thus exacerbating immunological fertility problems, and are commonly subclinical until a pregnancy attempt. It is the subclinical nature of RI and raised antibody levels/autoimmunity that has allowed extensive debate to continue over properly defining and categorising it to everyone's satisfaction. Dr Beer's list is used in this chapter as it affords a relatively simple explanation for the different categories. Having reviewed categories one and two under the genetics section, immunity to pregnancy, antibodies and high NK cells will now be considered.

Where autoimmunity is a factor, then raised antibody levels are a consequence. Autoimmunity can be triggered, especially where there is a genetic predisposition, by intestinal permeability. Intestinal permeability is in turn triggered by pathologies such as infection (Bischoff *et al.* 2014), stress (Heyman 2005), dietary factors such as gluten (Visser *et al.* 2009) and foods high in lectins (El Asmar *et al.* 2002), use of medications such as NSAIDs, alcohol (Bischoff *et al.* 2014) or antibiotics (Mårild *et al.* 2013), trauma (Bischoff *et al.* 2014), mucosal alterations (Bischoff *et al.* 2014) and ageing, all of which can mediate tight junctions, allowing material to pass through into systemic circulation, which can then precipitate an immune response that may be self-directed. Autoantibodies may not be creating any overt symptoms; however, some antibodies have been implicated as being associated with unexplained infertility.

How an autoimmune response specifically impacts on fertility will now be considered in relation to the following points; however, it should be noted that antibodies are a response to an antigen, so are just part of an infertility continuum, which also includes other immune reactions such as high NK cells, none of which is a sole cause of infertility but do all link to an abnormal T cell response that can be unsupportive of pregnancy: key antibodies such as the category three antibodies; anti-nuclear antibodies (ANAs) and category four antibodies; and anti-sperm antibodies. ANAs, which are antibodies to the nucleus of cells (in particular cellular DNA), have been particularly implicated in early miscarriage due to problems with placental development (Molazadeh, Karimzadeh and Azizi 2014). As their presence is commonly linked to category 5 factors and other autoimmune conditions, on their own they are unlikely to be an individual cause of infertility (Beer *et al.* 2006).

## Table 8.2 Overview of types of autoantibodies

**Anti-sperm antibodies**
These can impact on both men and women, and whilst in men they are linked with low sperm motility or no live sperm, in women IgG antibodies to sperm tails have been associated with miscarriage (Witkin and Chaudhry 1989).

## Antibodies to hormones

Hormones such as oestradiol, progesterone and human chorionic gonadotrophin (HCG) which are important for pregnancy can also be linked to an altered immune response, via antibodies generated by CD19+/5+ B lymphocytes. According to Dr Beer, any resulting lowered levels of progesterone as a result of high antibodies can lead to luteal phase defects, and inhibit implantation due to restricted development of the uterine lining (levels lower than 7mm are considered sub-optimal for pregnancy) (Beer *et al.* 2006).

## Antiphospholipid antibodies (APLAs)

These include lupus anticoagulant, anticardiolipin antibodies and anti-β2 glycoprotein, all of which have been identified in recurrent miscarriage and infertility studies (Li, Li and Tian 1998). Whilst a genetic polymorphism is important to consider, actual APLA levels should be tested. APLAs are found in around 10–20 per cent of women who experience recurrent miscarriage with loss being at higher risk beyond 10 weeks of pregnancy (Misita and Moll 2005), and association with increased risk of pre-eclampsia, placental insufficiency and pre-term delivery has also been identified (Al Abri, Vaclavinkova and Richens 2000). APLAs, associated with thrombophilic conditions such as antiphospholipid (Hughes' syndrome), have also been linked to autoimmunity as well as miscarriage. Anticardiolipin antibodies have been found to disrupt implantation by reacting against the trophoblast causing clots, thereby affecting placental development, as well as causing placental lesions (Al Abri *et al.* 2000). APLAs may be symptomless, which is why testing is important, and re-testing is also essential if the first test is negative as levels can vary over time. Successful pregnancy rates with antiphospholipid syndrome can be as high as 70 per cent with the right treatment (Ware Branch and Khamashta 2003). Whilst inherited thrombophilia is a key driving factor in APLAs, some medications such as hydralazine and phenytoin can precipitate their appearance, as can viruses (Beer *et al.* 2006).

### Anti-thyroglobulin and anti-thyroid peroxidase antibodies

Thyroid disease is associated with antibodies such as anti-thyroglobulin and anti-thyroid peroxidase, and it is important to note that whilst a thyroid condition may be being managed by medication, the underlying antibodies may still pose a risk in pregnancy. Around 30 per cent of women with recurrent miscarriage have tested positive for one or both of these thyroid antibodies (Dendrinos *et al.* 2000). Some studies have reported no clear link with thyroid antibodies and infertility (Kutteh, Schoolcraft and Scott 2000); however, a meta-analysis by Prummel and Wiersinga in 2004 showed a clear association between thyroid antibodies levels and miscarriage. The study stated that 'this association may be explained by a heightened autoimmune state affecting foetal allograft of which thyroid antibodies are just a marker' (Prummel and Wiersinga 2004), thus adding to the weight of evidence and opinion that antibodies are part of a bigger autoimmune infertility picture and not a sole cause.

### Other antibodies

- Serotonin is a key neurotransmitter, which is probably best known to be low in depression. However, it is also required for healthy uterine lining, as it regulates TNFa and relaxes blood vessels in the uterus to increase blood flow (Cohen and Wittenauer 1987), meaning that low serotonin levels, or antibodies to serotonin, can mediate fertility.

- Anti-laminin-1 autoantibodies are linked with endometriosis and may also be implicated in pregnancy failures (Inagaki *et al.* 2005).

- Anti-ovarian antibodies are linked to premature ovarian failure (Luborsky, Roussev and Coulam 2000). For more information on endometriosis see Chapter 5.

# 5. Impact of raised immune system markers on fertility

Raised immune system markers have been seen to mediate antibody levels, and antibody levels themselves in turn raise other immune markers. An example would be that CD19+/CD5+ B lymphocytes have been shown to mediate antiphospholipid antibodies, which in turn can trigger raised NK cell levels and TNFα (Beer, Kwak and Ruiz 1996).

## 5.1 Natural killer (NK) cells and killer-cell immunoglobulin-like receptors (KIR)

Having NK cells is of paramount importance to the immune system – usually they are protective, such as when they shield us from cancer, but low levels are linked to viral infection and tumour risk (Beer *et al.* 2006). However, in women with recurrent pregnancy loss and those with failed IV cycles, NK cell levels such as CD56+/CD16+ can be found to be high (Emmer *et al.* 2000). Women with thyroid antibodies have also been shown to have high levels of CD56+ NK cells and CD19+/5+ cells with additional T cell dysregulation (Hidaka *et al.* 1992). Dr Beer found that where CD56+ lymphocytes were in excess of 18 per cent this correlated with impending pregnancy loss (Beer, Kwak and Ruiz 1996). Uterine NK cells, in particular CD57, seem to correlate with a more aggressive immune response, but all of these cytokines can in turn trigger TNFα amongst other immune factors, which can cause the release of more cytokines, creating a 'cytokine storm' – something that is reported by women with immune-mediated infertility (Clark 2009), who can express symptoms such as flu-like aches, cramping, fever, fatigue and pruritis ahead of an early pregnancy loss (Beer *et al.* 2006).

TNFα, like NK cells, when within normal range is usually beneficial for us. However, when levels are high this can also be associated with pregnancy loss (Clark 2009), especially around the time of implantation (Lalitkumar, Sengupta and Ghosh 2005) and potentially increased if genetic predisposition is also evident. TNFα is part of a signalling cascade that triggers other cytokines, such as CD3, CD4 and CD8 T cells, and neutrophils and monocytes such as interleukin 1 and 6 (Beer *et al.* 2006). Again, it is this cascade/ continuum that is repeatedly shown to be at the very centre of RI studies. Studies also consistently point the finger at a further trigger, such as a viral cause, but this may be a little too reductionist.

It is likely that the final answer will be multifactorial and encompass viral, bacterial and environmental toxin factors at the very least, and even then also be individually expressed. It is therefore crucial to ensure that where no obvious reasons can be given for infertility and/or pregnancy failures, appropriate tests are prioritised to ascertain the underlying cause, and that full support is given to couples experiencing unexplained infertility (for further information on support for couples see Chapters 1 and 2).

Further research relating to unexplained infertility is ongoing. Novel aspects are coming to the fore on a regular basis, such as Shoenfeld *et al.*'s study showing that *Saccharomyces cerevisiae* antibodies can be linked with reproductive failure, including anti-saccharomyces cerivisiae antibody (ASCA) (Shoenfeld *et al.* 2006). Manohar *et al.*'s (2014) study regarding alteration of endometrial proteins in women with unexplained infertility is a further example. Novel treatments to mediate the immune system are also being researched, such as the anti-malarial treatment hydroxychloroquine, which in a 2010 study was shown to not only lower NK cells but also mediate prothrombotic mechanisms (Rand *et al.* 2010). The future will no doubt elicit even more information that will give additional answers and give names to new diagnostic markers and conditions, thereby reducing the 'unexplained' factors in infertility.

When factors are clearly identified then success rates go up. Treated endocrine disorders and APLAs now have a pregnancy success rate of 60–90 per cent (Ford and Shust 2009). Until factors are known it is down to each infertile couple to work with healthcare practitioners who are willing to go that additional mile to understand what is the most likely cause of their individual set of circumstances (their antecedents, triggers and mediators) that have led to their specific form of infertility. That support cannot be underestimated, and can often be life-changing.

## 6. Testing and treatment options

Review of gene markers to enable assessment of hetero or homozygosity:

- HLA histocompatibility (e.g. DQ, DR) and leukocyte antibody detection

- Factor V Leiden

- Protein C and Protein S deficiency

- Prothrombin G20120A

- Antithrombin deficiency (SERPINC1)

- TNFα

- Methylation genes (MTHFR – C677T or A1298C)

- MTR A2756G polymorphism is associated with uteroplacental insufficiency in mothers not supplementing with high dose B vitamins (Furness *et al.* 2008).

### 6.1 Typical reproductive immunology tests

NK ASSAYS, TJ6 PROTEIN AND KIR RECEPTORS

KIR receptors and TJ6 mediate NK cell activity, plus IVIg assay, usually as part of a wider immunophenotype test, which tests for cell designation (CD) levels, such as CD3+, CD4+, CD8+, CD19+, CD56+, CD3+/IL2-R, CD19+/CD5+, which are all types of NK cells.

### 6.2 Blood clotting markers

These are such as thrombophilia testing (antiphospholipid syndrome, lupus anticoagulant), anti-nuclear antibodies and anti-sperm antibody testing, as well as anti-DNA/histone antibodies.

OTHER ANTIBODIES

Thyroid antibodies, gluten and lectin antibodies and antibodies relating to intestinal permeability such as actomyosin, zonulin, occludin and lipopolysaccharides.

## 7. Treatment options (medical)

Medical treatment options are numerous and varied, depending on the cause of infertility. RI options include aspirin, hormone injections, low molecular weight heparin, corticosteroids, TNFα blocking agents, IVIg and intralipid infusions. Some information on these can be found in the case study in the next chapter. Other information can be found at the UK's HFEA website, which has dedicated information on RI (www.hfea.gov.uk/fertility-treatment-options-reproductive-immunology.html#4).

**UK doctors who specialise in RI at time of publication include:**

Dr Gorgy

Dr G. Ndukwe

Dr M. Taranissi

Both of the last two doctors studied under Dr Beer and pioneered RI in the UK.

**US doctors who specialise in RI include:**

Dr Kwak-Kim, Chicago

Dr Braverman, New York

Beer Clinic, California

For information on natural approaches, see Chapters 9, 10 and 11. For an overview of nutritional approaches, for example, immune modulators such as cordyceps and other common complementary approaches such as acupuncture, see Chapter 13.

## 8. Concluding remarks

With up to 15 per cent of couples now seeking support for infertility (Sharma *et al.* 2013) and three per cent experiencing multiple miscarriages (Molazadeh *et al.* 2014) it is important that answers are available to them in order that their reproductive fitness can be improved. Tiered support that takes into account the varied factors reviewed here must be offered. For example, for Gemma in the case study featured in Chapter 9, and who has gone through a successful pregnancy supported by measures included in this chapter, there is no doubt in her mind that she would not be holding even just one baby were it not for this level of personalised support.

A healthcare practitioner can work with a couple to ensure that they are satisfied that every avenue has been fully explored, as this will give them the best chance to make an informed decision about next steps (such as continuing with attempts to have their own baby, or considering other options such as surrogacy or adoption). It is therefore imperative that to explain unexplained infertility the right questions have to be asked for the answers to be given that give a couple the best chance of success.

## References

Al Abri, S., Vaclavinkova, V., and Richens, E.R. (2000) 'Outcome of pregnancy in patients possessing anticardiolipin antibodies.' *SQU Journal for Scientific Research 2*, 91–95.

Alfirevic, Z., Roberts, D., and Martlew, V. (2002) 'How strong is the association between maternal thrombophilia and adverse pregnancy outcome? A systematic review.' *European Journal of Obstetric and Gynaecological Reproductive Biology 101*, 6–14.

Anderson, K., Nisenblat, V., and Norman, R. (2010). 'Lifestyle factors in people seeking infertility treatment – a review.' *Australian and New Zealand Journal of Obstetrics and Gynaecology 50*, 1, 8–20.

Angell, R.R. (1994) 'Aneuploidy in older women. Higher rates of aneuploidy in oocytes from older women.' *Human Reproduction 9*, 1199–1200.

Baird, D.T., Collins, J., Egozcue, J., Evers, L.H., *et al.* (2005) 'Fertility and ageing.' *Human Reproduction Update 2*, 11, 261–276.

Balen, A.H., and Rutherford, A.J. (2007) 'Management of infertility.' *British Medical Journal 335*, 608.

Battinelli, E.M., Marshall, A., and Connors, J.M. (2013) 'The role of thrombophilia in pregnancy.' *Thrombosis*, 2013, 516420.

Beer, A.E., Kantecki, J., and Reed, J. (2006) *Is Your Body Baby Friendly?* USA: AJR Publishing. Available at www.ipgbook.com/is-your-body-baby-friendly--products-9780978507800.php?page_id=32&pid=AJR, accessed on 21 May 2015.

Beer, A.E., Kwak, J.Y.H., and Ruiz, J.E. (1996) 'Immunophenotypic profiles of peripheral blood lymphocytes in women with recurrent pregnancy losses and in infertile women with multiple failed in vitro fertilization cycles.' *American Journal of Reproductive Immunology 35*, 4, 376–382.

Bell, E.M., Hertz-Picciotto, I., and Beaumont, J.J. (2001) 'A case controlled study of pesticides and fetal death due to congenital abnormalities.' *Epidemiology 12*, 148–156.

Benedetto, C., Marozio, L., Tavella, A.M., Salton, L., Grivon, S., and Di Giampaolo, F. (2010) 'Coagulation disorders in pregnancy: acquired and inherited thrombophilias.' *Annals of the New York Academy of Sciences 1205*, 106–117.

Bischoff, S.C., Barbara, G., Buurman, W., Ockhuizen, T., *et al.* (2014) 'Intestinal permeability – a new target for disease prevention and therapy.' *BMC Gastroenterology 14*, 1, 189.

Boudjenah, R., Molina-Gomes, D., Torre, A., Boitrelle, F., et al. (2014) 'Associations between individual and combined polymorphisms of the TNF and VEGF genes and the embryo implantation rate in patients undergoing in vitro fertilization (IVF) programs.' PLoS ONE 9, 9, e108287.

Cardozo, E.R., Neff, L.M., Brocks, M.E., Ekpo, G.E., et al. (2012) 'Infertility patients' knowledge of the effects of obesity on reproductive health outcomes.' American Journal of Obstetrics and Gynaecology 207, 6, 509.

Carpenter, S. (2012) 'That gut feeling.' Monitor on Psychology 43, 8.

Chavarro, J.E., Rich Edwards, J.W., Rosner, B.A., and Willett, W.C. (2007) 'Diet and lifestyle in the prevention of ovulatory disorder infertility.' Obstet. Gynaecol. 110, 1050–1058.

Chavarro, J.E., Rich Edwards, J.W., Rosner, B.A., and Willett, W.C. (2008) 'Use of multivitamins, intake of B vitamins and risk of ovulatory infertility.' Fertility and Sterility 89, 3, 668–676.

Chu, S.Y., Kim, S.Y., Lau, J., Schmid, C.H., et al. (2007) 'Maternal obesity and risk of stillbirth: a meta analysis.' American Journal of Obstetric Gynaecology 197, 223–228.

Chuang, C.C., Chen, C.D., Chao, K.H., Chen, S.U., Ho, H.N., and Yang, Y.S. (2003) 'Age is a better predictor of pregnancy potential than basal follicle-stimulating hormone levels in women undergoing in vitro fertilization.' Fertility and Sterility 79, 63–68.

Clark, A.M., Thornley, B., Tomlinson, L., Galletley, C., and Norman, R.J. (1998) 'Weight loss in obese infertile women results in improvement in reproductive outcome for all forms of fertility treatment.' Human Reproduction 13, 1502–1505.

Clark, D.A. (2009) 'Should anti-TNF-α therapy be offered to patients with infertility and recurrent spontaneous abortion?' American Journal of Reproductive Immunology 61, 2, 107–112.

Clifford, K., Flanagan, A.M., and Regan, L. (1999) 'Endometrial CD56+ natural killer cells in women with recurrent miscarriage: a histomorphometric study.' Human Reproduction 14, 11, 2727–2730.

Cohen, M.L., and Wittenauer, L.A. (1987) 'Serotonin receptor activation of phosphoinositide turnover in uterine, fundal, vascular, and tracheal smooth muscle.' Journal of Cardiovascular Pharmacology 10, 2, 176–181.

Coulam, C.B., Jeyendran, R.S., Fishel, L.A., and Roussev, R. (2006) 'Multiple thrombophilic gene mutations rather than specific gene mutations are risk factors for recurrent miscarriage.' American Journal of Reproductive Immunology 55, 5, 360–368.

Dendrinos, S., Papasteriades, C, Tarassi, K., Christodoulakos, G., Prasinos, G., and Creatsas, G. (2000) 'Thyroid autoimmunity in patients with recurrent spontaneous miscarriages.' Gynaecological Endocrinology 14, 4, 270–274.

El Asmar, R., Panigrahi, P, Bamford, P., Berti, I., et al. (2002) 'Host-dependent zonulin secretion causes the impairment of the small intestine barrier function after bacterial exposure.' Gastroenterology 123, 5, 1607–1615.

Emmer, P.M., Nelen, W.L.D.M., Steegers, E.A.P., Hendricks, J.C.M., Veerhoek, M., and Joosten, I. (2000) 'Peripheral natural killer cytotoxicity and $CD56^{pos}CD16^{pos}$ cells increase during early pregnancy in women with a history of recurrent spontaneous abortion.' Human Reproduction 15, 5, 1163–1169.

Fedorcsak, P., Dale, P.O., Storeng, R., Ertzeid, G., et al. (2004) 'Impact of overweight and underweight on assisted reproduction treatment.' Human Reproduction 19, 2523–2528.

Flegal, K.M., Carroll, M.D., Ogden, C.L., and Curtin, L.R. (2010) 'Prevalence and trends in obesity among US adults, 1999–2008.' Journal of the American Medical Association 303, 235–241.

Ford, H.B., and Schust, D.J. (2009) 'Recurrent pregnancy loss: etiology, diagnosis and therapy.' Reviews in Obstetrics and Gynaecology 2, 2, 76–83.

Freizinger, M., Franko, D.L., Dacey, M., Okun, B., and Domar, A.D. (2010) 'The prevalence of eating disorders in infertile women.' *Fertility and Sterility 93*, 72–78.

Furness, D.L., Fenech, M.F., Khong, Y.T., Romero, R., and Dekker G.A. (2008) 'One-carbon metabolism enzyme polymorphisms and uteroplacental insufficiency.' *American Journal of Obstetrics and Gynaecology 199*, 3, 276, e1–e8.

Gerhard, I., Monga, B., Krähe, J., and Runnebaum, B. (1999) 'Chlorinated hydrocarbons in infertile women.' *Environmental Research 80*, 4, 299–310.

Gleicher, N., and El-Roeiy, A. (1988) 'The reproductive autoimmune failure syndrome.' *American Journal of Obstetrics and Gynaecology 159*, 1, 223–227.

Govindaiah, V., Naushad, S.M., Prabhakara, K., and Krishna, P.C. (2009) 'Association of parental hyperhomocysteinemia and C677T methylene tetrahydrofolate reductase (MTHFR) polymorphism with recurrent pregnancy loss.' *Clinical Biochemistry 42*, 4–5, 380–386.

Hakim, R.B., Gray, R.H., and Zacur, H. (1998) 'Alcohol and caffeine consumption and decreased fertility.' *Fertility and Sterility 70*, 632–637.

Heit, J.A., Kobbervig, C.E., James, A.H., Petterson, T.M., Bailey, K.R., and Melton, L.J., III. (2005) 'Trends in the incidence of venous thromboembolism during pregnancy or postpartum: a 30-year population-based study.' *Annals of Internal Medicine 143*, 10, 697–706.

Heyman, M. (2005) 'Gut barrier dysfunction in food allergy.' *European Journal of Gastroenterology Hepatology 17*, 1279–1285.

Hidaka, Y., Amino, N., Iwatani, Y., Kaneda, T., *et al.* (1992) 'Increase in peripheral natural killer cell activity in patients with autoimmune thyroid disease.' *Autoimmunity 11*, 4, 239–246.

Ho, H.N., Gill, T.J, Nsieh, R.P., Hsieh, H.J., and Lee, T.Y. (1990) 'Sharing of human leukocyte antigens in primary and secondary recurrent spontaneous abortions.' *American Journal of Obstetrics and Gynaecology 163*, 1 Pt 1, 178–188.

Homan, G.G., Davies, M., and Norman, R. (2007) 'The impact of lifestyle factors on reproductive performance in the general population and those undergoing infertility treatment: a review.' *Human Reproduction Update 13*, 3, 209–223.

Inagaki, J., Kondo, A., Lopez, L.R., Shoenfeld, Y., and Matsuura, E.A. (2005) 'Pregnancy loss and endometriosis: pathogenic role of anti-laminin-1 autoantibodies.' *New York Academy of Sciences 1051*, 174–184.

Jacques, P., Kalmbach, R., Bagley, P., *et al.* (2002) 'The relationship between riboflavin and plasma total homocysteine in the Framingham Offspring cohort is influenced by folate status and the C677T transition in the methylenetetrahydrofolate reductase gene.' *Journal of Nutrition 132*, 283–288.

James, A.H., Konkle, B.A., and Bauer, K.A. (2013) 'Prevention and treatment of venous thromboembolism in pregnancy in patients with hereditary antithrombin deficiency.' *International Journal of Women's Health 5*, 233–241.

Kim, S.Y., Park, S.Y., Choi, J.W., Kim do, J., *et al.* (2011) 'Association between MTHFR 1298A>C polymorphism and spontaneous abortion with fetal chromosomal aneuploidy.' *American Journal of Reproductive Immunology 66*, 4, 252–258.

Klonoff-Cohen, H., Natarajan, L., Marrs, R., and Yee, B. (2001) 'Effects of female and male smoking on success rates of IVF and gamete intra-Fallopian transfer.' *Human Reproduction 16*, 1382–1390.

Kutteh, W.H., Schoolcraft, W.B., and Scott, R.T., Jr. (2000) 'Antithyroid antibodies do not affect pregnancy outcome in women undergoing assisted reproduction.' *Human Reproduction 15*, 1046–1051.

Kwak-Kim, J., Kim, J.W., and Gilman-Sachs, A. (2000) *Immunology and Pregnancy Losses: HLA, Autoantibodies and Cellular Immunity.* Madame Curie Bioscience Database [Internet]. Austin, TX: Landes Bioscience. Available at www.ncbi.nlm.nih.gov/books/NBK6615, accessed on 21 May 2015.

Lalitkumar, P.G.L., Sengupta, J., and Ghosh, D. (2005) 'Endometrial tumor necrosis factor α (TNFα) is a likely mediator of early luteal phase mifepristone-mediated negative effector action on the preimplantation embryo.' *Reproduction 129*, 323–335.

Lee, B.E., Jeon, Y.J., Shin, J.E., Kim, J.H., *et al.* (2013) 'Tumor necrosis factor-α gene polymorphisms in Korean patients with recurrent spontaneous abortion.' *Reproductive Sciences 20*, 4, 408–413.

Li, Q., Li, H., and Tian, X. (1998) 'The study of autoantibodies in women with habitual abortion of unknown etiology.' *Zhonghua Fu Chan Ke Za Zhi 33*, 13–16.

Lipe, B., and Ornstein, D.L. (2011) 'Deficiencies of natural anticoagulants, protein C, protein S and antithrombin.' *Circulation 124*, e365–e368.

Luborsky, J., Roussev, B., and Coulam, C. (2000) 'Ovarian antibodies, FSH and inhibin B: independent markers associated with unexplained infertility.' *Human Reproduction 15*, 5, 1046–1051.

Manohar, M., Khan, H., Sirohi, V.K., Das, V., *et al.* (2014) 'Alteration in endometrial proteins during early- and mid-secretory phases of the cycle in women with unexplained infertility.' *PLoS ONE 9*, 11, e111687.

Mårild, K., Ye, W., Lebwohl, B., Green, P.H.R., *et al.* (2013) 'Antibiotic exposure and the development of coeliac disease: a nationwide case–control study.' *BMC Gastroenterology 13*, 109.

Martinelli, I., Taioli, E., Cetin, I., Marioni, A., *et al.* (2000) 'Mutations in coagulation factors in women with unexplained late fetal loss.' *New England Journal of Medicine 14*, 343, 1015–1018.

Martinelli, P., Troncone, R., Paparo, F., Torre, P., *et al.* (2000) 'Coeliac disease and unfavourable outcome of pregnancy.' *Gut 46*, 3, 332–335.

Meloni, G.F., Dessole, S., Vargiu, N., Tomasi, P.A., and Musumeci, S. (1999) 'The prevalence of coeliac disease in infertility.' *Human Reproduction 14*, 11, 2759–2761.

Metwally, M., Ong, K.J., Ledger, W.L., and Li, T.C. (2008) 'Does high body mass index increase the risk of miscarriage after spontaneous and assisted conception? A meta-analysis of the evidence.' *Fertility and Sterility 90*, 714–726.

Misita, C.P., and Moll, S. (2005) 'Antiphospholipid antibodies.' *Circulation 112*, e39–e44.

Moffett-King, A. (2002) 'Natural killer cells and pregnancy.' *National Review of Immunology. 2*, 9, 656–664.

Molazadeh, M., Karimzadeh, H., and Azizi, M.R. (2014) 'Prevalence and clinical significance of antinuclear antibodies in Iranian women with unexplained recurrent miscarriage.' *Iranian Journal of Reproductive Medicine 12*, 3, 221–226.

Munz, C., Holmes, N., King, A., Loke, Y.W., *et al.* (1997) 'Human histocompatibility leukocyte antigen (HLA)-G molecules inhibit NKAT3 expressing natural killer cells.' *Journal of Experimental Medicine 185*, 3, 385–391.

Murphy, M.M. (2007) 'Homocysteine: biomarker or cause of adverse pregnancy outcome?' *Biomarkers in Medicine 1*, 1, 145–157.

Mustafa, S., Mannhalter, C., Rintelen, C, Kyrle, P.A., *et al.* (1998) 'Clinical features of thrombophilia in families with gene defects in protein C or protein S combined with factor V Leiden.' *Blood Coagul. Fibrinolysis 9*, 1, 85–89.

Nasseri, A., and Grifo, J.A. (1998) 'Genetics, age, and infertility.' *Maturitas 30*, 189–192.

Ng, S.C., Gilman-Sachs, A., Thacker, P., Beaman, K.D., Beer, A.E., and Kwak-Kim, J. (2002) 'Expression of intracellular Th2 and Th2 cytokines in women with recurrent spontaneous abortion, implantation failures after IVF/ET or normal pregnancy.' *American Journal of Reproductive Immunology 48*, 77–86.

Onno, M., Guillaudeux, T. Amiot, L., *et al.* (1994) 'The HLA-G gene is expressed at a low mRNA level in different human cells and tissues.' *Human Immunology 41*, 1, 79–86.

Ornstein, D.L., and Cushman, M. (2003) 'Factor V Leiden.' *Circulation 107*, e94–e97.

Pastore, L., Hertz-Picciotto, I., and Beaumont, J.J. (1997) 'Risk of still birth from occupational and residential exposures.' *Occupational and Environmental Medicine 54*, 511–518.

Pellati, D., Mylonakis, I., Bertoloni G., Fiore, C., *et al.* (2008) 'Genital tract infections and infertility.' *European Journal of Obstetrics, Gynaecology and Reproductive Biology 140*, 1, 3–11.

Petrozza, J.C. (2014) *Recurrent Early Pregnancy Loss.* Medscape. Available at http://emedicine. medscape.com/article/260495-overview, accessed on 21 May 2015.

Pickell, L., Deqiang, L., Brown, K., Mikael, L.G., *et al.* (2009) 'Methylenetetrahydrofolate reductase deficiency and low dietary folate increase embryonic delay and placental abnormalities in mice.' *Birth Defects Research Part A: Clinical and Molecular Teratology 85*, 6, 531–541.

Poort, S.R., Rosendaal, F.R., Reitsma, P.H., and Bertina, R.M. (1996) 'A common genetic variation in the 3′-untranslated region of the prothrombin gene is associated with elevated plasma prothrombin levels and an increase in venous thrombosis.' *Blood 88*, 3698–3703.

Poppe, K., Glinoer, D., Van Steirteghem, A., Tournaye, F., *et al.* (2002) 'Thyroid dysfunction and autoimmunity in infertile women.' *Thyroid 12*, 11, 997–1001.

Prummel, M.F., and Wiersinga W.M. (2004) 'Thyroid autoimmunity and miscarriage.' *European Journal of Endocrinology 150*, 751–755.

Rand, J.H., Wu, X.X., Quinn, A.S., Ashton,W.A., *et al.* (2010) 'Hydroxychloroquine protects the annexin A5 anticoagulant shield from disruption by antiphospholipid antibodies: evidence for a novel effect for an old antimalarial drug.' *Blood 115*, 11, 2292–2299.

Rasch, V. (2003) 'Cigarette, alcohol, and caffeine consumption: risk factors for spontaneous abortion.' *Acta Obstetricia et Gynecologica Scandinavica 82*, 182–188.

Robertson, L,. Wu, O., Langhorne, P., Twaddle, S., *et al.* (2006) 'The Thrombosis: Risk and Economic Assessment of Thrombophilia Screening (TREATS) Study. Thrombophilia in pregnancy: a systematic review.' *British Journal of Haematology 132*, 2, 171–196.

Romero, P., Barnett, P.G., and Midtling, J.E. (1989) 'Congenital abnormalities with maternal exposure to oxydemeton-methyl.' *Environmental Research 50*, 2, 256–261.

Sharma, R., Biedenharn, K.R., Fedor, J.M., and Agarwal, A. (2013) 'Lifestyle factors and reproductive health: taking control of your fertility.' *Reproductive Biology and Endocrinology: RB&E 11*, 66.

Shoenfeld, Y., Carp, H.J., Molina, V., Blank, M., *et al.* (2006) 'Autoantibodies and prediction of reproductive failure.' *American Journal of Reproductive Immunology 56*, 5–6, 337–344.

Stephenson, M.D. (1996) 'Frequency of factors associated with habitual abortion in 197 couples.' *Fertility and Sterility 66*, 1, 24–29.

Sugiura-Ogasawara, M., Ozaki, Y, Sonta, S, Makino, T., and Suzumori, K. (2005) 'Exposure to bisphenol A is associated with recurrent miscarriage.' *Human Reproduction 20*, 2325–2329.

Ten Kate, M.K., and Van der Meer, J. (2008) 'Protein S deficiency: a clinical perspective.' *Haemophilia 14*, 6, 1222–1228.

Townsley, D.M. (2013) 'Hematologic complications of pregnancy.' *Seminars in Hematology 50*, 3, 222–231.

Vassiliadou, N., and Bulmer, J.N. (1996) 'Immunohistochemical evidence for increased numbers of 'classic' CD57+ natural killer cells in the endometrium of women suffering spontaneous early pregnancy loss.' *Human Reproduction 11*, 7, 1569–1574.

Visser, J., Rozing, J., Sapone, A., Lammers, K., and Fasano, A. (2009) 'Tight junctions, intestinal permeability, and autoimmunity celiac disease and type 1 diabetes paradigms.' *Annals of the New York Academy of Sciences 1165*, 195–205.

Walker, M.C., Garner, P.R., Keely, E.J., Rock, G.A., and Reis, M.D. (1997) 'Changes in activated protein C resistance during normal pregnancy.' *American Journal of Obstetrics and Gynaecology 177*, 1, 162–169.

Wang, J.X., Davies, M., and Norman, R.J. (2000) 'Body mass and probability of pregnancy during assisted reproduction treatment: retrospective study.' *British Medical Journal 321*, 1320–1321.

Ware Branch, D., and Khamashta, M.A. (2003) 'Antiphospholipid syndrome: obstetric diagnosis, management and controversies.' *Obstetrics and Gynaecology 101*, 1333–1344.

Weng, S.-L., Chiu, C.-M., Lin, F.-M., Huang, W.-C., *et al.* (2014) 'Bacterial communities in semen from men of infertile couples: metagenomic sequencing reveals relationships of seminal microbiota to semen quality.' *PLoS ONE 9*, 10.

Windham, G.C., Lee, D., Mitchell, P., Anderson, M., Petreas, M., and Lasley, B. (2005) 'Exposure to organochlorine compounds and effects on ovarian function.' *Epidemiology 16*, 2, 182–190.

Witkin, S.S., and Chaudhry, A.J. (1989) 'Association between recurrent spontaneous abortions and circulating IgG antibodies to sperm tails in women.' *Journal of Reproductive Immunology 15*, 2, 151–158.

Yin, Li-J., Zhang, Y., Lv, P.-P., He, W.-H., *et al.* (2012) 'Insufficient maintenance DNA methylation is associated with abnormal embryonic development.' *BMC Medicine 10*, 26.

Younglai, E.V., Holloway, A.C., and Foster, W.G. (2005) 'Environmental and occupational factors affecting fertility and IVF success.' *Human Reproduction Update 11*, 43–57.

Zammiti, W., Mtiraoui, N., Finan, R.R., Almawi, W.Y., and Mahjoub, T. (2009) 'Tumor necrosis factor alpha and lymphotoxin alpha haplotypes in idiopathic recurrent pregnancy loss.' *Fertility and Sterility 91*, 5, 1903–1908.

# Chapter 9

# A Reproductive Immunology Case History

*Justine Bold BA (Hons), PgCHE, Dip BCNH, NTCC, CNHC Senior Lecturer Institute of Health & Society, University of Worcester, UK*

## 1. Introduction

This chapter presents a case history where immunological issues were found to be a factor in pregnancy loss and infertility. The case study is of Gemma, who commenced assisted reproductive techniques (ART) in the UK at the age of 41 years. At the time of initial presentation to her general practitioner Gemma had several allergies (including reactions to both foods and drugs) and suffered with asthma, but overall was in good health and aged 39.

She and her partner had been trying to conceive for two years and she was nearing the cut-off age for funding of ART within her area in the UK. Gemma was told she would be over the cut-off age by the time she could be referred to a fertility specialist. The couple decided to fund private treatment; in many other countries this is the only option, hence funding is an important consideration in this area, as repeated ART failure is obviously very costly. It is a possibility that couples could place themselves under financial pressure, which may be repeated again and again; it is therefore a high consideration that immunological issues be investigated and identified as quickly as possible.

*Note:* In the UK, the National Institute for Clinical Excellence (NICE) guidelines were revised in 2013 and now recommend that one cycle of IVF treatment is funded in women aged 40–42. Previously the cut-off age in the UK for funded treatment was 39. However, in the UK routine investigation of immunological issues (other than thrombophilias) in those with ART failure is not currently recommended by NICE and couples who potentially have these issues are left to seek private treatment.

## 2. Case presentation

Before starting ART, Gemma had been trying to conceive with her current partner for nearly four years; this had unfortunately been unsuccessful. Gemma was ovulating and had a regular 28–38-day cycle. They were timing intercourse around ovulation, her hormone profiles were normal and she was in the healthy weight range with a BMI of 23. She reported some pain after intercourse and also noted that she often had swollen lymph glands in her groin after intercourse. This was brought to the attention of the initial specialist (a gynaecologist) treating the couple, though it was at the time deemed insignificant by that specialist. Gemma had a history of a missed miscarriage at 16 weeks with a previous partner (whilst aged 31 years). She reported that tests had been performed and no reasons had been identified for the loss of the pregnancy. This had been followed by a surgical procedure – an evacuation of retained products of conception (ERPC). During the procedure Gemma's cervix was damaged and stitched. Gemma had also had abnormal cervical cells some years previously, which had been treated via colposcopy and large loop excision of transformation zone (LLETZ). Her appendix had been removed when she was a teenager; this was thought significant as this type of abdominal surgery can be associated with fertility issues. Gemma reported being stressed at work and also stressed as a result of trying to conceive. Her partner had a teenage son from a previous relationship. They had both made several lifestyle and dietary modifications. Additionally, tests undertaken by the couple's general practitioner for sexually transmitted infections (STIs) were negative.

## 2.1 Initial clinical investigations

Gemma initially had a vaginal ultrasound scan and a laparoscopy. The scan identified two small intramural fibroids. These were not encroaching the uterine cavity. A small patch of endometriosis was found via laparoscopy on the outside of Gemma's womb; this was ablated. Otherwise the results were reassuring, as both Gemma's fallopian tubes appeared normal. Further blood tests were undertaken (full blood count, haemoglobin and thyroid function) – these were also all normal. Hormone blood tests taken on day two of the menstrual cycle reported follicle-stimulating hormone (FSH) level of of 6.3mIU/ml, luteinising hormone (LH) of 6.8mIU/ml. This was considered reassuring as elevations in FSH could indicate the onset of menopause and an LH above 7mIU/ml in the early stage of the menstrual cycle can be indicative of polycystic ovary syndrome.

## 2.2 Test results

An anti-Müllerian hormone (AMH) test was performed; this showed an ovarian reserve of 14.91pmol/l. This indicates low fertility; however, the fertility consultant/gynaecologist reported that this is roughly twice what might be normally expected in a woman aged 41 years.

## Table 9.1 AMH reference ranges

| Ovarian fertility potential | pmol/l |
|---|---|
| Optimal fertility | 28.6 pmol/l – 48.5 pmol/l |
| Satisfactory fertility | 15.7 pmol/l – 28.6 pmol/l |
| Low fertility | 2.2 pmol/l – 15.7 pmol/l |
| Very low/undetectable | 0.0 pmol/l – 2.2 pmol/l |
| High level | >48.5 pmol/l<br>? suspicion of polycystic ovarian disease/granulosa cell tumours |

*Source: The Doctors Lab (2008)*

### 2.2.1 CHLAMYDIA ANTIBODY TITRE

This was performed even though vaginal swabs had previously been taken for cell culture – producing a negative result. The serology was also negative. This was consistent with the results of the cell culture indicating that chlamydia infection was still thought unlikely.

### 2.2.2 PARTNER'S SEMEN ANALYSIS

Analysis identified that Gemma's partner's sample had good volume and motility; however, there were higher than normal levels of abnormally shaped sperm, that is, sperm with two heads, or tails or no tails.

## BOX 9.1 GEMMA'S PARTNER'S
··· SEMEN ANALYSIS RESULT ················································

This concluded her partner had a sub-optimal fertility potential. Results of the initial test were as follows:

| | | |
|---|---|---|
| Volume | 3ml | (ref > 2ml) |
| Concentration | 43m/ml | (ref >20) |
| Total count | 129 million | (ref >40 million) |
| Motility | 65 per cent | (ref >50%) |
| Normal forms | 4 | (ref >15%) |

## 2.3 Specialist's initial recommendations

The couple were told that the sperm problems, together with Gemma's age, were the most likely reasons for their failure to conceive. They were told that there was still a reasonable chance of natural conception and to continue trying to conceive naturally whilst considering ART as a future option if Gemma did not get pregnant.

## 2.4 Initial ART treatment

After several more months of trying naturally the couple asked to proceed with ART, aware of the reductions in success rates once women are over 42 years old. Intracytoplasmic sperm injection (ICSI) was recommended owing to the sperm issues and a long protocol using down regulation started. (For further information on types of ART, refer to Chapter 2.) However, before ovarian stimulation could commence Gemma had an allergic reaction to one of the drugs used for down regulation and the cycle was cancelled.

## 2.5 Next steps

A few months after this, Gemma started a gonadotrophin-releasing hormone (GnRH) antagonist protocol without any down regulation, using the drug Menopur to stimulate the ovaries and the drug Cetrotide (an LH antagonist – which suppresses the LH surge and thereby ovulation). Semen analysis at this stage showed only one per cent normal forms so IVF was deemed unsuitable.

## 2.6 Short protocol and ICSI

The cycle progressed well, with Gemma's ovaries responding to stimulation. Nine eggs were collected and ICSI was performed resulting in the creation of seven good quality embryos. Three were eventually transferred and four were frozen (at three days) for later use. Gemma was given progesterone pessaries to use after embryo transfer and told to take a pregnancy test after ten days. Gemma had some complications two days after embryo transfer; these resulted in her being admitted to hospital in severe pain. Tests were undertaken to rule out a pulmonary embolism and Gemma was released, having been diagnosed with costochondritis. This is an inflammatory condition, believed to be self-limiting and benign. It affects cartilage in the chest (Proulx and Zryd 2009) and it is believed to have either infectious or rheumatologic causes (Proulx and Zryd 2009). Doctors treating her at the time believed this to be unrelated to the ART or embryo transfer. Ten days after embryo transfer Gemma was given a negative pregnancy test result.

## 2.7 Frozen embryo transfer

After a review of the failed cycle the clinic treating Gemma was recommended to proceed with a frozen embryo transfer. It was recommended that this should be a natural cycle without progesterone support. Two of the four embryos initially frozen at day three survived the thaw-out. One was defrosted in good condition and grew in the laboratory overnight to 12 cells (grade AB), eventually being transferred after hatching and compacting, whilst the other had lost a few cells in the defrosting process (grade B). This round of treatment also produced a negative result and Gemma failed to get pregnant.

### ⋯ BOX 9.2 GEMMA'S STORY ⋯⋯⋯⋯⋯⋯⋯⋯⋯⋯⋯⋯⋯⋯⋯⋯⋯

'We were treated in a National Health Service clinic in the UK, but paid for treatment ourselves. Our first cycle was a "text book" near-perfect cycle as nine eggs were collected. I was told this was a great response and similar to a much younger woman. They said my ovaries were really good for a 41-year-old. ICSI produced seven really good embryos and three were transferred at day three after assisted hatching; the remaining four were frozen. After being told how good the embryos were, I was really confident I would get pregnant. But just two days later I was in crippling pain and was admitted to hospital. I had pains in my joints and in my chest; I couldn't breathe properly, which was very scary. I had to have CT scans on my lungs to rule out a pulmonary embolism; I was sobbing as the embryos were going to be exposed to radiation at a critical stage. I asked to wear a lead apron, but I am not sure that this helped. The CT scans ruled out an embolism and I was eventually discharged with the consultants saying they thought I had an inflammatory condition called costochondritis; they did not link it to the embryos.

'I spent the next ten days imagining I was pregnant and felt hopeful as I had started to feel sick. But the pregnancy test was negative and I was devastated. It took me weeks to stop crying. At our follow-up appointment I asked if they thought I might have had a reaction to the embryos; they said no. They recommended we proceed with a frozen transfer, but sadly after waiting two weeks to do a test, counting down the hours, this cycle too was negative. After this I started to read a lot and discovered that some internet forums were mentioning immunological factors in infertility in women. At another follow-up in our clinic to review our failed frozen cycles I asked if they thought immunological factors might be causing the problems. I was told there was no evidence that immunological treatments helped female infertility problems and told the main issue was probably just my age. I found this hard to reconcile with being told we had excellent quality embryos and that we had had a near-perfect cycle.

'This started a whole new journey for us, one that cost many tens of thousands of pounds. Eventually further privately funded tests showed that I had several immunological issues that were contributing to our issues... I wish I had been given a clear view of the evidence earlier in our journey, as by the time the immunological issues had been identified and treated I was another year older. I feel as though my concerns and questions were dismissed and I feel cross that I wasn't listened to or directed sooner to get the help we needed. In fact, I was made to feel foolish by asking if my immune system might be involved. I feel I was misinformed as there are plenty of papers published in respected journals linking immunological factors to IVF failure and early pregnancy loss; despite this I was told there was "no evidence".

'Once I had the first round of immune treatment I actually got pregnant naturally; unfortunately I lost this pregnancy too, but it at least gave me some renewed hope that with the right treatment I may be able to become a mother.'

## 2.8 Immune investigations and treatment

Gemma was concerned that the inflammatory problems after the first embryo transfer were related to their problems conceiving and found a new clinic in London offering immune investigations. They recommended that tests were undertaken to measure the levels of natural killer (NK) cells in Gemma's blood. They also did additional thyroid screening and recommended a thrombophilia profile, as well as measuring hormone levels through Gemma's menstrual cycle to confirm she was not peri-menopausal and to confirm ovulation. Most results were normal/negative; however, Gemma had raised anticardiolipin antibodies. This indicated she had a condition called antiphospholipid syndrome (APS) (originally known as Hughes' syndrome), which is associated with recurrent miscarriage amongst other problems.

This meant that Gemma would need anticoagulation therapy to maintain a pregnancy. She was informed that this was probably why she lost her initial pregnancy at 16 weeks. Results of the NK cell assays also pinpointed problems in particular high levels of TNF alpha (TNFα) and high levels of a type of NK cell (identified by surface marker CD56+). TNFα is a cytokine secreted mostly by macrophages; it is involved in controlling many biological processes and has been implicated in a number of diseases including autoimmune conditions. CD56+ NK cells have been linked to pregnancy loss and IVF treatment failure.

## BOX 9.3 OVERVIEW OF
··· ANTIPHOSPHOLIPID SYNDROME (APS) ·······················

In the 1980s, studies of patients with the autoimmune disorder systemic lupus erythematosus (SLE) showed an association with foetal loss, amongst other problems (Derksen, Khamashta and Branch 2004). The serologic entity was called APS (Derksen et al. 2004).

APS is a systemic autoimmune disorder, characterised by elevated titres of antiphospholipid antibodies or lupus anticoagulant (LAC), recurrent foetal loss, coagulation failure, repeated thromboembolic phenomena, and thrombocytopenia (Blank and Shoenfeld 2004).

APS can exist without other autoimmune disease and in this case is termed primary APS (Derksen et al. 2004).

The Miscarriage Association (n.d.) in the UK reports: 'In some women with antiphospholipid syndrome, in the first 13 weeks, the antibodies can prevent the pregnancy from embedding properly in the womb, increasing the chances of an early miscarriage. In the second and third trimesters of pregnancy (from 14 weeks gestation until birth), antiphospholipid syndrome in some women can cause blood clots in the placenta. This can lead to poor blood and oxygen supplies to the baby, causing poor growth, pre-eclampsia or even stillbirth.'

There are reports of associations with pregnancy problems such as subchorionic haematomas (Loi and Tan 2006) and pre-eclampsia (Branch *et al.* 1992), causing pre-term delivery and stillbirth (Loi and Tan 2006).

········································································································

## ··· BOX 9.4 OVERVIEW OF NK CELL CONTROVERSY ········

Numerous studies show associations between repeat miscarriage, often referred to as recurrent spontaneous abortion (RSA), and elevations in peripheral NK cells or NK cell activity (Kwak-Kim *et al.* 1995; Yamada *et al.* 2001; Yamada *et al.* 2003). They are also associated with infertility (Beer, Kwak and Ruiz 1996).

Case controlled studies were undertaken in 2012 by Karami *et al.* They concluded: 'the percentage of CD56(dim) cells and the level of peripheral blood NK cell cytotoxicity in RSA patients and women with IVF failure were significantly higher than in both the healthy multiparous and successful IVF control groups (P<0.001).'

However, much earlier studies have concluded that there is insufficient evidence about NK cell involvement to validate testing and justify treatments. For example, Moffett, Regan and Braude (2004) outline differences between uterine NK cells and those in peripheral blood and question how examination of peripheral blood NK cells relates to the uterus. They also describe how the functions of uterine NK cells are still not fully understood and describe how the percentage of CD56+ NK cells in peripheral blood in normal healthy individuals varies greatly (5% to 29%). They claim that this variation makes it very difficult to pinpoint what is normal.

········································································································

## 2.9 Natural pregnancy following immune treatment

Gemma was prescribed two doses of a drug to reduce levels of TNFα. There is now some research (though some studies are small-scale) suggesting that this is a treatment option where TNFα is raised (Clark 2010; Winger *et al.* 2011). This treatment was to be administered prior to commencing an ART cycle. (The drug is often used in treatment of rheumatoid arthritis. It is a monoclonal antibody inhibitor; the brand name of the drug is Humira.) Unfortunately, Gemma had an allergic reaction to the second dose, causing pronounced swelling at the injection site, and she experienced difficulty breathing. This allergic reaction resulted in another emergency hospital admission. As a result of this, Gemma was prescribed oral corticosteroids for two weeks (10mg a day of prednisolone).

Two weeks after this, prior to commencement of the ART cycle, the clinic treating her discovered she had become pregnant naturally. However, signs were that this pregnancy was struggling at the outset; levels of human chorionic gonadotrophin hormone (hCG) were low and NK cell tests showed marked increases in NK cells (CD56+). The clinic started further treatments to attempt to support the pregnancy. Intralipids and intravenous immunoglobulin (IVIg) were administered. She was advised to take 75mg aspirin and low molecular weight heparin injections twice a day. Gemma was also prescribed oral corticosteroids at a dose of 10mg prednisolone a day. Despite this, the pregnancy failed at approximately 10 weeks.

### ···  BOX 9.5 CD56+ NATURAL KILLER CELLS  ····················

- ▶ These NK cells are effective killers and more cytotoxic than other NK subsets.

- ▶ They express high levels of CD16 (this is a receptor that facilitates antibody dependent cellular cytotoxicity) and perforin (this is a protein that attacks and produces pores on target membrane).

- ▶ They are potent mediators of antibody dependent cellular toxicity, lymphokine-activated killer (LAK) activity or natural cytotoxicity.

(Kwak-Kim and Gilman-Sachs 2008)

## 2.10 Hysteroscopy and the next ART cycle

After the miscarriage, the clinic recommended a hysteroscopy and genetic karotype testing for herself and her partner. This was performed and results were normal. Another ART cycle commenced once Gemma's menstrual cycle resumed. This was approximately eight weeks after the miscarriage. Gemma again started oral corticosteroids; additionally intralipids were recommended. Ovarian stimulation produced 13 mature oocytes. ICSI was performed and 11 embryos were created. Four embryos out of the 11 progressed to blastocyst stage and three of these were transferred into Gemma's uterus on day five. This cycle produced an equivocal hCG result: hCG levels were not high enough for pregnancy to be confirmed, but were not negative either. The clinic recommended administration of intralipids and monitoring of hCG. Eventually levels of hCG fell and the possibility of pregnancy was excluded.

## 2.11 Next steps

After this, Gemma and her partner unsuccessfully tried intrauterine insemination (IUI). This was advised owing to improvements with her partner's sperm. After saving more money and trying to recover emotionally, Gemma and her partner tried again, using a clinic in Europe. The clinic reviewed their history and recommended a sample of menstrual blood undergo further chlamydia testing using polymerase chain reaction (PCR) detection and another hysteroscopy with dilatation and curettage (D&C). PCR uses DNA extraction and amplification and is now recognised as a very sensitive method of detecting microbial pathogens (Yamamoto 2002). Despite previous serological testing and cell culture indicating negative results for a chlamydia infection, findings of the PCR test indicated an infection. A specialist at the clinic expressed the view that immune issues such as Gemma's may well be a response to a 'silent' chlamydia infection.

The hysteroscopy revealed that Gemma had an endometrial polyp, which was removed, and it also showed that Gemma had a narrow cervix (the consultant said this was possibly from previous surgery). The surgeon stretched the cervix to aid embryo transfer in future cycles. As a result of the chlamydia PCR test result, Gemma and her partner were given antibiotics and the clinic also recommended a course of herbal supplements (cordyceps) for both her and her partner prior to commencement of the next round of fertility treatment. Gemma's general practitioner (GP) in the UK was unfamiliar with the use of PCR testing in the context of fertility treatment; however, the GP supported the use of antibiotics given Gemma's history. Other UK-based clinics previously consulted were confident that Gemma did not have chlamydia, given the previous test results.

The difference of opinion between the European clinic and UK-based clinics on the role of PCR testing in this context is interesting, but given the testing is low cost and the treatment very economical it could prove to be a valuable avenue of investigation in couples with recurrent ART failures. Cordyceps are a type of fungi that grow on insect larvae. They have a long history in Traditional Chinese Medicine (TCM) as a general health tonic and fertility aid (Holliday and Cleaver 2008). Immuno-modulating effects have also been noted (Holliday and Cleaver 2008) as well as positive effects on sperm parameters and reproductive hormone levels, though it must be noted that many studies are on animals. Gemma was also put on 10mg prednisolone and 75mg aspirin a month prior to treatment. Both of these are evidenced in women with autoimmune and implantation problems and additionally aspirin is recommended in women with antiphospholipid syndrome. Research from the late 1990s demonstrated improved implantation rates in such women with low dose aspirin and prednisolone (Hasegawa *et al.* 1998).

## 2.12 Successful cycle

After antibiotic treatment, semen analysis showed that Gemma's partner's sperm morphology issues had improved. The analysis showed morphology in normal parameters (15% normal forms) so the clinic then recommended IVF (without the use of ICSI). A GnRH antagonist protocol was used using the FSH drug Fostimon for ovarian stimulation. Six eggs were collected and two made it through to the blastocyst stage and were transferred. The clinic administered IV steroids at egg collection, owing to Gemma's drug allergies. Gemma also had intravenous intralipids a few days before embryo transfer. After transfer, Gemma was to take 10mg progesterone, oestrogen, low molecular weight heparin (Clexane), aspirin and antibiotics. An injection of hCG was recommended by the clinic; this was administered after embryo transfer and on days seven and nine post-transfer. Two days after embryo transfer Gemma started to experience the same problems as with her first embryo transfer. She had pains in her chest and joints. At this point the clinic increased her steroid dosage to 40mg prednisolone a day, and eventually the pains subsided. Nine days after transfer Gemma got a positive pregnancy test result via a home test using a urine sample. She remained on 40mg prednisolone until 12 weeks pregnant, then started tapering the dose down. Intravenous intralipids were administered bi-weekly until the eighteenth week of pregnancy.

Gemma is now a mother to a healthy baby but the pregnancy was complicated throughout, owing to a sub-chorionic haematoma forming in early pregnancy and pre-term premature rupture of membranes (PPROM), which caused Gemma to go into labour at 30 weeks pregnant.

## BOX 9.6 THERAPEUTIC OPTIONS ··· FOR IMPLANTATION FAILURE ····································

A 2013 paper in the *Journal of Human Reproductive Sciences* (Kumar and Mahajan 2013) outlines the role of hCG and progesterone as therapeutic options for implantation failure and cites that the two treatments offered 'excellent outcomes'; however, it cautions that hCG was associated with an increased risk of ovarian hyperstimulation syndrome (OHSS).

## 3. Concluding remarks

Gemma and her partner's case is complex. There were obviously issues with her partner's sperm and Gemma was over 41 years old when she started ART. Moreover, Gemma and her partner spent more than two years trying natural methods before seeking advice regarding ART. With the benefit of hindsight Gemma believes she wasted valuable time and should have started ART and investigations sooner, given declining success rates when a woman is over 40. Yet, despite her age and issues with her partner's sperm, Gemma had several immunological issues that needed identification and management in order for ART to have the best chance of success. Without this, Gemma believes she would not have become a mother. Gemma's issues included the autoimmune problem APS, but in addition she had other problems with raised levels of NK cells (CD56+). Medical management of the immune issues was required for her to achieve and maintain a pregnancy.

## References

Beer, A.E., Kwak, J.Y., and Ruiz, J.E. (1996) 'Immunophenotypic profiles of peripheral blood lymphocytes in women with recurrent pregnancy losses and in infertile women with multiple failed in vitro fertilisation cycles.' *American Journal Reproductive Immunology 35*, 376–382.

Blank, M., and Shoenfeld, Y. (2004) 'Antiphosphatidylserine antibodies and reproductive failure.' *Lupus 13*, 661–665.

Branch, D.W., Silver, R.M., Blackwell, J.L., Reading, J.C., and Scott, J.R. (1992) 'Outcome of treated pregnancies in women with antiphospholipid syndrome: an update of the Utah experience.' *Obstetrics & Gynaecology 80*, 614–620.

Clark, D.A. (2010) 'Anti-TNFalpha therapy in immune-mediated subfertility: state of the art.' *Journal of Reproductive Immunology 85*, 1, 15–24.

Derksen, R., Khamashta, M., and Branch, D. (2004). 'Management of obstetric Antiphospholipid Syndrome.' *Arthritis & Rheumatism 50*, 4, 1028–1039.

Hasegawa, I., Yamanoto, Y., Suzuki, M., Murakawa, H., *et al.* (1998) 'Prednisolone plus low-dose aspirin improves the implantation rate in women with autoimmune conditions who are undergoing in vitro fertilization.' *Fertility & Sterility 70*, 6, 1044–1048.

Holliday, J., and Cleaver, M. (2008) 'Medicinal value of the caterpillar fungi species of the genus cordyceps (fr.) link (ascomycetes). A review.' *International Journal of Medicinal Mushrooms 10*, 3, 219–234.

Karami, N., Boroujerdnia, M.G., Nikbakht, R., and Khodadadi, A. (2012) 'Enhancement of peripheral blood CD56(dim) cell and NK cell cytotoxicity in women with recurrent spontaneous abortion or in vitro fertilization failure.' *Journal of Reproductive Immunology 95*, 1–2, 87–92.

Kumar, P., and Mahajan, S. (2013) 'Preimplementation and postimplementtation therapy for the treatment of reproductive failure.' *J. Hum. Reprod. Sci. 6*, 2, 88–92.

Kwak-Kim, J., and Gilman-Sachs, A. (2008) 'Clinical implication of natural killer cells and reproduction.' *American Journal of Reproductive Immunology 59*, 388–400.

Kwak-Kim, J.Y., Beaman, K.D., Gilman-Sachs, A., Ruiz, J.E., Schweitz, D., and Beer, A.E. (1995) 'Up-regulated expression of CD56+, CD56+/CD16+ and CD19+ cells in peripheral blood lymphocytes in pregnant women with recurrent pregnancy losses.' *American Journal of Reproductive Immunology 34*, 93–99.

Loi, K., and Tan, K. (2006) 'Massive pre-placental and subchorionic haematoma.' *Singapore Medical Journal 47*, 12, 1084–1086.

Miscarriage Association (n.d.) *Antiphospholipid Syndrome and Pregnancy Loss.* Available at www.miscarriageassociation.org.uk/wp/wp-content/leaflets/Antiphospholipid-syndrome-and-pregnancy-loss.pdf, accessed on 22 May 2015.

Moffett, A., Regan, L., and Braude, P. (2004) 'Natural killer cells, miscarriage, and infertility.' *British Medical Journal 329*, 7477, 1283–1285.

National Institute of Clinical Excellence (2013) *Fertility: Assessment and Treatment for People with Fertility Problems.* Available at www.nice.org.uk/guidance/cg156/chapter/recommendations, accessed on 22 May 2015.

Proulx, A.M., and Zryd, T.W. (2009) 'Costochondritis: diagnosis and treatment.' *American Family Physician 80*, 6, 617–620.

The Doctors Lab (2008) Available online at www.tdlpathology.com, accessed 24 August 2009.

Winger, E.E., Reed, J.L., Ashoush, S., El-Toukhy, T., Ahuja, S., and Taranissi, M. (2011) 'Degree of TNF-α/IL-10 cytokine elevation correlates with IVF success rates in women undergoing treatment with Adalimumab (Humira) and IVIG.' *American Journal of Reproductive Immunology 65*, 6, 610–618.

Yamada, H., Kato, E.H., Kobashi, G., Ebina, Y., *et al.* (2001) 'High NK cell activity in early pregnancy correlates with subsequent abortion with normal chromosomes in women with recurrent abortion.' *American Journal of Reproductive Immunology 46*, 132–136.

Yamada, H., Morikawa, M., Kato, E.H., Shimada, S., Kobashi, G., and Minakami, H. (2003) 'Pre-conceptional natural killer cell activity and percentage as predictors of biochemical pregnancy and spontaneous abortion with normal chromosome karyotype.' *American Journal of Reproductive Immunology 50*, 351.

Yamamoto, Y. (2002) 'PCR in diagnosis of infection: detection of bacteria in cerebrospinal fluids.' *Clinical and Diagnostic Laboratory Immunology 9*, 3, 508–514.

## Chapter 10

# Dietary Factors, Key Micronutrients and Nutritional Support

*Karen MacGillivray-Fallis*
*BA Hons, FIPD, MSc (Nut. Th), MBANT, CNHC*

*To Jonathan and Daniel – for all your love, support and encouragement.*

## 1. Overview

It is widely accepted that a healthy diet is fundamental for optimum health and wellbeing. There already exists a large body of evidence which links nutrition to a wide variety of detrimental health conditions (Reilly *et al.* 2003; Bowen and Beresford 2002) and increasingly several studies have shown that dietary factors can have an impact on fertility and pregnancy outcomes (Lim, Noakes and Norman 2007; Gardiner *et al.* 2008; Sharma *et al.* 2013).

A large-scale prospective study found that women with high fertility diet scores had lower rates of infertility due to ovulation disorders. This diet was characterised by higher monounsaturated to trans-fat ratio (that is, more good fats than bad fats), increased vegetable over animal protein, high-fat intake over low-fat dairy, a decreased glycaemic load (lower sugar load), and an increased intake of iron and multivitamins (Chavarro *et al.* 2007b). Another study suggested that adherence to a pre-conception diet as recommended by the Netherlands Nutrition Centre increased the chance of pregnancy in women undergoing in vitro fertilisation (IVF) (Twigt *et al.* 2012). The recommendations referred to in this study included at least four slices of wholewheat bread daily (or servings of other wholegrain cereals), the use of monounsaturated or polyunsaturated oils, 200g or more vegetables every day, two or more pieces of fruit daily, three or fewer servings of meat or meat replacers weekly and one or more portion of fish weekly (Twigt *et al.* 2012).

High adherence to the Mediterranean diet (characterised by consumption of vegetables, fruits, beans, whole grains, olive oil and fish) has been associated with a 40 per cent increased chance of biochemical pregnancy on day 15 after embryo transfer (Vujkovic *et al.* 2010). Some studies have suggested that users of micronutrient supplements achieve higher pregnancy rates (Chavarro *et al.* 2008b). It has been suggested that particular supplement brands may be effective in both male and female fertility (Westphal, Polan and Trant 2006; Abed 2013). One study examined the efficacy of a supplement containing B vitamins, zinc, vitamin E, N-acetylcysteine and a proprietary extract of opuntia fig fruit extract and found that it may improve the outcomes in both natural and assisted reproduction (Dattilo *et al.* 2014). However, despite this, it should be noted that human studies relating to how particular nutrients can influence fertility are limited (Homan, Davies and Norman 2007; Rooney and Domar 2014).

The literature can often be confusing because of contradictory and conflicting results. Current guidelines from the National Institute for Clinical Excellence (NICE), US Department of Health and Human Services (HHS), the National Institute of Child Health and Human Development (NIH), the American College of Obstetricians and Gynaecologists (ACOG) and the American Society for Reproductive Medicine (ASRM) are sparse in terms of nutritional guidance. Recommendations include eating a nutritious and well-balanced diet, to be a healthy weight, to not smoke and to limit alcohol consumption (NICE 2012). However, it is not clear to what extent this information is communicated effectively to those trying to conceive. Indeed, information given by health professionals is often seen as inadequate as it is either not given or suggestions are vague and general (Curtis *et al.* 2006; Porter and Bhattacharya 2008). This may be further highlighted in studies which have shown that knowledge of lifestyle and nutrition risk factors among those trying to conceive is often absent (Hammiche *et al.* 2011; Frey and Files 2006; Cardozo *et al.* 2012). The aim of this chapter, therefore, is to explore which nutrients may be beneficial for reproductive health both within the general population and those undergoing assisted reproductive techniques (ART) while using an evidenced-based approach.

## 2. Calorific intake

In the UK, the general population recommendations for estimated average energy requirements are 2000 calories for females age 19–50 and 2500 calories for males in the same age group (NHS 2014a). In the United States, the guidance is 1800–2400 calories for females and 2200–3000 calories for males depending on age and activity levels (Health and Human Services 2010). Calorie intake is associated with weight gain/loss and therefore obesity and low body weight can have a negative impact on reproductive potential through interference with hormonal and metabolic mechanism (Jokela, Elovainio and Kivimäki 2008; Moragianni, Jones and Ryley 2012). Body mass index (BMI) is a simple calculation that is commonly used to indicate whether an individual is a healthy weight in relation to height. (Further information on BMI can be found in Chapter 3.) The recommended BMI by the World Health Organisation (WHO) is in the range of 18.5–24.9 while a BMI greater than 30 is classed as obese (WHO 2015). While there are validity issues with BMI as an effective measurement tool (Okorodudu *et al.* 2010), the increased chance of delayed conception/infertility has been acknowledged (Anderson, Nisenblat and Norman 2010; Hawkins *et al.* 2014). Women with a BMI less than 19 or greater than 29 have had a greater time to conception (Hassan and Killick 2004; Bolúmar *et al.* 2000) although it should be noted that the Bolúmar study found that an increased time to conception for those with a high BMI was only amongst those that smoked. Obesity has also shown to have a negative effect on assisted reproductive outcomes (Chavarro *et al.* 2012; Shah *et al.* 2011; Pinborg *et al.* 2011).

A systematic review found that overweight and obese women undergoing IVF needed higher doses of gonadotrophins, have a lower chance of pregnancy and also an increased miscarriage rate (Maheshwari, Stofberg and Bhattacharya 2007). In a retrospective study of 2349 women, obesity increased the risk of pregnancy loss/ spontaneous abortion (Wang, Davies and Norman 2002). In a further retrospective cohort study of 4609 patients, obesity had a significant negative effect on ART outcomes. Patients with BMI >30 had up to 68 per cent lower odds of having a live birth following their first ART cycle compared with women with BMI <30 (Moragianni *et al.* 2012). The distribution of body fat may also impact on reproductive performance, although the mechanism for this is unclear (Norman *et al.* 2006). In comparison, the number of studies investigating male obesity and fertility are limited (MacDonald *et al.* 2010). Some have suggested a link between obesity and time to conception (Hassan and Killick 2004; Jensen *et al.* 2004) while a meta-analysis concluded that there was insufficient evidence to demonstrate an association between obesity and semen parameters (MacDonald *et al.* 2010). Another study suggested that, while there were major differences in reproductive hormone levels with increasing body weight, only extreme levels of obesity may negatively influence male reproductive potential (Chavarro *et al.* 2010). Some of the studies in this area are investigated more in Chapter 3.

Insufficient calorie intake may be associated with depleted nutrients, which in turn impacts on reproductive health (Wong *et al.* 2002; Winter *et al.* 2002). Low body weight may disturb the hypothalamic–pituitary axis resulting in ovulatory disorders. However, studies examining the impact of low BMI on IVF outcomes have shown conflicting results with some demonstrating lower pregnancy rates (Li *et al.* 2013) and others showing no difference compared to normal weight women (Moragianni *et al.* 2012; Pinborg *et al.* 2011). One study did not find any significant impact of underweight on clinical pregnancy or live birth rates after IVF, but found a significantly higher proportion of cancelled ART cycles among underweight women (Fedorcsak *et al.* 2004).

## 3. Protein

Protein is a building block for cellular growth. Its primary functions are to build and repair body tissues, create new cells, and produce hormones (BNF 2014). The Reference Nutrient Intake in both the UK and the United States is around 46g for women and 56g for men (NHS 2014a; Health and Human Services 2010). Dietary proteins and amino acids are important modulators of glucose metabolism and insulin sensitivity. Insulin sensitivity is an important determinant of ovulatory function and fertility (Taylor and Marsden 2000) and impaired insulin sensitivity is associated with polycystic ovary syndrome (PCOS) (Rondanelli *et al.* 2014). However, the type of protein rather than the quantity has been shown to modulate insulin resistance (Tremblay *et al.* 2007). In a retrospective study involving 18,555 women, replacing carbohydrates with animal protein was demonstrated to be detrimental to ovulatory fertility. Adding just one serving of meat was correlated with a 32 per cent higher chance of developing ovulatory infertility, particularly if the meat was chicken or turkey. However, replacing carbohydrates with vegetable protein demonstrated a protective effect. The study found that consuming 5 per cent of total energy intake as vegetable protein rather than animal protein was associated with a 50 per cent lower risk of ovulatory infertility (Chavarro *et al.* 2008a). Proteins derived from fish might also have desirable effects on insulin sensitivity and this will be examined more fully later.

It is not clear to what extent protein consumption affects sperm quality. One study involving 30 men with poor semen quality and 31 normospermic men found that frequent intakes of meat and dairy products may detrimentally affect semen quality (Mendiola *et al.* 2009). The reason for this is not clear but the study suggests that the results are consistent with other research, which proposes that poor semen quality may be associated with a higher intake of products that incorporate xenobiotics, mainly xenoestrogens or certain anabolic steroids (Swan *et al.* 2007). Xenoestrogens are highly lipophilic substances that can accumulate in fat-rich foods such as meat or milk, and are suspected as partially responsible for the decline in semen quality (Santti *et al.* 1998). In some fertility clinics, whey protein is suggested to couples to support egg and sperm health. Whey protein is a complete protein as it contains all the essential and non-essential amino acids (Murray and Pizzorno 2010). It has high concentrations of glutamine, which is a precursor for the synthesis of proteins, nucleotides, glutathione and other important molecules (Murray and Pizzorno 2010). Glutathione supplementation was found to help with sperm motility in a pilot study involving 11 men (Lenzi et al. 1994) although recent research is lacking. There are currently no clinical trials relating to the role of whey protein in ART.

## 3.1 L-arginine

L-arginine is a semi-essential amino acid and is a key precursor to nitric oxide (NO), a small molecule that is responsible for relaxing blood vessels and promoting circulation which helps promote blood flow to the uterus, ovaries and genitals. This may result in an increase of endocervical secretions during the ovulatory phase in women. In a study involving 34 patients undergoing IVF, of the 17 receiving L-arginine supplementation, two became pregnant while there were no pregnancies in the control group (Battaglia et al. 1999). A double-blind placebo study involving 93 women suggested that a nutritional supplement containing L-arginine may aid fertility in some women (Westphal et al. 2006). However, one study of 32 patients found that L-arginine supplementation may be detrimental to embryo quality and pregnancy rates during controlled ovarian hyperstimulation cycles (Battaglia et al. 2002) This study suggested that the use of L-arginine resulted in quick, intense and incongruent follicular growth, which has previously been shown may have a negative influence on the outcome of gamete intra-Fallopian transfer cycles (Eldar-Geva et al.1998).

L-arginine may benefit men by increasing sperm health, count and motility, although if the sperm count is less than 20 million per millilitre it is less likely to be of benefit (Pizzorno, Murray and Joiner-Bey 2008). In an earlier study involving 40 infertile men, L-arginine supplementation increased sperm motility over a six-month period (Scibona et al. 1994). In order for it to be effective, the dosage should be at least 4g a day for three months (Murray and Pizzorno 2010) and should be taken on an empty stomach. However, it should be noted that as the herpes virus utilises arginine, a diet high in arginine in people who harbour the herpes virus may lead to reactivation. It is therefore essential to be mindful of this when supplementing arginine and to balance the intake of arginine with an increased intake of lysine (Murray 1996).

## 4. Carbohydrates

Dietary carbohydrates play a central role in human nutrition because they provide the primary source of energy. Simple carbohydrates are either monosaccharide, composed of one sugar molecule, or disaccharides, which are composed of two sugar molecules. Complex carbohydrates are composed of many simple sugars joined together by chemical bonds. The more complex a carbohydrate is, the slower it is to break down (Mann and Truswell 2007). Another way of labelling carbohydrates is to consider glycaemic index and glycaemic load. Glycaemic index provides a numerical value that expresses the rise of blood glucose after consuming a particular food. The glycaemic load gives a more accurate picture as it also takes into account the amount of carbohydrate in the food (Murray and Pizzorno 2010).

As previously mentioned, insulin sensitivity appears to have a critical relationship to androgen modulation (Jones 2005). It is suggested that a high dietary glycaemic index is positively related to ovulatory infertility, and the amount and quality of carbohydrate may be important determinants in reproductive health. A retrospective study found that greater carbohydrate intake and dietary glycaemic load were associated with an increased risk of infertility due to anovulation; and that dietary glycaemic index was positively related to this condition among women who have not been able to carry a pregnancy beyond 20 weeks (Chavarro et al. 2009a). However, it should be noted that the increase in carbohydrate intake was at the expense of naturally occurring fats and therefore ovulatory fertility may be associated more with the beneficial effect of consuming natural fats. Other studies have suggested that a low glycaemic diet may improve insulin sensitivity in women with PCOS (Barr et al. 2013; Rondanelli et al. 2014) and a reduction in carbohydrates has shown numerous beneficial effects on the metabolic profile of women suffering from this condition (Gower et al. 2013; Douglas et al. 2006). PCOS and associated hormonal balances are dealt with in more detail in Chapter 3.

## 5. Fats

Dietary fat plays a number of important roles in the body. It is the most concentrated source of calories, is the preferred energy source of the body and forms the structural components in cell membranes (Mann and Truswell 2007). The consumption of trans-unsaturated fats has been associated with a greater risk of ovulatory infertility. Trans-fats are considered to be 'bad fats'; they occur naturally in the fat of meat and milk, but are also produced artificially by food manufacturers and found in foods such as biscuits, crackers, baked goods and margarine. A large-scale prospective study of 18,555 women found that every two per cent increase in energy from trans-unsaturated fats as opposed to carbohydrates was associated with a 73 per cent greater risk of ovulatory infertility (Chavarro et al. 2007a). Higher intake of saturated fats, which are found predominantly in animal products, has also been associated with the retrieval of fewer fertilised eggs (Chavarro et al. 2012). Indeed, consumption of monosaturated polyunsaturated fatty acids (PUFAs) (found in olive oil, avocado and nuts such as almonds) may be correlated with higher implantation and pregnancy rates (Jungheim et al. 2013; Chavarro et al. 2012).

The long chain polyunsaturated fatty acids (LC-PUFAs) are essential compounds of cell membranes and after activation by hormones and growth factors they become precursors of eicosanoids, which are important in immune-mediated responses (Hammiche et al. 2011). These can be distinguished as omega-3, 6 and 9. Several studies have suggested a link with omega-3 intake and reproductive outcomes. Omega-3 comprises alpha-linoleic acid (ALA), eicosapentaenoic acid (EPA) and docosahexaenoic acid (DHA). In one study, LC-PUFAs, in particular ALA and DHA, had a positive effect on the number of follicles and embryo morphology (Hammiche et al. 2011). It has also been suggested that omega-3 may possibly increase uterine blood flow and facilitate pregnancy by increasing the prostacyclin/thromboxane ratio (Saldeen and Saldeen 2004). Supplementation with omega-3 fatty acids (FA) during pregnancy lowers the risk of premature birth and can increase the length of pregnancy and birthweight by altering the balance of eicosanoids involved in labour and promote foetal growth by improving placental blood flow (Saldeen and Saldeen

2004). Omega-3 fatty acids are found in oily fish such as sardines, salmon and trout, and walnuts and linseeds (otherwise known as flax).

As with females, fat consumption in males may have an effect on reproductive health. The consumption of trans-fatty acids may be inversely related to sperm count in healthy men while the consumption of omega-3 may have a beneficial effect (Chavarro *et al.* 2014; Safarinejad 2012). Omega-3 may be important in male fertility as it is involved in the production of prostaglandins, which are important in sperm formation (BNF 2014). In a preliminary cross-sectional study involving 99 men, dietary analysis and semen quality were measured. High intakes of saturated fats were negatively correlated to sperm concentrations whereas higher intakes of omega-3 fats were positively related to sperm morphology (Attaman *et al.* 2012).

## 6. Alcohol

It is acknowledged that alcohol may be detrimental to reproductive health and ART (NICE 2012; Human Fertilisation and Embryology Authority 2010). However, the mechanisms by which alcohol can affect conception are not clear. It is suggested that alcohol may result in a rise in oestrogen, which reduces FSH secretion suppressing folliculogenesis and ovulation (Homan *et al.* 2007). It may also have an effect on ovum maturation, ovulation, blastocyst development and implantation (Eggert, Theobald and Engfeldt 2004). An 18-year study involving 7393 individuals found that high alcohol consumption was associated with increased risk of infertility (Eggert *et al.* 2004). Moderate levels of alcohol consumption have also been associated with reduced fertility (Jensen *et al.* 1998). Female alcohol consumption is associated with fewer oocytes obtained, lower pregnancy rates, and a 2.21 times increased risk of miscarriage (Klonoff-Cohen, Lam-Kruglick and Gonzalez 2003; Hassan and Killick 2004). In another study, IVF patients who stopped consuming alcohol and caffeine prior to their IVF cycle had higher clinical pregnancy and live birth rates than those who did not. However, it should be acknowledged that these women may also have adopted other healthy lifestyle practices (Huang *et al.* 2012). In a study that examined the pre-conception alcohol consumption of 1042 women who had recently given birth,

80 per cent reported drinking alcohol (Tough *et al.* 2006). While it is not clear whether any had issues with fertility, it does question to what extent alcohol impedes fertility. While there are bias issues with self-reporting behaviours and recall in this study, the exact mechanisms involved in how alcohol may affect fertility and ART need to be further explored. Studies have not fully examined whether particular types of alcohol have a more significant effect than others, and clearly further research is needed. Alcohol consumption and its effect on fertility is covered in more detail in Chapter 11.

Deterioration of sperm quality has been associated with alcohol consumption (Gaur, Talekar and Pathak 2010). A Danish study of 1221 men found that even modest habitual alcohol consumption of more than five units per week had adverse effects on semen quality, although most pronounced associations were seen in men who consumed more than 25 units per week (Jensen *et al.* 2014). However, the research is not conclusive as it is not clear what level of alcohol consumption affects fertility and there are individual genetic characteristics that may influence alcohol metabolism (Homan *et al.* 2007).

## 7. Caffeine

There is no consistent advice given to couples trying to conceive with regard to caffeine consumption, both within the general population and those undergoing ART, as studies have demonstrated conflicting results. Some associate consumption of caffeinated beverages with reduced fecundity (Bolúmar *et al.* 1997) while others have not found a link (Hakim, Gray and Zacur 1998; Chavarro *et al.* 2009b; Hatch *et al.* 2012). Some research indicates that caffeine intake of more than 50mg/day is linked to lower pregnancy rates in IVF patients (Klonoff-Cohen, Bleha and Lam-Kruglick 2002). A study of over 600 women reviewed the effect of coffee and tea on IVF and found that increased caffeine serum levels adversely affected the number of eggs, coffee consumption was correlated with the number of miscarriages and high tea consumption resulted in a decline in the number of good embryos (Al-Saleh 2010). However, another study, involving 201 women who had been trying to conceive for less than three months, suggested that drinking half a cup of tea doubled the chances of conception (Caan,

Quesenberry and Coates 1998). Tea contains anti-oxidants so this may in part be why a different effect is seen; obviously this is an area for future research to clarify. The reasons for inconclusive findings with regard to caffeine consumption are unclear and may suggest other methodological shortcomings, issues with recall, variations in caffeine metabolism or issues with accounting for other lifestyle factors. Table 10.1 shows the caffeine content of popular drinks, though note that the caffeine amount can vary depending on brand, how it is manufactured and brewing time.

### Table 10.1 Caffeine content (Mayo Clinic 2015)

| Beverage | Serving | Caffeine |
|---|---|---|
| Coffee – instant | 237ml | 27–173mg |
| Coffee – brewed | 237ml | 95–200mg |
| Decaffeinated coffee – Instant | 237ml | 2–12mg |
| Tea | 237ml | 14–70mg |
| Decaffeinated tea | 237ml | 0–12mg |
| Green tea | 237ml | 24–25mg |
| Coke | 335ml | 23–35mg |
| Diet Coke | 335ml | 23–47mg |
| Red Bull | 248ml | 75–80mg |

## 8. Oxidative stress and the role of anti-oxidants

Oxidative stress can be multifactorial and the resultant overproduction of free radicals alongside the reduction in anti-oxidant activity is implicated in infertility (Poston et al. 2011; Agarwal and Saleh 2014; Ruder et al. 2014; Wright, Milne and Leeson 2014). In males, exposure to increased levels of free radicals may result in abnormal sperm and impaired motility (Tremellen 2008) and it has been suggested that anti-oxidants may play a protective role (Showell et al. 2011; Imhof *et al.* 2012). Indeed, subfertile men have been identified as having lower levels of anti-oxidant in their semen compared with fertile men (Tremellen *et al.* 2007). A study involving 30 men attending a fertility clinic found that a low intake of anti-oxidant nutrients was associated with poor semen quality (Mendiola *et al.* 2010). A systematic review of the effect of oral anti-oxidant supplementation on male infertility indicates a possible improvement in sperm quality and pregnancy rates. This review examined the results of 17 randomised trials and included assessment of vitamins C and E, zinc, selenium, folate, carnitine and carotenoids (Ross *et al.* 2010).

A Cochrane Database Systematic Review examined 34 trials and concluded that anti-oxidant supplementation in subfertile males may improve outcomes of live births and pregnancy rates in couples undergoing ART cycles (Showell *et al.* 2011). However, it should be noted that many of the studies examined focused on improvements in sperm health and motility and not necessarily increased birth rates (Agarwal *et al.* 2004; Jensen *et al.* 2011). In females, the effect of oxidative stress on oocytes and reproductive functions is less clear as studies have tended to be in vitro or animal based (Agarwal *et al.* 2012). However, some suggest that the intake of anti-oxidants may help (Buhling and Grajecki 2013; Ruder *et al.* 2014) and some studies have commented that time to pregnancy may be shorter with certain supplementation (Ruder *et al.* 2014; Westphal *et al.* 2006). This is in contrast to a Cochrane Database Systematic Review which included 28 trials and judged the quality of evidence to be low as the variation in the type of anti-oxidant administered meant that comparison was difficult (Showell *et al.* 2013).

## 9. Vitamin A and carotenes

Vitamin A is a fat-soluble vitamin and is important for growth and development, and for the maintenance of the immune system; it is an anti-oxidant so may play a role in reducing oxidative stress. It comes in two forms, retinol and carotenoids, beta carotene being the most abundant (BNF 2014). Vitamin A deficiency can result in male infertility while in females there are low rates of conception and high rates of stillbirths (Mann and Truswell 2007) although the precise mechanisms are unclear. However, excess vitamin A consumption by women in pregnancy can cause congenital defects and should be avoided (NICE 2012).

Carotenes found in orange, red and yellow fruits and vegetables exert significant anti-oxidant activity; and beta carotene, in particular, may affect fertility as the corpus luteum has the highest concentration of beta carotene in any organ measured and inadequate function is linked to infertility (Murray 1996). In one study, time to pregnancy was shorter for women with a BMI greater than 25 who increased beta carotene intake, and for those younger than 35, increasing both beta carotene and vitamin C also decreased time to pregnancy (Ruder *et al.* 2014). Beta carotene and vitamin C may also play a role in maintaining the health of amniotic membranes (Murray 1996). Lycopene, a lipid soluble carotenoid, exhibits great anti-oxidant qualities and is positively associated with improved semen quality (Mendiola *et al.* 2010).

## 10. B vitamins

B vitamins are involved in energy release in the body and play a vital role in detoxification, hormonal balance and fertility (BNF 2014).

### 10.1 Pyridoxine (B6)

B6 (pyridoxine) is involved in the formation of proteins and structural compounds, chemical transmitters, red blood cells and prostaglandins. It is also critical in maintaining proper hormone balance (Murray 1996). In a study of 364 women in China, poor B6 vitamin status appeared to decrease the possibility of conception and contribute to the risk of early pregnancy loss (Ronnenberg *et al.* 2007).

### 10.2 Folic acid (B9)

B9 (folic acid) is involved in cellular division as it is necessary in DNA synthesis. It is widely recommended that folic acid supplementation of 400 micrograms is taken by women planning to conceive as it has been shown to reduce the risk of neural tube damage (NHS 2014b; Centers for Disease Control and Prevention 2014). A retrospective study of 18,555 women suggests that intake of folic acid is inversely related to the risk of ovulatory infertility (Chavarro et al. 2008b). Although currently unknown, it is possible that ovarian response to endogenous FSH pulses is also decreased in low folate conditions which can be overcome by greater intake of folic acid (Chavarro et al. 2008b). There may be a correlation between follicular fluid homocysteine concentration and oocyte maturity. Homocysteine is a metabolite of the amino acid methionine and is involved in sulphurylation and methylation metabolic pathways and has been proposed to have pro-oxidant effects (Sekhon et al. 2010). In one study, homocysteine concentration in follicular fluid and serum was significantly lower in the group who received folic supplementation. Those women who had received folic acid supplementation also had better quality oocytes compared with the control group (Szymański and Kazdepka-Ziemińska 2003). However, a recent study commented that folic acid supplementation or good folate status did not have a positive effect on pregnancy outcome following infertility treatment in women with unexplained infertility (Murto et al. 2014).

### 10.3 Cobalamin (B12)

Cobalamin (B12), like the other B vitamins, is important for metabolism (Mann and Truswell 2007) and it has been suggested that, as with folic acid, a B12 deficiency may lead to increased homocysteine levels which in turn could be detrimental to fertility (Szymański and Kazdepka-Ziemińska 2003). It is critically involved in cellular replication and a deficiency may lead to reduced sperm count and motility (Murray 1996) although one study found little to support the idea that low folate/B12 can impact on idiopathic infertility (Murphy et al. 2011). Vitamin B12 deficiency has also been linked to recurrent foetal loss. In a small study of 14 patients with vitamin B12 deficiency, foetal loss occurred in eleven women (Bennett 2001).

## 11. Ascorbic acid

Ascorbic acid (vitamin C) is involved in immune function, the manufacture of certain nerve transmitting substances and hormones, and carnitine synthesis and is an important anti-oxidant (BNF 2014).

As an anti-oxidant it may play an important part in protecting sperm DNA from damage and may reduce the number of agglutinated sperm which occur when antibodies produced by the immune system bind to the sperm (Murray 1997). Some studies have shown that increasing vitamin C consumption may improve sperm count and motility (Akmal *et al.* 2006; Mínguez-Alarcón *et al.* 2012) although the exact amount of vitamin C is unclear. A review of the literature suggests that the data may demonstrate that dietary anti-oxidants can be beneficial in reducing sperm DNA damage, particularly in men with high levels of DNA fragmentation, although the mechanism is unclear and trials have been small (Zini, San Gabriel and Baazeem 2009). In an earlier study, where dietary vitamin C was reduced from 250 milligrams to 5 milligrams, sperm DNA damage increased by 91 per cent (Fraga *et al.* 1991).

In females, the role of vitamin C in reproductive health is less clear. Ovarian vitamin C is an essential cofactor for the biosynthesis of collagen, which is required for the high rates of tissue remodelling that attends follicle growth, ovulation and corpus luteum development. In one study, women with a BMI less than 25 had a shorter time to pregnancy when vitamin C intake was increased and when combined with beta carotene; for women under 35, the same applied (Ruder *et al.* 2014). It is claimed that when given to women undergoing ART, vitamin C can significantly increase success rates (Infertility Network 2014) although research is conflicting. A prospective, randomised, placebo-controlled, group comparative, double-blind study to evaluate the impact of different doses of ascorbic acid as additional support during luteal phase in infertility treatment found no benefit (Griesinger *et al.* 2002).

## 12. Vitamin D

Vitamin D is most widely recognised for its role in stimulating the absorption of calcium (BNF 2014).There are two major food sources of Vitamin D: vitamin D2 (ergocalciferol) and vitamin D3 (cholecalciferol). Ergocalciferol is most commonly used in nutritional supplements (Murray 1997); however, the role it may have in reproductive health is unclear and study findings are conflicting. A study involving 84 infertile women showed that women with higher vitamin D levels in their serum and follicular fluid were significantly more likely to achieve clinical pregnancy (Ozkan *et al.* 2010). However, other studies have shown that vitamin D deficiency is not an indicator of ART outcome (Aleyasin *et al.* 2011*).* A randomised, double-blind trial looking at 52 patients found no significant difference between IVF cycle outcomes for patients taking vitamin D supplements for a month compared with the control group (Polak de Fried *et al.* 2013). Indeed, one study of 101 women undergoing IVF found that women with sufficient vitamin D had poorer outcomes than those who were deficient (Anifandis *et al.* 2010). In men, vitamin D is positively associated with semen quality and androgen status although there are no randomised control trials on the effect of vitamin D supplementation on semen quality (Lerchbaum and Obermayer-Pietsch 2012).

## 13. Alpha-tocopherol

Alpha-tocopherol (an active form of vitamin E) functions primarily as an anti-oxidant, protecting cell membranes from oxidative damage (BNF 2014). While there are eight natural forms of vitamin E (Mann and Truswell 2007), most studies at present focus primarily on the role of alpha-tocopherol. As oxidative stress may be implicated in infertility, its role as an anti-oxidant may be beneficial (Agarwal *et al.* 2012). Higher dietary vitamin E intake may also be associated with lower fasting glucose (Ley *et al.* 2013).

Studies examining the effects of vitamin E on female fertility are limited. Recent research found that those over the age of 35 had a shorter time to pregnancy by increasing their vitamin E intake (Ruder *et al.* 2014). A pilot study showed that vitamin E supplementation of 600mg may aid in increasing the thickness of the endometrium in women with thin uterine lining (Takasaki *et al.* 2010). In males, studies have shown that vitamin E may increase sperm health and motility (Greco *et al.* 2005). In one study involving 690 infertile men, supplementation of vitamin E (dose 400 international units) and selenium (dose 200μg) for 100 days may have had a beneficial and a protective effect especially on sperm motility (Moslemi and Tavanbakhsh 2011). In a study where participants took a supplement containing vitamin E (12mg) amongst other nutrients, a positive effect on sperm oxidative stress occurred (Dattilo *et al.* 2014). However, another study demonstrated that neither vitamin E nor selenium had significant effects on semen quality (Mendiola *et al.* 2010). It should be noted that few of these studies examined pregnancy rates and many examined combined supplementation, so it is difficult to isolate the specific benefit of a particular nutrient.

## 14. Zinc

Zinc is extensively used in many enzyme and body functions and is necessary for proper immune system function. It is important for metabolism and thyroid function as it is one of the cofactors for iodothyronine iodinase enzyme which is involved in the conversion of thyroxine to triiodothyronine (Murray 1997). Zinc is critical to male sex hormone and prostate function and is used in hormone metabolism, sperm formation and sperm motility. Zinc levels are typically much lower in infertile men with low sperm counts, indicating that a low zinc status may be a contributory factor in infertility (Murray and Pizzorno 2005). Zinc and folic acid supplement therapy have shown to have a positive effect on total sperm count and acrosomal integrity (Azizollahi *et al.* 2013; Wong *et al.* 2002). In another study, anti-oxidant supplementation including zinc resulted in a significant improvement in viable pregnancy rates in 60 couples undergoing ART (Tremellen *et al.* 2007). As previously mentioned, Dattilo *et al.* examined the efficacy of a supplement containing 12.5mg of zinc amongst other nutrients and found that it may improve reproductive outcomes (Dattilo *et al.* 2014).

As zinc is essential for cell division, it has a key role in foetal development (Murray 1997). Women need zinc to ensure correct oocyte formation, maintain follicular fluid and regulate hormones. A deficiency can lead to hormone imbalance, abnormal ovarian development and menstrual irregularity (Murray 1997). Low levels of zinc may be linked to premature births and foetal development. In a study of African-American women who had low levels of zinc plasma, they were given either a supplementation of 25mg of zinc sulphate or a placebo. The zinc-supplemented group demonstrated greater body weight and head circumference compared with the placebo group (Goldenberg *et al.* 1995).

## 15. Selenium

Selenium, in the form of selenocysteine, is incorporated in the body into a range of enzymes (selenoproteins), which are crucial to human health (BNF 2014). The best known of these is glutathione peroxidase, which plays an important role in protecting cell membranes from damage by free radicals and therefore may help to protect both eggs and sperm (Murray and Pizzorno 2005). It may also be an essential element for normal testicular development, spermatogenesis, and spermatozoa motility and function (Moslemi and Tavanbakhsh 2011).

Selenium plays a key role in thyroid hormone metabolism and studies have shown that women with thyroid autoimmunity have a significant increased risk of infertility (Poppe *et al.* 2003). Indeed, it is suggested that the presence of thyroid antibodies increases the risk of miscarriage in both natural and ART pregnancies (Prummel and Wiersinga 2004; Negro *et al.* 2007). However, the extent to which selenium deficiency contributes to miscarriage is unclear. In a small study of 40 women, selenium deficiency was associated with a higher rate of miscarriage (Barrington *et al.* 1996). However, in another study, while there was evidence of selenium deficiency in women with recurrent miscarriages compared with a control group with a good reproductive performance, this difference was only seen in hair samples and not serum samples. This study concluded that the importance of selenium deficiency in miscarriage still needs to be determined (Al-Kunani *et al.* 2001). There have been few studies that have examined the role of selenium supplementation on its own in reproductive health. It has been suggested that anti-oxidants may work better in combination because they protect each other from oxidation and preclude the need for large single doses which may be harmful (Westphal *et al.* 2006).

In an earlier small study, six women with unexplained infertility received two months' supplementation of 200mg selenium and six months' supplementation of 600mg magnesium. All six women produced normal, healthy babies within eight months of completing the trial (Howard, Davies and Hunnisett 1994). In a double-blind, placebo-controlled pilot study, the efficacy of a multivitamin containing selenium was examined. Thirty women who had not been able to become pregnant after at least six months of attempts were randomly assigned to receive the supplement or placebo for three months. The supplement, FertilityBlend, contained chasteberry, green tea extracts, L-arginine, vitamin B6, vitamin B12, folate, iron, magnesium, zinc and selenium although the study does not state specific dosage information. After five months, 33 per cent of the women in the supplement group and none in the control group had achieved a pregnancy (Westphal *et al.* 2004). This study was repeated with 93 women and 14 out of 53 in the supplement group conceived compared with 4 out of 40 in the control group (Westphal *et al.* 2006).

It has been suggested that supplementation with zinc, copper and selenium may improve female fertility (Bedwal and Bahuguna 1994). However, Mistry *et al.* (2012) concluded that there still remains inadequate information from the available small intervention studies to inform public health strategies and that selenium's role in infertility has yet to be fully explored.

The effectiveness of selenium in male reproductive health is also not clear. Some studies have found that selenium supplementation may increase sperm health. One trial suggested that selenium supplementation in subfertile men with low selenium status can improve sperm motility and the chance of successful conception (Scott *et al.* 1998). However, not all patients responded, with only 56 per cent showing a positive response to treatment. In another small study involving 20 men, selenium improved sperm quality in contrast to B vitamins and vitamin E (Keskes-Ammar *et al.* 2003).

The effect of vitamin E and selenium on sperm quality is disputed. One study involving 690 men with idiopathic asthenoteratospermia received daily supplementation of selenium (200μg) in combination with vitamin E (400 units) for at least 100 days. There was a 52.6 per cent total improvement in sperm motility, morphology, or both (Moslemi and Tavanbakhsh 2011). Other studies have found that neither vitamin E nor selenium had significant effects on semen quality (Hawkes and Turek 2001; Mendiola *et al.* 2010).

A double controlled blind study was conducted on the efficacy of selenium and N-acetylcysteine (NAC) for the treatment of male infertility. The results indicated that supplemental selenium and NAC may improve semen quality (Safarinejad and Safarinejad 2009).

## 16. Magnesium

Magnesium is critical to many cellular functions including energy production, cellular replication and protein formation (BNF 2014). Its role in infertility has not been fully explored but a small trial studied 12 women with unexplained infertility – or early miscarriage – who had deficient magnesium levels. Six restored their magnesium levels after six months of magnesium supplementation while the remainder did not. The women who had failed to restore their magnesium levels were found to have significantly lower activity levels of the potent anti-oxidant (glutathione) and were prescribed a further two months of supplementation with selenium and magnesium. All 12 women produced normal, healthy babies within eight months of restoring their red blood cell (RBC) magnesium levels (Howard *et al.* 1994).

The role of magnesium in male infertility is also unclear, although one study which compared zinc, copper, iron and magnesium in seminal plasma in both infertile men and a control group surmised that both zinc and magnesium may be important for spermatogenesis (Abed 2013).

Magnesium requirements increase during pregnancy and a deficiency may be linked to complications during pregnancy including pre-eclampsia, pre-term delivery and foetal growth retardation (Pathak and Kapil 2004). However, a Cochrane Database Systematic Review concluded that there was insufficient high quality evidence to show that dietary magnesium was beneficial during pregnancy (Makrides and Crowther 2014).

## 17. Iodine

Iodine is a trace element required in the manufacture of thyroid hormones and a deficiency can affect the entire endocrine system. Its role in fertility is not clear as, while thyroid dysfunction is associated with ovulatory dysfunction and adverse pregnancy outcome (Negro *et al.* 2007; Prummel and Wiersinga 2004), ovulation and conception can still occur (Poppe, Velkeniers and Glinoer 2008).

## 18. Iron

Iron is important in the haemoglobin molecule of red blood cells. It also functions in several key enzymes in energy production and metabolism including the synthesis of DNA (Murray and Pizzorno 2005). There are two forms of dietary iron. Heme is found in animal products while non-heme is present in plant foods. Heme is most efficiently absorbed in the body. It is not clear to what extent iron directly influences fertility, although some studies suggest that it may have an important role to play in ovulatory function and fertility.

In a double-blind, placebo-controlled pilot study, the efficacy of a multivitamin containing iron was examined. Thirty women who had not been able to become pregnant after at least six months of attempts were randomly assigned to receive the supplement or placebo for three months. The supplement FertilityBlend contained chasteberry, green tea extracts, L-arginine, vitamin B6, vitamin B12, folate, iron, magnesium, zinc and selenium. After five months, 33 per cent of the women in the supplement group and none in the control group had achieved a pregnancy (Westphal *et al.* 2004).

In a retrospective study, women who consumed iron supplements and iron from non-heme sources were less likely to be at risk of ovulatory infertility (Chavarro *et al.* 2006).

## 19. Carnitine

Carnitine is a vitamin-like compound that transports long-chain fatty acids into the mitochondria. In humans, high carnitine levels are critical to sperm energy metabolism and are found in high concentrations in the epididymis of the testes, where sperm mature and acquire their motility (Murray 1996). Some studies suggest that carnitine supplements may increase sperm count and mobility (Balercia *et al.* 2005; Lenzi *et al.* 2004). A systematic review compared carnitine and L-carnitine with placebo treatments and found improvements in pregnancy rates and sperm motility (Zhou, Liu and Zhai 2007) although others have found no clinical or statistical effect on sperm quality or motility (Sigman *et al.* 2006).

L-carnitine has also been reported to increase sperm health by providing the protection the body needs to counteract free radical damage. However, many of these studies lack placebo and double-blind design making it difficult to reach a definite conclusion (Agarwal *et al.* 2014).

## 20. Calcium

Calcium is important for building and maintaining bones and teeth as well as being essential to enzyme activity. While animal studies suggest the role that calcium plays particularly in sperm function (Munire *et al.* 2004), there are no human studies which demonstrate the influence calcium intake may have on natural and assisted reproduction.

## 21. Coenzyme Q10

Coenzyme Q10 (CoQ10) is a vital element of the mitochondrial respiratory chain and plays a crucial role in energy metabolism (Murray 1996). CoQ10 is also an anti-oxidant and may protect egg and sperm cells from oxidative and toxic damage (Agarwal *et al.* 2004). In one study, CoQ10 content was measured in follicular fluid obtained from 20 infertile women undergoing ovarian stimulation programme for IVF. CoQ10/protein levels resulted significantly higher in mature vs. dysmorphic oocytes and, similarly, CoQ10/cholesterol was significantly higher in grading I–II vs. grading III–IV embryos (Turi *et al.* 2012). This suggests that the role of CoQ10 needs to be further explored.

It has been shown that CoQ10 supplementation in men with idiopathic oligoasthenoteratozoospermia may result in improved sperm parameters (Mancini and Balercia 2011; Safarinejad 2012) although others have found no benefit (Nadjarzadeh *et al.* 2011).

## 22. N-acetyl cysteine

NAC is a powerful anti-oxidant that may have a very protective effect on egg quality as women age, although this as yet has only been demonstrated in an animal study which showed that NAC may reduce the signs of oocyte ageing (Liu *et al.* 2012). In studies, women with PCOS who were treated with clomiphene citrate plus NAC for another cycle had increased ovulation rates compared with those who were treated with clomiphene citrate alone (Badawy, State and Abdelgawad 2007; Rizk *et al.* 2005).

As an anti-oxidant, NAC may be effective in improving semen parameters (Ciftci *et al.* 2009). In a randomised trial, both NAC and selenium supplementation indicated a beneficial effect on semen quality (Safarinejad and Safarinejad 2009).

## 23. Resveratrol

Resveratrol is a member of a group of plant compounds called polyphenols. It may help with insulin resistance (Murray 1997). Its role in human fertility is yet unexplored, although animal-based studies have suggested it may improve the number and quality of oocytes (Liu *et al.* 2013; Kong *et al.* 2011).

## Table 10.2 An overview (BNF 2014; Nutritiondata 2015)

| Nutrient | Role | Dietary Source |
|---|---|---|
| Vitamin A – retinol and carotenoids | Anti-oxidant, embryonic development, growth and cellular differentiation | Retinol: liver, whole milk, cheese, butter, margarine<br><br>Carotenoids: green leafy vegetables, orange-coloured fruit, carrots |
| Lycopene | Anti-oxidant | Tomatoes, red peppers, asparagus, cabbage |
| Pyridoxine (B6) | Hormonal balance, maintains homocysteine levels | Poultry, white fish, milk, eggs, whole grains |
| Folic acid (B9) | Embryo development | Green leafy vegetables, brown rice, peas, oranges, bananas |
| Cobalamin (B12) | Metabolism, maintains homocysteine levels | Meat, fish, milk, cheese, eggs, yeast extract |
| Ascorbic acid (vitamin C) | Immune function, anti-oxidant | Fresh fruits especially citrus fruits and berries, green vegetables, peppers and tomatoes |
| Vitamin D | Calcium absorption | Green leafy vegetables, tinned salmon, tinned sardines, dairy products |
| Vitamin E | Anti-oxidant function | Vegetable oils, nuts and seeds |
| Zinc | Growth and tissue repair, immune function | Meat, milk, cheese, eggs, shellfish, wholegrain cereals, nuts and pulses |

| Nutrient | Role | Dietary Source |
|---|---|---|
| Selenium | Anti-oxidant function, thyroid hormone production, immune system and reproductive function | Brazil nuts, mushrooms, garlic fish, meat and eggs |
| Magnesium | Enzyme activation, cellular replication, parathyroid hormone secretion | Green leafy vegetables, nuts, quinoa, figs, seeds, brown rice |
| Iodine | Thyroid hormone production | Seafoods |
| Iron | Haemoglobin formation | Liver, red meat, pulses, nuts, eggs, dried fruits, poultry, fish, whole grains and dark green leafy vegetables |
| Carnitine | Energy production | Meat, fish, poultry |
| Calcium | Enzyme activity | Milk, cheese and other dairy products |
| Coenzyme Q10 | Anti-oxidant, energy metabolism | Ubiquitous but dietary sources may be insufficient to produce clinical effects |
| N-acetyl cysteine (NAC) | Anti-oxidant | Meat, fish, cruciferous vegetables |
| Resveratrol | Insulin resistance | Red grapes, red wine, peanuts |

## 24. Concluding remarks

The relationship between nutrition and reproduction is increasingly acknowledged (Homan *et al.* 2007; Sharma *et al.* 2013; Rooney and Domar 2014) and a number of studies have identified a range of dietary factors which may positively influence fertility in both males and females. Indeed, a fertility diet may be characterised by appropriate calorific intake; limiting consumption of animal proteins, trans-fatty acids and refined carbohydrates; increasing intake of vegetable proteins and monounsaturated fats; and reducing alcohol and caffeine. The extent to which individual macro- and micro-nutrients may influence conception and ART is still unclear as there is limited conclusive evidence and many studies demonstrate methodological shortcomings.

It is often difficult to isolate the benefits of an individual nutrient as most studies examine the effect of combined dietary factors and nutraceuticals on reproductive health, therefore making comparison problematic (Westphal *et al.* 2004; Dattilo *et al.* 2014; Ruder *et al.* 2014). However, it may be that it is the combinations that are effective as they may protect each other from oxidation and preclude the need for large doses of single nutrients, which may result in toxicity (Westphal *et al.* 2006).

The case for supplementation seems gender-specific. In the case of male infertility, the evidence suggests that anti-oxidant supplementation may positively impact on semen parameters and pregnancy rates (Showell *et al.* 2011) while the case for the use of anti-oxidants in female fertility is less convincing (Showell *et al.* 2013; Ruder *et al.* 2014). While no definitive link has yet been established for many nutrients, the consumption of a nutritious and well-balanced diet may be essential for improving fertility for both men and women in both natural and assisted reproduction. Given the financial, social and emotional burden faced by couples wishing to conceive, optimising dietary intake should be considered as a key strategy in an integrated clinical approach.

# References

Abed, A.A. (2013) 'Essence of some trace elements in seminal fluid and their role in infertility.' *International Journal of Chemical and Life Sciences 2*, 06, 1179–1184.

Agarwal, A., and Saleh, R.A. (2014) *Chapter Oxidative Stress and DNA Damage in Human Sperm: The Cleveland Clinic Story.* Available at www.researchgate.net/publication/259873884_Chapter_Oxidative_Stress_and_DNA_Damage_in_Human_Sperm_The_Cleveland_Clinic_Story, accessed on 27 May 2015.

Agarwal, A., Aponte-Mellado, A., Premkumar, B.J., Shaman, A., and Gupta, S. (2012) 'The effects of oxidative stress on female reproduction: a review.' *Reprod. Biol. Endocrinol. 10*, 1, 49.

Agarwal, A., Nallella, K.P., Allamaneni, S.S., and Said, T.M. (2004) 'Role of antioxidants in treatment of male infertility: an overview of the literature.' *Reproductive Biomedicine Online 8*, 6, 616–627.

Akmal, M., Qadri, J.Q., Al-Waili, N.S.,Thangal S., Haq, A., and Saloom, K.Y. (2006) 'Improvement in semen quality after oral supplementation of vitamin C.' *Journal of Medicinal Food 9*, 3, 440–442.

Aleyasin, A., Hosseini, M.A., Mahdavi, A., Safdarian, L. *et al.* (2011) 'Predictive value of the level of vitamin D in follicular fluid on the outcome of assisted reproductive technology.' *European Journal of Obstetrics & Gynaecology and Reproductive Biology 159*, 1, 132–137.

Al-Kunani, A.S., Knight, R., Haswell, S.J., Thompson, J.W., and Lindow, S.W. (2001) 'The selenium status of women with a history of recurrent miscarriage.' *British Journal of Obstetrics and Gynaecology 108*, 10, 1094–1097.

Al-Saleh, I., El-Doush, I., Grisellhi, B., and Coskun, S. (2010). The effect of caffeine consumption on the success rate of pregnancy as well various performance parameters of in-vitro fertilization treatment. *Medical Science Monitor Basic Research, 16*(12), CR598-CR605.

Anderson, K., Nisenblat, V., and Norman, R. (2010) 'Lifestyle factors in people seeking infertility treatment – a review.' *Australian and New Zealand Journal of Obstetrics and Gynaecology 50*, 1, 8–20.

Anifandis, G.M., Dafopoulos, K., Messini, C.I., Chalvatzas, N., *et al.* (2010) 'Prognostic value of follicular fluid 25-OH vitamin D and glucose levels in the IVF outcome.' *Reproductive Biology and Endocrinology 8*, 1, 91.

Attaman, J.A., Toth, T.L., Furtado, J., Campos, H., Hauser, R., and Chavarro, J.E. (2012) 'Dietary fat and semen quality among men attending a fertility clinic.' *Human Reproduction 27*, 5, 1466–1474.

Azizollahi, G., Azizollahi, S., Babaei, H., Kianinejad, M., Baneshi, M.R., and Nematollahi-mahani, S.N. (2013) 'Effects of supplement therapy on sperm parameters, protamine content and acrosomal integrity of varicocelectomized subjects.' *Journal of Assisted Reproduction and Genetics 30*, 4, 593–599.

Badawy, A., State, O., and Abdelgawad, S. (2007) 'N acetyl cysteine and clomiphene citrate for induction of ovulation in polycystic ovary syndrome: a cross-over trial.' *Acta Obstetricia et Gynecologica Scandinavica 86*, 2, 218–222.

Balercia, G., Regoli, F., Armeni, T., *et al.* (2005) 'Placebo-controlled double-blind randomized trial on the use of l-carnitine, l-acetylcarnitine, or combined l-carnitine and l-acetylcarnitine in men with idiopathic asthenozoospermia.' *Fertility Sterility 84*, 662–671.

Barr, S., Reeves, S., Sharp, K., and Jeanes, Y.M. (2013) 'An isocaloric low glycemic index diet improves insulin sensitivity in women with polycystic ovary syndrome.' *Journal of the Academy of Nutrition and Dietetics 113*, 11, 1523–1531.

Barrington, J.W., Lindsay, P., James, D., *et al.* (1996) 'Selenium deficiency and miscarriage: a possible link?' *Br. J. Obst. Gynaecol. 103*, 130–132.

Battaglia, C., Regnani, G., Marsella, T., Facchinetti, F., *et al.* (2002) 'Adjuvant L-arginine treatment in controlled ovarian hyperstimulation: a double-blind, randomized study.' *Human Reproduction 17*, 3, 659–665.

Battaglia, C., Salvatori, M., Maxia, N., Petraglia, F., Facchinetti, F., and Volpe, A. (1999) 'Adjuvant L-arginine treatment for in-vitro fertilization in poor responder patients.' *Human Reproduction 14*, 7, 1690–1697.

Bedwal, R.S., and Bahuguna, A. (1994) 'Zinc, copper and selenium in reproduction.' *Experientia 50*, 7, 626–640.

Bennett, M. (2001) 'Vitamin B12 deficiency, infertility and recurrent fetal loss.' *Journal of Reproductive Medicine 46*, 3, 209–212.

Bolúmar, F., Olsen, J., Rebagliato, M., and Bisanti, L. (1997) 'Caffeine intake and delayed conception: a European multicenter study on infertility and subfecundity.' *American Journal of Epidemiology 145*, 4, 324–334.

Bolúmar, F., Olsen, J., Rebagliato, M., Sáez-Lloret, I., and Bisanti, L. (2000) 'Body mass index and delayed conception: a European multicenter study on infertility and subfecundity.' *American Journal of Epidemiology 151*, 11, 1072–1079.

Bowen, D.J., and Beresford, S.A. (2002) 'Dietary interventions to prevent disease.' *Annual Review of Public Health 23*, 1, 255–286.

British Nutrition Foundation (BNF) (2014) *Nutrition Science.* Available at www.nutrition. org.uk, accessed on 27 May 2015.

Buhling, K.J., and Grajecki, D. (2013) 'The effect of micronutrient supplements on female fertility.' *Current Opinion in Obstetrics and Gynaecology 25*, 3, 173–180.

Caan, B., Quesenberry Jr, C.P., and Coates, A.O. (1998) 'Differences in fertility associated with caffeinated beverage consumption.' *American Journal of Public Health 88*, 2, 270–274.

Cardozo, E.R., Neff, L.M., Brocks, M.E., Ekpo, G.E., *et al.* (2012) 'Infertility patients' knowledge of the effects of obesity on reproductive health outcomes.' *American Journal of Obstetrics and Gynaecology 207*, 6, 509.e1–509.e10.

Centers for Disease Control and Prevention (2014) *Folic Acid.* Available at www.cdc.gov/ ncbddd/folicacid/index.html, accessed on 27 May 2015.

Chavarro, J.E., Ehrlich, S., Colaci, D.S., Wright, D.L., *et al.* (2012) 'Body mass index and short-term weight change in relation to treatment outcomes in women undergoing assisted reproduction.' *Fertility and Sterility 98*, 1, 109–116.

Chavarro, J.E., Mínguez-Alarcón, L., Mendiola, J., Cutillas-Tolín, A., López-Espín, J.J., and Torres-Cantero, A.M. (2014) 'Trans fatty acid intake is inversely related to total sperm count in young healthy men.' *Human Reproduction 29*, 3, 429–440.

Chavarro, J.E., Rich-Edwards, J.W., Rosner, B.A., and Willett, W.C. (2006) 'Iron intake and risk of ovulatory infertility.' *Obstetrics & Gynaecology 108*, 5, 1145–1152.

Chavarro, J.E., Rich-Edwards, J.W., Rosner, B.A., and Willett, W.C. (2007a) 'Dietary fatty acid intakes and the risk of ovulatory infertility.' *American Journal of Clinical Nutrition 85*, 1, 231–237.

Chavarro, J.E., Rich-Edwards, J.W., Rosner, B.A., and Willett, W.C. (2007b) 'Diet and lifestyle in the prevention of ovulatory disorder infertility.' *Obstetrics & Gynaecology 110*, 5, 1050–1058.

Chavarro, J.E., Rich-Edwards, J.W., Rosner, B.A., and Willett, W.C. (2008a) 'Protein intake and ovulatory infertility.' *American Journal of Obstetrics and Gynaecology 198*, 2, 210-e1.

Chavarro, J.E., Rich-Edwards, J.W., Rosner, B.A., and Willett, W.C. (2008b) 'Use of multivitamins, intake of B vitamins, and risk of ovulatory infertility.' *Fertility and Sterility 89*, 3, 668–676.

Chavarro, J.E., Rich-Edwards, J.W., Rosner, B.A., and Willett, W.C. (2009a) 'A prospective study of dietary carbohydrate quantity and quality in relation to risk of ovulatory infertility.' *European Journal of Clinical Nutrition 63*, 1, 78–86.

Chavarro, J.E., Rich-Edwards, J.W., Rosner, B.A., and Willett, W.C. (2009b) 'Caffeinated and alcoholic beverage intake in relation to ovulatory disorder infertility.' *Epidemiology (Cambridge, Mass.) 20*, 3, 374.

Chavarro, J.E., Toth, T.L., Wright, D.L., Meeker, J.D., and Hauser, R. (2010) 'Body mass index in relation to semen quality, sperm DNA integrity, and serum reproductive hormone levels among men attending an infertility clinic.' *Fertility and Sterility 93*,7, 2222–2231.

Ciftci, H., Verit, A., Savas, M., Yeni, E., and Erel, O. (2009) 'Effects of N-acetylcysteine on semen parameters and oxidative/antioxidant status.' *Urology 74*, 1, 73–76.

Curtis, M., Abelman, S., Schulkin, J., Williams, J.L., and Fassett, E.M. (2006) 'Do we practice what we preach? A review of actual clinical practice with regards to preconception care guidelines.' *Maternal and Child Health Journal 10*, 1, 53–58.

Dattilo, M., Cornet, D., Amar, E., Cohen, M., and Menezo, Y. (2014) 'The importance of the one carbon cycle nutritional support in human male fertility: a preliminary clinical report.' *Reproductive Biology and Endocrinology 12*, 71.

Douglas, C.C., Gower, B.A., Darnell, B.E., Ovalle, F., Oster, R.A., and Azziz, R. (2006) 'Role of diet in the treatment of polycystic ovary syndrome.' *Fertility and Sterility 85*, 3, 679–688.

Eggert, J., Theobald, H., and Engfeldt, P. (2004) 'Effects of alcohol consumption on female fertility during an 18-year period.' *Fertility and Sterility 81*, 2, 379–383.

Eldar-Geva, T., Lowe, P.J.M., MacLachlan, V., Rombauts, L., and Healy, D.L. (1998) 'Different influence of incongruent follicular development on in vitro fertilization–embryo transfer and gamete intrafallopian transfer pregnancy rates.' *Fertility and Sterility 70*, 1039–1043.

Fedorcsak, P., Dale, P.O., Storeng, R., Ertzeid, G., *et al.* (2004) 'Impact of overweight and underweight on assisted reproduction treatment.' *Human Reproduction 19*, 11, 2523–2528.

Fraga, C.G., Motchnik, P.A., Shigenaga, M.K., Helbock, H.J., Jacob, R.A., and Ames, B.N. (1991) 'Ascorbic acid protects against endogenous oxidative DNA damage in human sperm.' *Proceedings of the National Academy of Sciences 88*, 24, 11003–11006.

Frey, K.A., and Files, J. A. (2006) 'Preconception healthcare: what women know and believe.' *Maternal and Child Health Journal 10*, 1, 73–77.

Gardiner, P.M., Nelson, L., Shellhaas, C.S., Dunlop, A.L., *et al.* (2008) 'The clinical content of preconception care: nutrition and dietary supplements.' *American Journal of Obstetrics and Gynaecology 199*, 6, S345–S356.

Gaur, D.S., Talekar, M.S., and Pathak, V.P. (2010) 'Alcohol intake and cigarette smoking: impact of two major lifestyle factors on male fertility.' *Indian Journal of Pathology and Microbiology 53*, 1, 35–40.

Goldenberg, R.L., Tamura, T., Neggers, Y., Copper, R.L., *et al.* (1995) 'The effect of zinc supplementation on pregnancy outcome.' *JAMA 274*, 6, 463–468.

Gower, B.A., Chandler-Laney, P.C., Ovalle, F., Goree, L.L., *et al.* (2013) 'Favourable metabolic effects of a eucaloric lower carbohydrate diet in women with PCOS.' *Clinical Endocrinology 79*, 4, 550–557.

Greco, E., Iacobelli, M., Rienzi, L., Ubaldi, F., Ferrero, S., and Tesarik, J. (2005) 'Reduction of the incidence of sperm DNA fragmentation by oral antioxidant treatment.' *Journal of Andrology 26*, 3, 349–353.

Griesinger, G., Franke, K., Kinast, C., Kutzelnigg, A., *et al.* (2002) 'Ascorbic acid supplement during luteal phase in IVF.' *Journal of Assisted Reproduction and Genetics 19*, 4, 164–168.

Hakim, R.B., Gray, R.H., and Zacur, H. (1998) 'Alcohol and caffeine consumption and decreased fertility.' *Fertility and Sterility 70*, 4, 632–637.

Hammiche, F., Laven, J.S.E., van Mil, N., de Cock, M., *et al.* (2011) 'Tailored preconception dietary and lifestyle counselling in a tertiary outpatient clinic in the Netherlands.' *Human Reproduction 26*, 9, 2432–2441.

Hassan, M.A.M., and Killick, S.R. (2004) 'Negative lifestyle is associated with a significant reduction in fecundity.' *Fertility and Sterility 81*, 2, 384.

Hatch, E.E., Wise, L.A., Mikkelsen, E.M., Christensen, T., *et al.* (2012) 'Caffeinated beverage and soda consumption and time to pregnancy.' *Epidemiology (Cambridge, Mass.) 23*, 3, 393.

Hawkes, W.C., and Turek, P.J. (2001) 'Effects of dietary selenium on sperm motility in healthy men.' *Journal of Andrology 22*, 5, 764–772.

Hawkins, L.K., Rossi, B.V., Correia, K.F., Lipskind, S.T., Hornstein, M.D., and Missmer, S.A. (2014) 'Perceptions among infertile couples of lifestyle behaviors and in vitro fertilization (IVF) success.' *Journal of Assisted Reproduction and Genetics 31*, 3, 255–260.

Health and Human Services (2010) *Dietary Guidelines for Americans*. Available at www. health.gov/dietaryguidelines/dga2010/dietaryguidelines2010.pdf, accessed on 27 May 2015.

Homan, G.F., Davies, M., and Norman, R. (2007) 'The impact of lifestyle factors on reproductive performance in the general population and those undergoing infertility treatment: a review.' *Human Reproduction Update 13*, 3, 209–223.

Howard, J., Davies, S., and Hunnisett, A. (1994) 'Red cell magnesium and glutathione peroxidase in infertile women – effects of oral supplementation with magnesium and selenium.' *Magnesium Research: Official Organ of the International Society for the Development of Research on Magnesium 7*, 1, 49–57.

Huang, H., Karl, R., Hansen, K.R., Factor-Litvak, P., *et al.* (2012) National Institute of Child Health and Human Development Cooperative Reproductive Medicine Network. 'Predictors of pregnancy and live birth after insemination in couples with unexplained or male-factor infertility.' *Fertility and Sterility 97*, 4, 959–967.e5.

Human Fertilisation and Embryology Authority (HFEA) (2010) *Improve Your Chances – Lifestyle and Health*. Available at www.hfea.gov.uk/getting-pregnant.html, accessed on 27 May 2015.

Imhof, M., Lackner, J., Lipovac, M., Chedraui, P., and Riedl, C. (2012) 'Improvement of sperm quality after micronutrient supplementation.' *e-SPEN Journal 7*, 1, e50–e53.

Infertility Network (2014) *Infertility Network UK Factsheets*. Available at www. infertilitynetworkuk.com/information/factsheets, accessed on 27 May 2015.

Jensen, M.B., Bjerrum, P.J., Jessen, T.E., Nielsen, J.E., Joensen, U.N., Olesen, I.A., and Jørgensen, N. (2011). Vitamin D is positively associated with sperm motility and increases intracellular calcium in human spermatozoa. *Human reproduction 26*, 6, 1307–1317.

Jensen, T.K., Andersson, A.M., Jørgensen, N., Andersen, A.G., Carlsen, E., and Skakkebaek, N.E. (2004) 'Body mass index in relation to semen quality and reproductive hormones among 1558 Danish men.' *Fertility and Sterility 82*, 4, 863–870.

Jensen, T.K., Gottschau, M., Madsen, J.O.B., Andersson, A.M., *et al.* (2014) 'Habitual alcohol consumption associated with reduced semen quality and changes in reproductive hormones; a cross-sectional study among 1221 young Danish men.' *British Medical Journal Open 4*, 9, e005462.

Jensen, T.K., Hjollund, N.H.I., Henriksen, T.B., Scheike, T., *et al.* (1998) 'Does moderate alcohol consumption affect fertility? Follow up study among couples planning first pregnancy.' *British Medical Journal 317*, 7157, 505–510.

Jokela, M., Elovainio, M., and Kivimäki, M. (2008) 'Lower fertility associated with obesity and underweight: the US National Longitudinal Survey of Youth.' *American Journal of Clinical Nutrition 88*, 4, 886–893.

Jones, D.S. (2005) *Textbook of Functional Medicine.* Gig Harbor, WA: Institute of Functional Medicine.

Jungheim, E.S., Macones, G.A., Odem, R.R., Patterson, B.W., and Moley, K.H. (2011) 'Elevated serum alpha-linolenic acid levels are associated with decreased chance of pregnancy after in vitro fertilization.' *Fertility and Sterility 96*, 4, 880–883.

Jungheim, E.S., Frolova, A I., Jiang, H., and Riley, J.K. (2013) 'Relationship between serum polyunsaturated fatty acids and pregnancy in women undergoing in vitro fertilization'. *Journal of Clinical Endocrinology and Metabolism*, 98, 8, E1364–E1368.

Keskes-Ammar, L., Feki-Chakroun, N., Rebai, T., Sahnoun, Z., *et al.* (2003) 'Sperm oxidative stress and the effect of an oral vitamin E and selenium supplement on semen quality in infertile men.' *Systems Biology in Reproductive Medicine 49*, 2, 83–94.

Klonoff-Cohen, H., Bleha, J., and Lam-Kruglick, P. (2002) 'A prospective study of the effects of female and male caffeine consumption on the reproductive endpoints of IVF and gamete intra-Fallopian transfer.' *Human Reproduction 17*, 7, 1746–1754.

Klonoff-Cohen, H., Lam-Kruglick, P., and Gonzalez, C. (2003) 'Effects of maternal and paternal alcohol consumption on the success rates of in vitro fertilization and gamete intrafallopian transfer.' *Fertility and Sterility 79*, 330–339.

Kong, X.X., Fu, Y.C., Xu, J.J., Zhuang, X.L., Chen, Z.G., and Luo, L.L. (2011) 'Resveratrol, an effective regulator of ovarian development and oocyte apoptosis.' *Journal of Endocrinological Investigation 34*, 11, e374–e381.

Lenzi, A., Picardo, M., Gandini, L., Lombardo, F., *et al.* (1994) 'Glutathione treatment of dyspermia: effect on the lipoperoxidation process.' *Human Reproduction 9*, 11, 2044–2050.

Lenzi, A., Sgro, P., Salacone, P., Paoli, D., *et al.* (2004) 'A placebo-controlled double-blind randomized trial of the use of combined l-carnitine and l-acetyl-carnitine treatment in men with asthenozoospermia.' *Fertility and Sterility 81*, 6, 1578–1584.

Lerchbaum, E., and Obermayer-Pietsch, B. (2012) 'Mechanisms in endocrinology: vitamin D and fertility: a systematic review.' *European Journal of Endocrinology 166*, 5, 765–778.

Ley, S.H., Hanley, A.J., Sermer, M., Zinman, B., and O'Connor, D.L. (2013) 'Lower dietary vitamin E intake during the second trimester is associated with insulin resistance and hyperglycemia later in pregnancy.' *European Journal of Clinical Nutrition 67*, 11, 1154–1156.

Li, N., Liu, E., Guo, J., Pan, L., *et al.* (2013) 'Maternal prepregnancy body mass index and gestational weight gain on pregnancy outcomes.' *PLoS ONE 8*, 12, e82310.

Lim, S.S., Noakes, M., and Norman, R.J. (2007) 'Dietary effects on fertility treatment and pregnancy outcomes.' *Current Opinion in Endocrinology, Diabetes and Obesity 14*, 6, 465–469.

Liu, J., Liu, M., Ye, X., Liu, K., *et al.* (2012) 'Delay in oocyte aging in mice by the antioxidant N-acetyl-L-cysteine (NAC).' *Human Reproduction 27*, 5, 1411–1420.

Liu, M., Yin, Y., Ye, X., Zeng, M., *et al.* (2013) 'Resveratrol protects against age-associated infertility in mice.' *Human Reproduction 28*, 3, 707–717.

MacDonald, A.A., Herbison, G.P., Showell, M., and Farquhar, C.M. (2010) 'The impact of body mass index on semen parameters and reproductive hormones in human males: a systematic review with meta-analysis.' *Human Reproduction Update 16*, 3, 293–311.

Maheshwari, A., Stofberg, L., and Bhattacharya, S. (2007) 'Effect of overweight and obesity on assisted reproductive technology – a systematic review.' *Human Reproduction Update 13*, 5, 433–444.

Makrides, M., and Crowther, C. A. (2014) 'Magnesium supplementation in pregnancy.' *Cochrane Database of Systematic Reviews 4*, CD000937.

Mancini, A., and Balercia, G. (2011) 'Coenzyme Q10 in male infertility: physiopathology and therapy.' *Biofactors 37*, 5, 374–380.

Mann, J., and Truswell, A.S. (2007) *Essentials of Human Nutrition*. Oxford: Oxford University Press.

Mayo Clinic (2015) *Nutrition and Healthy Eating*. Available at www.mayoclinic.org/healthy-living/nutrition-and-healthy-eating/in-depth/caffeine/art-20049372, accessed on 27 May 2015.

Mendiola, J., Torres-Cantero, A.M., Moreno-Grau, J.M., Ten, J., *et al.* (2009) 'Food intake and its relationship with semen quality: a case-control study.' *Fertility and Sterility 91*, 3, 812–818.

Mendiola, J., Torres-Cantero, A.M., Vioque, J., Moreno-Grau, J.M., *et al.* (2010) 'A low intake of antioxidant nutrients is associated with poor semen quality in patients attending fertility clinics.' *Fertility and Sterility 93*, 4, 1128–1133.

Mínguez-Alarcón, L., Mendiola, J., López-Espín, J. J., Sarabia-Cos, L., *et al.* (2012) 'Dietary intake of antioxidant nutrients is associated with semen quality in young university students.' *Human Reproduction 27*, 9, 2807–2814.

Mistry, H.D., Pipkin, F.B., Redman, C.W., and Poston, L. (2012) 'Selenium in reproductive health.' *American Journal of Obstetrics and Gynaecology 206*, 1, 21–30.

Moragianni, V.A., Jones, S.M.L., and Ryley, D.A. (2012) 'The effect of body mass index on the outcomes of first assisted reproductive technology cycles.' *Fertility and Sterility 98*, 1, 102–108.

Moslemi, M.K., and Tavanbakhsh, S. (2011) 'Selenium–vitamin E supplementation in infertile men: effects on semen parameters and pregnancy rate.' *International Journal of General Medicine 4*, 99.

Munire, M., Shimizu, Y., Sakata, Y., Minaguchi, R., and Aso, T. (2004) 'Impaired hyperactivation of human sperm in patients with infertility.' *Journal of Medical and Dental Sciences 51*, 1, 99–104.

Murphy, L.E., Mills, J.L., Molloy, A.M., Qian, C., *et al.* (2011) 'Folate and vitamin B12 in idiopathic male infertility.' *Asian Journal of Andrology 13*, 6, 856.

Murray, M.T. (1996) *Encyclopaedia of Nutritional Supplements*. New York: Three Rivers Press.

Murray, M.T., and Pizzorno J. (2005, reprinted 2008 and 2010) *The Encyclopaedia of Healing Foods*. London: Piatkus.

Murto, T., Skoog Svanberg, A., Yngve, A., Nilsson, T.K., *et al.* (2014) 'Folic acid supplementation and IVF pregnancy outcome in women with unexplained infertility.' *Reproductive Biomedicine Online 28*, 6, 766–772.

Nadjarzadeh, A., Sadeghi, M.R., Amirjannati, N., Vafa, M.R., *et al.* (2011) 'Coenzyme Q10 improves seminal oxidative defense but does not affect on semen parameters in idiopathic oligoasthenoteratozoospermia: a randomized double-blind, placebo controlled trial.' *Journal of Endocrinological Investigation 34*, 8, e224–e228.

Negro, R., Greco, G., Mangieri, T., Pezzarossa, A., Dazzi, D., and Hassan, H. (2007) 'The influence of selenium supplementation on postpartum thyroid status in pregnant women with thyroid peroxidase autoantibodies.' *Journal of Clinical Endocrinology & Metabolism 92*, 4, 1263–1268.

NHS (2014a) *What Should My Daily Intake of Calories Be?* Available at www.nhs.uk/chq/pages/1126.aspx?categoryid=51, accessed on 27 May 2015.

NHS (2014b) *Infertility*. Available at www.nhs.uk/conditions/infertility, accessed on 27 May 2015.

NICE (2012) *Fertility: Assessment and Treatment for People with Fertility Problems.* Update May 2012. Available at www.nice.org.uk/guidance/cg156/documents/fertility-update-nice-version2, accessed on 27 May 2015.

Norman, R.J., Homan, G., Moran, L., and Noakes, M. (2006) 'Lifestyle choices, diet, and insulin sensitizers in polycystic ovary syndrome.' *Endocrine 30*, 1, 35–43.

Nutritiondata (2015) *Nutrition Search Tool.* Available at http://nutritiondata.self.com/tools/nutrient-search, accessed on 27 May 2015.

Okorodudu, D.O., Jumean, M.F., Montori, V.M., Romero-Corral, A., *et al.* (2010) 'Diagnostic performance of body mass index to identify obesity as defined by body adiposity: a systematic review and meta-analysis.' *International Journal of Obesity 34*, 5, 791–799.

Ozkan, S., Jindal, S., Greenseid, K., Shu, J., *et al.* (2010) 'Replete vitamin D stores predict reproductive success following in vitro fertilization.' *Fertility and Sterility 94*, 4, 1314–1319.

Pathak, P., and Kapil, U. (2004) 'Role of trace elements zinc, copper and magnesium during pregnancy and its outcome.' *Indian Journal of Pediatrics 71*, 11, 1003–1005.

Pinborg, A., Gaarslev, C., Hougaard, C.O., Andersen, A.N., *et al.* (2011) 'Influence of female bodyweight on IVF outcome: a longitudinal multicentre cohort study of 487 infertile couples.' *Reproductive Biomedicine Online 23*, 4, 490–499.

Pizzorno Jr, J.E., Murray, M.T., and Joiner-Bey, H. (2008) *The Clinician's Handbook of Natural Medicine.* Oxford: Elsevier Health Sciences.

Polak de Fried, E., Bossi, N.M., Notrica, J.A., and Vazquez Levin, M.H. (2013) 'Vitamin-D treatment does not improve pregnancy rates in patients undergoing ART: a prospective, randomized, double-blind placebo controlled trial.' *Fertility and Sterility 100 (Suppl.)*, S493–S494.

Poppe, K., Glinoer, D., Tournaye, H., Devroey, P., *et al.* (2003) 'Assisted reproduction and thyroid autoimmunity: an unfortunate combination?' *Journal of Clinical Endocrinology & Metabolism 88*, 9, 4149–4152.

Poppe, K., Velkeniers, B., and Glinoer, D. (2008) 'The role of thyroid autoimmunity in fertility and pregnancy.' *Nature Clinical Practice Endocrinology & Metabolism 4*, 7, 394–405.

Porter, M., and Bhattacharya, S. (2008) 'Helping themselves to get pregnant: a qualitative longitudinal study on the information-seeking behaviour of infertile couples.' *Human Reproduction 23*, 3, 567–567.

Poston, L., Igosheva, N., Mistry, H.D., Seed, P.T., *et al.* (2011) 'Role of oxidative stress and antioxidant supplementation in pregnancy disorders.' *American Journal of Clinical Nutrition 94*, 6 Suppl., 1980S–1985S.

Prummel, M.F., and Wiersinga, W.M. (2004) 'Thyroid autoimmunity and miscarriage.' *European Journal of Endocrinology 150*, 6, 751–755.

Reilly, J.J., Methven, E., McDowell, Z.C., Hacking, B., *et al.* (2003) 'Health consequences of obesity.' *Archives of Disease in Childhood 88*, 9, 748–752.

Rizk, A.Y., Bedaiwy, M.A., and Al-Inany, H.G. (2005) 'N-acetyl-cysteine is a novel adjuvant to clomiphene citrate in clomiphene citrate-resistant patients with polycystic ovary syndrome.' *Fertility and Sterility 83*, 2, 367–370.

Rondanelli, M., Perna, S., Faliva, M., Monteferrario, F., Repaci, E., and Allieri, F. (2014) 'Focus on metabolic and nutritional correlates of polycystic ovary syndrome and update on nutritional management of these critical phenomena.' *Arch. Gynaecol. Obstet. 290*, 6, 1079–1092.

Ronnenberg, A.G., Venners, S.A., Xu, X., Chen, C., *et al.* (2007) 'Preconception B-vitamin and homocysteine status, conception, and early pregnancy loss.' *American Journal of Epidemiology 166*, 3, 304–312.

Rooney, K.L., and Domar, A.D. (2014) 'The impact of lifestyle behaviors on infertility treatment outcome. *Current Opinion in Obstetrics and Gynaecology 26*, 3, 181–185.

Ross, C., Morriss, A., Khairy, M., Khalaf, Y., *et al.* (2010) 'A systematic review of the effect of oral antioxidants on male infertility.' *Reproductive Biomedicine Online 20*, 6, 711–723.

Ruder, E.H., Hartman, T.J., Reindollar, R.H., and Goldman, M.B. (2014) 'Female dietary antioxidant intake and time to pregnancy among couples treated for unexplained infertility.' *Fertility and Sterility 101*, 3, 759–766.

Safarinejad, M.R. (2012) 'The effect of coenzyme Q10 supplementation on partner pregnancy rate in infertile men with idiopathic oligoasthenoteratozoospermia: an open-label prospective study.' *International Urology and Nephrology 44*, 3, 689–700.

Safarinejad, M.R., and Safarinejad, S. (2009) 'Efficacy of selenium and/or N-acetyl-cysteine for improving semen parameters in infertile men: a double-blind, placebo controlled, randomized study.' *Journal of Urology 181*, 2, 741–751.

Saldeen, P., and Saldeen, T. (2004) 'Women and omega-3 fatty acids.' *Obstetrical & Gynaecological Survey 59*, 10, 722–730.

Santti, R., Mäkelä, S., Strauss, L., Kokman, J., and Kostian, M.L. (1998) 'Phytoestrogens: potential endocrine disruptors in males.' *Toxicol. Ind. Health 14*, 223–237.

Scibona, M., Meschini, P., Capparelli, S., Pecori, C., Rossi, P., and Menchini, F. G. (1994) '[L-arginine and male infertility.]' *Minerva urologica e nefrologica [The Italian Journal of Urology and Nephrology] 46*, 4, 251–253.

Scott, R., MacPherson, A., Yates, R.W.S., Hussain, B., and Dixon, J. (1998) 'The effect of oral selenium supplementation on human sperm motility.' *British Journal of Urology 82*, 1, 76–80.

Sekhon, L., Gupta, S., Kim, Y., and Agarwal, A. (2010) 'Female infertility and antioxidants.' *Current Women's Health Reviews 6*, 2, 84–95.

Shah, D.K., Missmer, S.A., Berry, K.F., Racowsky, C., and Ginsburg, E.S. (2011) 'Effect of obesity on oocyte and embryo quality in women undergoing in vitro fertilization.' *Obstetrics & Gynaecology 118*, 1, 63–70.

Sharma, R., Biedenharn, K.R., Fedor, J.M., and Agarwal, A. (2013) 'Lifestyle factors and reproductive health: taking control of your fertility.' *Reprod. Biol. Endocrinol. 11*, 66, 1–15.

Showell, M.G., Brown, J., Clarke, J., and Hart, R.J. (2013) 'Antioxidants for female subfertility.' *Cochrane Database of Systematic Reviews 8*, CD007807.

Showell, M.G., Brown, J., Yazdani, A., Stankiewicz, M.T., and Hart, R.J. (2011) 'Antioxidants for male subfertility.' *Cochrane Database of Systematic Reviews 1*, CD007411.

Sigman, M., Glass, S., Campagnone, J., and Pryor, J.L. (2006) 'Carnitine for the treatment of idiopathic asthenospermia: a randomized, double-blind, placebo-controlled trial.' *Fertility and Sterility 85*, 5, 1409–1414.

Swan, S.H., Liu, F., Overstreet, J.W., Brazil, C., and Skakkebaek, N.E. (2007) 'Semen quality of fertile US males in relation to their mothers' beef consumption during pregnancy.' *Hum. Reprod. 22*, 1497–1502.

Szymański, W., and Kazdepka-Ziemińska, A. (2003) '[Effect of homocysteine concentration in follicular fluid on a degree of oocyte maturity.]' *Ginekologia polska 74*, 10, 1392–1396.

Takasaki, A., Tamura, I., Kizuka, F., Lee, L., Maekawa, R., Asada, H., *et al.* (2011). Luteal blood flow in patients undergoing GnRH agonist long protocol. *J Ovarian Res, 4*(2). Available online at www.biomedcentral.com/content/pdf/1757-2215-4-2.pdf, accessed 17 September 2015.

Taylor, R., and Marsden, P. J. (2000) 'Insulin sensitivity and fertility.' *Human Fertility 3*, 1, 65–69.

Tough, S., Tofflemire, K., Clarke, M., and Newburn-Cook, C. (2006) 'Do women change their drinking behaviours while trying to conceive? An opportunity for preconception counselling.' *Clinical Medicine & Research 4*, 2, 97–105.

Tremblay, F., Lavigne, C., Jacques, H., and Marette, A. (2007) Role of dietary proteins and amino acids in the pathogenesis of insulin resistance. *Annu. Rev. Nutr. 27*, 293–310.

Tremellen, K. (2008) 'Oxidative stress and male infertility – a clinical perspective.' *Human Reproduction Update 14*, 3, 243–258.

Tremellen, K., Miari, G., Froiland, D., and Thompson, J. (2007) 'A randomised control trial examining the effect of an antioxidant (Menevit) on pregnancy outcome during IVF-ICSI treatment.' *Aust. N.Z. J. Obstet. Gynaecol. 47*, 3, 216–221.

Turi, A., Giannubilo, S.R., Brugè, F., Principi, F., *et al.* (2012) 'Coenzyme Q10 content in follicular fluid and its relationship with oocyte fertilization and embryo grading.' *Archives of Gynaecology and Obstetrics 285*, 4, 1173–1176.

Twigt, J.M., Bolhuis, M.E.C., Steegers, E.A.P., Hammiche, F., *et al.* (2012) 'The preconception diet is associated with the chance of ongoing pregnancy in women undergoing IVF/ICSI treatment.' *Human Reproduction 27*, 8, 2526–2531.

Vujkovic, M., de Vries, J.H., Lindemans, J., Macklon, N.S., *et al.* (2010) 'The preconception Mediterranean dietary pattern in couples undergoing in vitro fertilization/intracytoplasmic sperm injection treatment increases the chance of pregnancy.' *Fertility and Sterility 94*, 6, 2096–2101.

Wang, J.X., Davies, M., and Norman, R.J. (2002) 'Obesity increases the risk of spontaneous abortion during infertility treatment.' *Obesity Research 10*, 6, 551–554.

Westphal, L.M., Polan, M.L., and Trant, A.S. (2006) 'Double-blind, placebo-controlled study of FertilityBlend®: a nutritional supplement for improving fertility in women.' *Clinical and Experimental Obstetrics and Gynaecology 33*, 4, 205.

Westphal, L.M., Polan, M.L., Trant, A.S., and Mooney, S.B. (2004) 'A nutritional supplement for improving fertility in women.' *J. Reprod. Med. 49*, 4, 289–293.

WHO (2015) *Obesity and Overweight.* Available at www.who.int/mediacentre/factsheets/fs311/en, accessed on 27 May 2015.

Winter, E., Wang, J., Davies, M.J., and Norman, R. (2002) 'Early pregnancy loss following assisted reproductive technology treatment.' *Hum. Reprod. 17*, 3220–3223.

Wong, W.Y., Merkus, H.M., Thomas, C.M., Menkveld, R., Zielhuis, G.A., and Steegers-Theunissen, R.P. (2002) 'Effects of folic acid and zinc sulfate on male factor subfertility: a double-blind, randomized, placebo-controlled trial.' *Fertility and Sterility 77*, 3, 491–498.

Wright, C., Milne, S., and Leeson, H. (2014) 'Sperm DNA damage caused by oxidative stress: modifiable clinical, lifestyle and nutritional factors in male infertility.' *Reproductive Biomedicine Online 28*, 6, 684–703.

Zhou, X., Liu, F., and Zhai, S. (2007) 'Effect of L-carnitine and/or L-acetyl-carnitine in nutrition treatment for male infertility: a systematic.' *Asia Pac. J. Clin. Nutr. 16*, 1, 383–390.

Zini, A., San Gabriel, M., and Baazeem, A. (2009) 'Antioxidants and sperm DNA damage: a clinical perspective.' *Journal of Assisted Reproduction and Genetics 26*, 8, 427–432.

# Chapter 11

# Lifestyle and Nutritional Factors Affecting Male and Female Fertility

*Susan Bedford BSc (Hons), PGCE, MSc (Nut. Th), mBANT, CNHC*

## 1. Introduction

This chapter reviews the evidence surrounding key lifestyle factors and their effects on both genders. Lifestyle factors are thought to influence fertility in both men and women (Grodstein, Goldman and Cramer 1994; Mello 1988). Medical history, age, consultant expertise and experience, stress levels, alcohol and diet are all recognised as factors affecting fertility and the success of assisted reproduction (Templeton, Morris and Parslow 1996). It is thought that this may be because some lifestyle factors may induce changes in genetic material affecting the gametes and thus impact upon the embryo's development if conception occurs (Nafee *et al.* 2008; Steeghers Theunissen 2003). Other factors such as smoking and endocrine disruptors are also thought to impact on fertility (Pasqulotto 2004). Endocrine disruptors, such as environmental oestrogens, are chemicals that are able to affect the way in which hormones work (Rogan and Chen 2005). These will be explored in more depth later in this chapter. Although there is limited data available, exercise is also believed to have an impact on fertility in certain groups of people. The findings of these studies are considered below.

## 2. Exercise

Exercise is of great importance to humans for a variety of reasons, including prevention of diseases, improving stamina, improving mood, reducing stress, strengthening and toning, helping to control weight and assisting sleep (Wilmore and Knuttgen 2003). However, the relationship between exercise and fertility (also success at assisted reproduction) appears not to be straightforward. Exercise is important for fertility as it helps to balance blood sugar levels and regulate hormones and thus ovulation (Rich-Edwards *et al.* 2002). It is also important in relation to BMI as exercise helps to maintain a healthy weight. A BMI below 18.5 is considered to be underweight, whereas a BMI over 25 is considered to be overweight, and both of these extremes may have consequences for fertility (Health Canada 2009).

### 2.1 Exercise in women

In a study conducted by Rich-Edwards *et al.* in 2002, it was discovered that, among women, both being underweight and overweight affected fertility as did the level and the type of exercise. The study also reported that a higher rate of ovulatory infertility can be linked to being overweight and a sedentary lifestyle than to overexertion and being underweight. With regard to a low BMI, from the current research that is available it is known that the fertility of top female athletes can be affected by strenuous exercise if they have low body fat, or a low BMI to begin with. It is thought that it may negatively impact on ovulation and may also affect implantation (De Souza *et al.* 2003; Frisch 2002, Rich-Edwards *et al.* 2002; Warren and Perlroth 2001). In a study involving 3628 Danish women aged 18–40 conducted by Wise *et al.* in 2012 that investigated the association between physical activity and time to achieve a pregnancy, it was discovered that in normal-weight women, higher levels of strenuous exercise (defined as swimming, running, fast cycling or gymnastics for more than five hours per week) appeared to delay conception; however, moderate exercise led to a faster conception rate in all categories of women. It was also concluded in the findings of this study that exercise of any kind may improve fertility among overweight and obese women.

A study conducted in the United States (Morris *et al.* 2006) investigated the effect of exercise on IVF success. The researchers reported that women who exercise regularly prior to IVF may negatively affect their chance of success. It was also discovered that those women who exercised for between one and nine years for four hours or more per week before beginning the IVF process had the least success (Morris *et al.* 2006). In this study, 2232 patients were prospectively enrolled between 1994 and 2003. These patients were about to begin their first IVF treatment cycle in three clinics in the United States. Researchers examined end points of fertility treatment including healthy live birth, cancellation of cycles, fertilisation and implantation failures and miscarriage. A questionnaire was completed prior to starting IVF treatment. Participants were asked about exercise history including the type, frequency and duration of exercise as well as medical history, environmental and lifestyle factors.

The researchers discovered that women who exercised for four or more hours a week were 40 per cent less likely to have been successful at IVF (OR=0.6; CI=0.4–0.8) and the chance of having the IVF cycle cancelled (OR=2.8; CI=1.5–5.3) than women who did not exercise at all. It is important to bear in mind that the misreporting of exercise history could be a limiting factor in terms of the findings generated by this study. Also, it was difficult to quantify type, intensity, frequency and duration of exercise, so the authors were unable to study the differences between two two-hour exercise sessions per week vs. four one-hour sessions or eight 30-minute sessions. The study also indicated that the type of exercise undertaken can have an impact on IVF success, with exercise such as walking only having no effect, to strenuous exercise having a marked negative impact on success (Morris *et al.* 2006).

Obviously, further research is needed into this area to ascertain why exercise, and different types of exercise, can have such a marked effect on IVF success rates (Hofman, Davies and Norman 2007; Morris *et al.* 2006). Possible mechanisms include the loss of body fat and subsequent leanness, which may interfere with the hypothalamus's release of gonadotrophin-releasing hormone (GnRH), which results in a hypo-oestrogenic state (Morris *et al.* 2006).

## 2.2 Exercise in men

A healthy amount of exercise in men may be beneficial to fertility (Sharma *et al.* 2013). In a study conducted by Vaamonde *et al.* in 2009 it was noted that men who are physically active, exercising at least three times per week for one hour, typically scored higher in almost all sperm parameters in comparison with men who engaged in rigorous and more frequent exercise. It was discovered that in men who were moderately physically active, sperm morphology was significantly better in comparison with men who played competitive sport or were elite athletes. The other factors considered in this study were sperm concentration, number and velocity, all of which showed a similar trend but to a lesser degree (Vaamonde *et al.* 2009). Endurance exercise in men seems to affect male reproductive hormonal profiles, such as basal and total testosterone concentrations without concurrent LH elevations. Men displaying these symptoms have been considered as exhibiting the 'exercise-hypogonadal male condition' (Hackney 2008). Again, this area requires further research (Hackney 2008). In a study conducted on rats it was concluded that exercise combined with diet in obese male rats showed there to be an increase to both sperm morphology and sperm motility, along with a decrease in reactive oxygen species (ROS) and sperm DNA damage (Palmer *et al.* 2012).

Overall, exercise is important for good health; and normal exercise does not seem to negatively affect fertility in most cases. It may also help to alleviate stress and assist in maintaining a healthy weight, both of which are important factors when trying to conceive, either naturally or through ART. Research suggests that exercise which is too vigorous or which causes a low BMI in females may well affect ovulation and thus fertility. If a person is overweight or obese, exercise may in fact improve fertility due to weight loss improving the regulation of blood sugar levels and insulin, thus lowering the level of testosterone in the blood and improving menstrual regularity and ovulation (Chavarro, Willett and Skerrett 2009). Exercise is also thought to help those with polycystic ovary syndrome (PCOS) for this reason along with others (see Box 11.1).

## BOX 11.1 POSSIBLE BENEFITS OF EXERCISE FOR ··· THOSE WITH PCOS (HARRISON *ET AL.* 2011) ················

▶ Improved insulin sensitivity

▶ Improved frequency of ovulation

▶ Lowering of cholesterol levels

▶ Improved body composition.

## 3. Smoking

Cigarettes contain more than seventy carcinogenic compounds and release over four thousand chemicals when burnt (US Environmental Protection Agency 1993). Smoking can affect fertility in males and females, so that they take longer to conceive than non-smokers (Shiverick 2011). The mixture of chemicals found in cigarettes is thought to affect fertility in women by disrupting hormone levels, affecting ovulation (Augood, Duckitt and Templeton 1998). In men, smoking can lead to lower sperm count and cause motility issues (Li *et al.* 2011).

### 3.1 Smoking in women

It has also been discovered that smoking can have an adverse effect on ovarian function in women undergoing assisted reproduction cycles (Voorhis *et al.* 1996). Smoking has been found to have a significant negative effect on fertility and ART success by affecting live birth outcome, with a higher risk of miscarriage and ectopic pregnancy in those women that smoke (Klonoff-Cohen, Marrs and Yee 2001; Waylen, Metwally and Jones 2009). Smoking may affect ovarian age and cause it to age more quickly in a smoker than a non-smoker. Sharara *et al.* (1994) discovered that a reduced ovarian reserve was significantly higher in women who smoked than in non-smokers of the same age (12.31% and 4.83%, respectively), and that the fertilisation and pregnancy rates were of a similar pattern. Smoking disrupts hormones and alters uterine functioning (Sharma *et al.* 2013). Soares *et al.* (2007) found that whilst using donor eggs, women who smoked between zero and ten cigarettes per day had a higher pregnancy rate (52.2%) than women who smoked ten or more cigarettes each day (34.1%), suggesting that the uterine environment had been affected by the cigarette smoke and possibly was responsible for the lower pregnancy rate found in smokers. Smoking may affect the oviducts and the transport of embryos, leading to infertility, ectopic pregnancies or a longer time to conception (Talbot and Riveles 2005).

Smoking has also been found to have a negative impact on success at IVF by affecting egg maturation and numbers (Klonoff-Cohen *et al.* 2001). In a large Dutch study published in 2005, it was discovered that women who smoked were much less likely to succeed at IVF compared with those who did not. 'Our study found that the effect of smoking more than one cigarette a day for a year reduced women's chances of having a live birth through IVF by 28 per cent – that's the same percentage disadvantage that occurs between a 20-year-old woman and a 30-year-old woman,' says Didi Braat, Professor of Gynaecology at the University Medical Centre in Nijmegen, where the study was undertaken. Braat and colleagues analysed medical data and questionnaire responses from nearly 8500 women aged 20 to 45, who had undergone IVF treatment at centres in The Netherlands between 1983 and 1995. More than 40 per cent of the women were smokers and at least seven per cent were overweight – with a BMI of $27 \text{kg}/\text{m}^2$ or higher – at the time of their first IVF attempt (Linsten *et al.* 2005). The women's subfertility was attributed to one of four causes: fallopian tube problems; male partner subfertility; unexplained subfertility; and other causes – mainly PCOS or endometriosis. 'Smoking had the greatest effect on those women with unexplained fertility problems, where IVF treatment led to 20.7 per cent of non-smokers achieving a live birth, compared with just 13.4 per cent of smokers,' says Braat. 'These results indicate that smoking may actually be causing the infertility problems these women were experiencing.' The researchers concluded that it is not known exactly how smoking affects fertility; however, the toxins in the smoke may have a toxic effect on the lining of the uterus, or the zona pellucida (the glycoprotein membrane that surrounds the plasma membrane of the oocyte) may be affected and become harder and thicker (Linsten *et al.* 2005).

## 3.2 Smoking in men

Smoking has also been found to have a negative impact on male fertility, in terms of affecting sperm production, motility and morphology (Monoski, Nudell and Lipschultz 2002). In males, smoking can cause a higher chance of infertility due to damage caused to the DNA in the sperm (Sepaniak *et al.* 2006). There is increasing evidence that the carcinogens found in cigarette smoke kill sperm cells (Agarwal, Prabakaran and Said 2005). Smoking increases the intake of cadmium, as a result of the tobacco plant absorbing the metal. Cadmium is chemically similar to zinc (Valko, Morris and Cronin 2005) and may replace the zinc in the DNA polymerase, which plays a very important role in sperm production, and lead to damage to the testes affecting sperm (Emsley 2001). Endocrine function in men may also be affected by smoking, due to the fact that an increase in the serum levels of follicle-stimulating hormone (FSH) and LH and decreases in testosterone have been recorded (Terzioglu 2001).

# 4. Alcohol

## 4.1 Alcohol consumption in women

Alcohol affects fertility in a number of ways. In research conducted by Eggert, Theobald and Engfeldt in 2004, it was discovered that women who drink large amounts of alcohol seem to have a greater chance of experiencing an infertility examination than moderate drinkers or women who consume low amounts of alcohol. Alcohol consumption has been linked to hormonal and ovulatory abnormalities (Eggert *et al.* 2004; Gill 2000), although the exact level of consumption associated with risk is unclear (Gill 2000).

Heavy consumption of alcohol can hinder insulin sensitivity, which can affect ovulation and thus fertility. This is because excessive sugar consumption contributes to hormonal imbalances, insulin resistance, yeast infection, vitamin and mineral deficiency and lowered immunity (Grodstein *et al.* 1994), all of which may impair fertility for both men and women. It can also lead to fewer eggs being collected during assisted reproduction (Groll and Groll 2006; Klonoff-Cohen, Lam-Kruglick and Gonzalez 2003).

Alcohol may have a direct effect on egg maturation and lead to elevated oestrogen levels, thus reducing FSH secretion (Hofman *et al.* 2007). A 40 per cent and 70 per cent reduced fecundity has been reported in women consuming any alcohol and those with intakes above ten drinks per week, respectively (Jensen *et al.* 1998). Social alcohol use revealed an approximately 60 per cent reduced fecundity rate (Hakim, Gray and Zacur 1998). In a study conducted by Klonoff-Cohen *et al.* in 2003 on 221 couples with female infertility, the relationship between IVF success and alcohol consumption was considered and similar results were found. Female alcohol consumption during the IVF process affected success rates. This study also discovered that having one drink per day in the month prior to IVF caused the risk of not achieving a pregnancy to rise by 2.86 times. This was the first study to examine the effect of alcohol directly on IVF success.

In a more recent study by Rossi Berry *et al.* in 2011, 2545 couples undergoing 4729 IVF cycles were studied over a nine-year period in three IVF clinics in the United States, and the effects of alcohol on IVF success were investigated. The couples filled in a questionnaire before the first IVF cycle. The couples were asked to record the type of alcohol that they consumed, the amount of alcohol, and how often they consumed it. The study discovered that in women who had more than four drinks of alcohol a week there was a 16 per cent decrease in live births after IVF in comparison with women who consumed fewer than four alcoholic drinks a week. For the couples in which both partners had at least four alcoholic drinks per week, the chance of a live birth occurring were 21 per cent lower compared with couples in which both had fewer than four drinks per week (OR=0.79; CI=0.66–0.96). Overall, the research concluded that alcohol consumption in men and women just prior to the start of the IVF process can have a negative effect on IVF success. Although the study does find that alcohol affects success at IVF it must be taken into account, on deeper analysis, that 10.7 per cent of the women and 17.2 per cent of the men in the study were obese after their BMI had been calculated, 25.4 per cent of the women and 34.3 per cent of the men were over the age of forty at the start of the first IVF cycle (which is the age when IVF success begins to decrease rapidly), and 10 per cent of the women and men in the study smoked. Other limitations of the study are that alcohol consumed was not recorded during the IVF cycle itself or in the subsequent pregnancy if success occurred; it was only recorded prior to IVF.

Rossi Berry et al. (2011) also concluded that the women who drank wine became pregnant much more quickly than those who drank spirits or beer. They found further that drinking white wine had a greater effect on the IVF process than red wine in that fewer eggs were collected at egg collection in women who had between one and seven drinks of white wine per week. This is interesting as there are higher amounts of the anti-oxidant levels in red wine.

However, in a study conducted by Juhl et al. in 2003 no distinction was found in the effect of drinking red or white wine and becoming pregnant, though the study did not concentrate solely on IVF.

Another study, carried out by Bellver (2008), found alcohol consumption either to have no effect on IVF success or the results to be inconclusive.

## 4.2 Alcohol consumption in men

In men, consuming alcohol can lead to a reduced sperm count (Muthusami and Chinnaswamy 2005). It can also affect sperm quality and embryo quality (Grodstein et al. 1994; Klonoff-Cohen et al. 2003). Alcohol seems to negatively affect both sperm motility and sperm morphology (Gaur, Talekar and Pathak 2010). Alcohol has been linked to an increase in oxidative stress (Cederbaum, Lu and Wu 2009). Further research is required to determine whether there is a link between alcohol and sperm oxidative stress (Kefer, Agarwal and Sabanegh 2009).

## 5. Stress

Stress, unfortunately, is an unavoidable part of everyday life. Stress takes many forms: psychological, physical or social (Schneiderman, Ironson and Siegel 2005). Infertility can also exert considerable stress and pressure for many reasons, such as emotional, financial, social and failure pressures (Anderheim *et al.* 2005; McQuillian *et al.* 2003). Stress can affect the hypothalamic–pituitary–adrenal (HPA) axis, which is involved in the production of cortisol, and this affects the hypothalamic–pituitary–gonadal (HPG) axis (Nepomnaschy *et al.* 2007). Production of cortisol can affect the HPG axis by affecting the pituitary release of FSH and LH (Erickson 1993). This in turn can negatively affect development and release of the egg in the ovary (Erickson 1993).

The research to date on the effect of stress on IVF success has largely focused on stress levels and the effect of stress throughout the IVF process treatment itself, not daily stress prior to IVF treatment and its effect on success (Anderheim *et al.* 2005; Harlow *et al.* 1996; Milad *et al.* 1998). Everyday stress (baseline stress) needs to be addressed before IVF treatment begins (Klonoff-Cohen *et al.* 2001). However, in a study conducted by Ebbesen *et al.* (2009) the effect of stressful life events in the twelve months prior to IVF were investigated and it was discovered that major events in the year prior to IVF may reduce success at IVF due to fewer eggs being retrieved at egg collection.

In research conducted by Anderheim *et al.* in 2005 involving 166 women undergoing their first cycle of IVF, stress was measured using the Psychological General Wellbeing Index and the psychological effects of infertility were measured by 14 items. The study investigated the effect of psychological stress before and after IVF treatment. The results of the study found there to be no evidence to suggest that psychological stress affected IVF success; other studies have found similar results (Harlow *et al.* 1996; Milad *et al.* 1998).

Other research, conducted by Sanders and Bruce in 1999 and Klonoff-Cohen in 2005, has found there to be a link between stress, coping mechanisms, personality traits and resilience to IVF outcomes and that these factors may contribute to an inability to get pregnant before any fertility treatment is considered.

A study conducted by Ebbeson *et al.* in 2009 was the first study to investigate the effect of stress in the twelve months prior to IVF. Their study involved 809 women all embarking on their first IVF attempt, with a mean age of 31.2 years. Participants completed a questionnaire that aimed to measure perceived stress and depressive symptoms. Researchers discovered that the women who were successful at their first IVF attempt had recorded fewer negative life events unrelated to infertility in the twelve months prior to IVF than those who were unsuccessful. The women who were more successful also had more eggs retrieved at egg collection and so the researchers concluded that chronic stress may not only affect IVF success but also the number of eggs retrieved. This research used a relatively large sample in comparison to other studies researching psychological factors and their effect on IVF, which mainly involve fewer than fifty participants. There were some limitations, in that the questionnaires were handed out by clinic staff, so the researchers themselves could not record non-responses. They also found there to be differences in hormone doses when examining clinic records in that the participants in the study seemed to require higher doses of drugs prior to egg collection than the rest of their cohort. The researchers state that this may have been due to a smaller proportion of patients following the mild hormone stimulation protocol amongst the participants, but they did not have any information on this particular aspect in relation to the non-participating part of the cohort so cannot draw further conclusions on this result. They were also unable to include any measure of alcohol consumption and so were unable to ascertain whether this factor was a possible mediator in stress from infertility.

It is clear that the experience of infertility is a major stress in itself, undergoing ART adds to this further and in many cases disappointment from unsuccessful treatment only compounds an already difficult situation. Many couples also experience financial worries and pressure when attempting to fund treatment privately. Being mindful of this, it is imperative that healthcare professionals and practitioners support patients sensitively throughout the whole process, especially in the scenario of failed treatment or pregnancy loss (Anderson, Niesenblat and Norman 2010).

## 6. Endocrine disruptors

The balance of the endocrine system is very important in the human body, especially in females, due to the fact that the menstrual cycle and fertility are very sensitive to hormone imbalances (Nicolopoulou-Stamati and Pitsos 2001). Human fertility in both men and women may be at particular risk from endocrine disruptors (Bergman *et al.* 2012). We encounter many threats to fertility in everyday life from agents such as viruses, radiation and chemicals (Smedley, Dick and Sadhra 2007). Endocrine-disrupting chemicals are found in many everyday products such as pesticides, paints, detergents and cosmetics (Bergman *et al.* 2012). Many of these chemicals affect the way in which hormones work in the body and are thus known as endocrine disruptors (Rogan and Chen 2005). Mimicking natural hormones, impeding normal hormone activity, and varying regulation and function of the endocrine system are a few of the many ways that endocrine disruptors affect the human body (Ritz *et al.* 2007). Exposure to endocrine-disrupting chemicals can affect organisms during critical periods of development such as during foetal maturation or puberty (Bergman *et al.* 2012). This may lead to situations such as low birthweight or pre-term birth (Bergman *et al.* 2012).

Organochlorides, although found in very low levels naturally in the environment, are thought to be one of the main endocrine disruptors. These are formed when carbon and chlorine combine chemically. Humans and animals are unable to detoxify these substances and thus if an organism is continually exposed, bioaccumulation occurs in the fatty tissues of the body (Warhurst 1995). This build-up has led to a decrease in fertility and sperm quality in animals and humans (Safe 2005; Rogan and Chen 2005).

Over the last few decades, there has been increasing concern about the use of chemicals with hormone-disrupting properties and various wildlife species such as fish and mice have been affected by exposure to endocrine-disrupting chemicals (EDCs) (Diamanti-Kandarakis *et al.* 2009). Chemical substances containing 'oestrogenic' properties such as those contained in pesticides, plastics and paints, and their effect on the endocrine system, have been of particular concern. These chemical substances seem to mimic the effects of oestrogens or block the action of androgens and thus can affect reproduction in animals (Greenpeace 2003). There are up to eight hundred chemicals used worldwide with potential or known endocrine-disrupting properties; however, only a small proportion of these have been specifically tested to determine whether they produce an effect in intact organisms (Bergman *et al.*

2012). Table 11.1 shows the different classes and some examples of endocrine-disrupting chemicals used worldwide.

## Table 11.1 Classes and examples of endocrine-disrupting chemicals (EDCs) (Bergman *et al.* 2012)

| Classification | Specific examples of EDCs |
| --- | --- |
| **Persistent and bioaccumulative halogenated chemicals** | |
| Persistent Organic Pollutants (POPs) (Stockholm Convention) (section 3.1.1.1) Other Persistent and Bioaccumulative Chemicals (section 3.1.1.2) | Polychlorinated dibenzo-p-dioxins (PCDD) Polychlorinated dibenzofurans (PCDF) Polychlorinated biphenyls (PCB) Hexachlorobenzene (HCB) Perfluorooctanesulfonic acid (PFOS) Polybrominated diphenyl ethers (PBDE) Polybrominated biphenyls (PBB) Chlordane Mirex Toxaphene Dichlorodiphenyltrichloroethane (DDT) Lindane Endosulfan Hexabromocyclododecane (HBCDD) Octachlorostyrene PCB methyl sulfones |

| Classification | Specific examples of EDCs |
|---|---|
| **Less persistent and less bioaccumulative chemicals** | |
| Plasticisers and Other Additives in Materials and Goods (section 3.1.1.3) Polycyclic Aromatic Chemicals (PACs) including PAHs (section 3.1.1.4) Halogenated Phenolic Chemicals (HPCs) (section 3.1.1.5) Non-halogenated Phenolic Chemicals (Non-HPCs) (section 3.1.1.5) | Phthalate esters, Triphenyl phosphate, Bis(2-ethylhexyl) adipate, n-Butylbenzene, Triclocarban, Butylated hydroxyanisole Benzo(a)pyrene, Benzo(a) anthracene, Pyrene, Anthracene 2,4-Dichlorophenol, Pentachlorophenol, Hydroxy-PCBs, Hydroxy-PBDEs, Tetrabromobisphenol A, 2,4,6-Tribromophenol, Triclosan Bisphenol A, Bisphenol F, Bisphenol S, Nonylphenol, Octylphenol, Resorcinol |
| **Pesticides, pharmaceuticals and personal care product ingredients** | |
| Current-use Pesticides (section 3.1.1.6) Pharmaceuticals, Growth Promoters, and Personal Care Product Ingredients (section 3.1.1.7) | 2,4-D, Atrazine, Carbaryl, Malathion, Mancozeb, Vinclozolin, Procloraz, Procymidone, Chlorpyrifos, Fenitrothion, Linuron Endocrine active (e.g. Diethylstilbestrol, Ethinylestradiol, Tamoxifen, Levonorgestrel), Selective serotonin reuptake inhibitors (SSRIs; e.g. Fluoxetine), Flutamide, 4-Methylbenzylidene camphor, Octyl-methoxycinnamate, Parabens, Cyclic methyl siloxanes (D4, D5, D6), Galaxolide, 3-Benzylidene camphor |

### Other chemicals

| | |
|---|---|
| Metals and Organometallic Chemicals (section 3.1.1.8) | Arsenic, Cadmium, Lead, Mercury, Methylmercury Tributyltin, Triphenyltin |
| Natural Hormones (section 3.1.1.9) | 17β-Estradiol, Estrone, Testosterone |
| Phytoestrogens (section 3.1.1.9) | Isoflavones (e.g. Genistein, Daidzein), Coumestans (e.g. Coumestrol), Mycotoxins (e.g. Zearalenone), Prenylflavonoids (e.g. 8-prenylnaringenin) |

In a recent study which examined the effect of rainbow fish being exposed to oestrogenic compounds it was concluded that 'exogenous oestrogens may lead to effects on sex differentiation, sexual behaviour and reproductive cycles in this fish' (Shanthanagouda and Patil 2013). In an earlier study it was concluded that if male embryos of rats or mice are exposed to chemicals such as BPA (many plastic products used in baby care are marketed as being without this), DDT or vinclozilin (a fungicide), such exposure can negatively affect the development of male sex organs (Skakkebaek, Meyts and Main 2001).

Studies carried out in Scotland, Belgium and Paris indicated that human sperm counts had declined over the previous twenty years at a rate of two per cent per year and that the sperm count of a twenty-year-old at the time of the study was lower than it would have been at the same age twenty years previously (Auger *et al.* 1995, Van Waeleghem *et al.* 1996, Irvine *et al.* 1996). The studies also concluded that other indicators of sperm quality had also declined, for example the percentage of motile sperm had decreased and the numbers of abnormal sperm had increased.

A study conducted in Finland concluded that 'deteriorating sperm production may explain why sperm counts are declining' (Pajarinen *et al.* 1997). Male factors in infertility and pregnancy loss are explained in detail in Chapter 6. It is important to consider environmental factors alongside these.

## 6.1 Endocrine disruptors and conditions that affect fertility

Endometriosis (discussed in depth in Chapter 5) is an endocrine and autoimmune disease and is thought to affect around 10 per cent of women in reproductive years (Eskenazi and Warner 1997). It has been suggested that there may be a link between the incidence of endometriosis, with exposure to PCB or to dioxin. It is thought (from studies on monkeys) that both of these chemicals may increase the severity of endometriosis due to the impact they have on the immune system (Rier *et al.* 1995). It appears that the incidence of endometriosis is highest in the industrialised countries (Koninckx *et al.* 1994). It has been suggested that avoidance of fatty foods (e.g. red meat), which may contain high levels of PCB and dioxins, may help to reduce the exposure of women with endometriosis to these chemicals (Rier *et al.* 1995).

## 7. Sleep

Recent studies have suggested that the amount of sleep a woman has may affect her fertility (Morris 2008). The quantity and quality of sleep affects hormones, mood, health and fertility. Sleep is important as it is during this time that our bodies can repair cells, regenerate cells and regulate our hormone levels.

Leptin is a hormone, secreted by fat cells into the bloodstream, which works by modulating the size of the adipose tissues in the body. The level of plasma leptin falls when fat mass decreases so that appetite is stimulated until the fat mass is recovered (Moschos, Chan and Mantzoros 2002). Energy expenditure is also reduced and body temperature decreases. However, levels of plasma leptin increase when fat mass increases, resulting in appetite being suppressed and consequent weight loss. In this way leptin regulates fat stores and energy intake so that weight is maintained within quite a narrow range. A lack of sleep reduces the amount of serum leptin (Seaborg 2007).

Leptin is thought to affect fertility, as a lack of sleep has been linked with irregular ovulation (Morris 2008). Leptin is important in appetite and weight regulation (Friedman and Halaas 1998). A lack of leptin can affect the appetite, which can disrupt the menstrual cycle

(Morris 2008). Leptin levels that are too high or too low can affect egg quality and success during IVF (Anifandis *et al.* 2005).

Scientists believe that there may be a link between fertility and amount of sleep, due to the circadian rhythm's influence on the endocrine system and thus hormone production. A recent study conducted by a team of researchers in Korea, led by Dr Daniel Park, examined the sleeping habits of 656 women about to begin IVF treatment. They divided the women into those who had between four and six hours sleep a night, those who had between seven and eight hours sleep a night and those who had nine to eleven hours sleep a night. They found that those who had between seven and eight hours sleep a night were more likely to become pregnant (56% pregnancy rate) than those who got four to six hours sleep a night (46% pregnancy rate) or nine hours or more (43% pregnancy rate). The study did not take into account weight or stress levels. The researchers presented their findings in 2013 at the American Society for Reproductive Medicine's annual meeting.

Infertility can cause considerable stress that can affect eating habits, sleep and mood. When cortisol levels rise, sleep patterns may be affected which in turn may affect fertility. Stress has been shown to decrease pregnancy rates and increase miscarriage rates (Nakamura, Sheps and Arck 2008).

Disturbed sleep affects sperm counts in men, according to a recent study conducted by Jensen *et al.* in 2013 at the University of Southern Denmark. The researchers carried out a cross-sectional study of 953 men between 2008 and 2011. Each participant completed a questionnaire on their lifestyle that included questions on sleep disturbances, particularly on sleep patterns over the four most recent weeks. The men also provided blood samples and semen samples and were given a physical examination. According to Jensen *et al.*: 'Sleep disturbances showed an inverse U-shaped association with sperm concentration, total sperm count, percent motile and percent morphologically normal spermatozoa, and testis size.' It was discovered that the men who experienced a higher level of sleep disturbance (less than six hours sleep a night) had a 29 per cent lower adjusted sperm concentration and 1.6 per cent fewer morphologically normal sperm (Jensen *et al.* 2013). At the time of writing, further research is required on the relationship between sleep and fertility, such as to ascertain if there is a link between improvement of sleep quality and fertility.

··· BOX 11.2 TIPS FOR A GOOD NIGHT'S SLEEP ···············

▶ Make sure that the room is not too hot or too cold.

▶ Remove all distractions from the toom which may affect restful sleep such as phones, TVs, mobile devices/tablets/ laptops.

▶ Try a warm bath before bed with lavender oil.

▶ Do not eat a main meal immediately before bedtime (try to leave at least two hours after eating).

▶ Do not go to sleep stressed or upset.

▶ Try to aim for 7–8 hours sleep.

▶ Make your bedroom a relaxing place to sleep in.

▶ Listen to some calming music before sleep.

# References

Agarwal, A., Prabakaran, S., and Said, T. (2005) 'Prevention of oxidative stress injury to sperm.' *Journal of Andrology 26*, 6, 654–660.

Anderheim, L., Holter, H., Bergh, C., and Moller, A. (2005) 'Does psychological stress affect the outcome of in vitro fertilization?' *Human Reproduction 20*, 10, 2969–2975.

Anderson, K., Niesenblat, V., and Norman, R. (2010) 'Lifestyle factors in people seeking infertility treatment – a review.' *Australian and New Zealand Journal of Obstetrics and Gynaecology 50*, 8–20.

Anifandis, G., Koutselini, E., Louridas, K., Liakopoulos, V., *et al.* (2005) 'Estradiol and leptin as conditional prognostic IVF markers.' *Reproduction 129*, 4, 531–534.

Auger J., Kuntsmann J., Czyglik, F., and Jouannet P. (1995) 'Decline in semen quality among fertile men in Paris during the past 20 years.' *New England Journal of Medicine 332*, 5, 281–285.

Augood, C., Duckitt, K., and Templeton, A. (1998) 'Smoking and female infertility: a systematic review and meta-analysis.' *Human Reproduction 13*,1532–1539.

Bellver, J. (2008) 'Impact of bodyweight and lifestyle on IVF outcome.' *Expert Review of Obstretrics and Gynaecology 3*, 5, 607–625.

Bergman, A., Heindel, J., Jobling, S., Kidd, K., and Zoeller, T. (eds) (2012) *State of the Science of Endocrine Disrupting Chemicals*. Geneva: United Nations Environment Programme and the World Health Organisation. Available at www.who.int/ceh/publications/endocrine/en/index.html, accessed on 28 May 2015.

Cederbaum, A., Lu, Y., and Wu, D. (2009) 'Role of oxidative stress in alcohol-induced liver injury.' *Archives of Toxicology 83*, 519–548.

Chavarro, J., Willett, W., and Skerrett, P. (2009) *Fertility Diet: Groundbreaking Research Reveals Natural Ways to Boost Ovulation and Improve Your Chances of Getting Pregnant*. New York: McGraw Hill.

De Souza, M., Van Heest, J., Demers, L., and Lasley, B. (2003) 'Luteal phase deficiency in recreational runners: evidence for a hypometabolic state.' *Journal of Clinical Endocrinology and Metabolism 88*, 337–346.

Diamanti-Kandarakis, E., Bourguignon, J., Giudice, L., Hauser, R., *et al.* (2009) 'Endocrine-disrupting chemicals: an Endocrine Society scientific statement.' *Endocrine Reviews 30*, 293–342.

Ebbesen, S., Zachariae, R., Mehlsen, M., Thomsen, D., Hojgaard, A., and Ottosen, L. (2009) 'Stressful life events are associated with a poor in-vitro fertilization (IVF) outcome.' *Human Reproduction 22*, 543–547.

Eggert, J., Theobald, H., and Engfeldt, P. (2004) Effects of alcohol consumption on female fertility during an 18-year period. *Fertility and Sterility 81*, 379–383.

Emsley, J. (2001) *Nature's Building Blocks: An A–Z Guide to the Elements*. Oxford: Oxford University Press.

Erickson, G. (1993) 'Normal regulation of ovarian androgen production.' *Seminars in Reproductive Endocrinology 11*, 307–312.

Eskenazi, B., and Warner, M. (1997). 'Epidemiology of endometriosis.' *Obstetrics and Gynaecology Clinics of North America 24*, 2, 235–258.

Friedman, J., and Halaas, J. (1998) 'Leptin and the regulation of body weight in mammals.' *Nature 395*, 6704, 763–770.

Frisch, R. (2002) *Female Fertility and the Body Fat Connection*. Chicago: University of Chicago Press.

Gaur, D., Talekar, M., and Pathak, V. (2010) 'Alcohol intake and cigarette smoking: impact of two major lifestyle factors on male fertility.' *Indian Journal of Pathology and Microbiology 53*, 35–40.

Gill, J. (2000) 'The effects of moderate alcohol consumption on female hormone levels and reproductive function.' *Alcohol 35*, 417–423.

Greenpeace UK (October 2003). *Human Impacts of Man-made Chemicals*. Available at www.greenpeace.org.uk/toxics, accessed on 28 May 2015.

Grodstein, F., Goldman, M., and Cramer, D. (1994) 'Infertility in women and moderate alcohol use.' *American Journal of Public Health 84*, 1429–1432.

Groll, J., and Groll, L. (2006) *Fertility Foods: Optimise Ovulation and Conception Through Food Choices*. New York: Fireside Books.

Hackney, A. (2008) 'Effects of endurance exercise on the reproductive system of men: the exercise-hypogonadal male condition.' *Journal of Endocrinological Investigation 31*, 10, 932–938.

Hakim, R., Gray, R., and Zacur, H. (1998) 'Alcohol and caffeine consumption and decreased fertility.' *Fertility and Sterility 70*, 632–637.

Harlow, C., Fahy, U., Talbot, W., Wardle, P., and Hull, M. (1996) 'Stress and stress-related hormones during in-vitro fertilization treatment.' *Human Reproduction 11*, 274–279.

Harrison, C., Lombard, C., Moran, L., and Teede, H. (2011) 'Exercise therapy in polycystic ovary syndrome: a systematic review.' *Human Reproduction Update 14*, 2, 171–183.

Health Canada (2009) *Prenatal Nutrition Guidelines for Health Professionals: Gestational Weight Gain*. Available at www.hc-sc.gc.ca/fn-an/nutrition/prenatal/ewba-mbsa-eng.php, accessed on 28 May 2015.

Hofman, G., Davies, M., and Norman, R. (2007) 'The impact of lifestyle factors on reproductive performance in the general population and in those undergoing fertility treatment: a review.' *Human Reproductive Update 13*, 209–223.

Irvine, S., Cawood, E., Richardson, D., MacDonald, E., and Aitken, J. (1996) 'Evidence of deteriorating semen quality in the United Kingdom: birth cohort study in 577 men in Scotland over 11 years.' *British Medical Journal 312*, 467–471.

Jensen, T., Andersson, A., Skakkebaek, N., Joensen, U., *et al.* (2013) 'Association of sleep disturbances with reduced semen quality.' *American Journal of Epidemiology 177*, 10, 1027–1037.

Jensen, T., Hjollund, N., Henriksen, T., Scheike, T., *et al.* (1998) 'Does moderate alcohol consumption affect fertility? Follow up study among couples planning first pregnancy.' *British Medical Journal 317*, 505–510.

Juhl, M., Olsen, J., Anderson, A., and Gronbaek, M. (2003) 'Intake of wine, beer and spirits and waiting time to pregnancy.' *Human Reproduction 18*, 1967–1971.

Kefer, J., Agarwal, A., and Sabanegh, E. (2009) 'Role of antioxidants in the treatment of male infertility.' *International Journal of Urology 16*, 449–457.

Klonoff-Cohen, H. (2005) 'Female and male lifestyle habits and IVF: what is known and unknown.' *Human Reproduction Update 11*, 180–204.

Klonoff-Cohen, H., Lam-Kruglick, M., and Gonzalez, C. (2003) 'Effects of maternal and paternal alcohol consumption on the success rates of in vitro fertilization and gamete intrafallopian transfer.' *Fertility and Sterility 79*, 330–339.

Klonoff-Cohen, H., Marrs, R., and Yee, B. (2001) 'Effects of female and male smoking on success rates of IVF and gamete intra-Fallopian transfer.' *Human Reproduction 16*, 7, 1382–1390.

Koninckx, P., Braet, P., Kennedy, S.H., and Barlow, D.H. (1994) 'Dioxin pollution in and endometriosis in Belgium.' *Human Reproduction 9*, 6, 1001–1002.

Li, Y., Lin, H., Li, Y., and Cao, J. (2011) 'Association between socio-psycho-behavioral factors and male semen quality: systematic review and meta-analyses.' *Fertility and Sterility 95*, 116–123.

Linsten, A., Pasker-de-Jong, P., de Boer, E., Burger, C., *et al.* (2005) 'Effects of subfertility cause, smoking and body weight on the success rate of IVF.' *Human Reproduction 2*, 7, 1867–1875.

McQuillian, J., Greil, A., White, L., and Jacob, M. (2003) 'Frustrated fertility: infertility and psychological distress among women.' *Journal of Marriage and Family 65*, 4, 1007–1018.

Mello, N. (1988) 'Effects of alcohol abuse on reproductive function in women.' *Recent Developments in Alcoholism 6*, 253–276.

Milad, M., Klock, S., Moses, S., and Chatterton, R. (1998)' Stress and anxiety do not result in pregnancy wastage.' *Human Reproduction 13*, 2296–2300.

Monoski, M., Nudell, D., and Lipshultz, L. (2002) 'Effects of medical therapy, alcohol, and smoking on male fertility.' *Contemporary Urology*, 57–63.

Morris, R. (June 2008) *Could Leptin be the Next Fertility Medication?* IVF1. Available at www.ivf1.com/leptin, accessed on 28 May 2015.

Morris, S., Missmer, S., Cramer, D., Powers, D., McShane, P., and Mark, D. (2006) 'Effects of lifetime exercise on the outcome of in vitro fertilisation.' *Obstetrics & Gynaecology 108*, 4, 938–945.

Moschos, S., Chan, J., and Mantzoros, C. (2002) 'Leptin and reproduction: a review.' *Fertility and Sterility 77*, 433–444.

Muthusami, K., and Chinnaswamy, P. (2005) 'Effect of chronic alcoholism on male fertility hormones and semen quality.' *Fertility and Sterility 84*, 919–924.

Nafee, T., Farrell, W., Carroll, W., Fryer, A., and Ismail, K. (2008) 'Epigenetic control of fetal gene expression.' *International Journal of Obstetrics & Gynaecology 115*, 2, 158–168.

Nakamura, K., Sheps, S., and Arck, P. (2008). 'Stress and reproductive failure: past notions, present insights and future directions.' *Journal of Assisted Reproduction and Genetics 25*, 47.

Nepomnaschy, P., Schneider, E., Mastorakos, G., and Arck, P. (2007) 'Stress, immune function, and women's reproduction.' *Annals of the New York Academy of Sciences 1113*, 350–364.

Nicolopoulou-Stamati, P., and Pitsos, M. (2001) 'The impact of endocrine disruptors on the female reproductive system.' *Human Reproduction Update 7*, 3, 323–330.

Pajarinen, J., Laippala, P., Penttila, A., and Karhunen, P. (1997) 'Incidence of disorders of spermatogenesis in middle aged Finnish men, 1981–91: two necropsy series.' *British Medical Journal 314*, 13–18.

Palmer, N., Bakos, H., Owens, J., Setchell, B., and Lane, M. (2012) 'Diet and exercise in an obese mouse fed a high-fat diet improve metabolic health and reverse perturbed sperm function.' *American Journal of Physiology, Endocrinology and Metabolism 302*, E768–E780.

Pasqulotto, F. (2004) 'Effects of medical therapy, alcohol, smoking, and endocrine disruptors on male infertility.' *Revista do Hospital das Clínicas da Faculdade de Medicina da Universidade de São Paulo 59*, 6, 375–382.

Rich-Edwards, J., Spiegelman, D., Garland, M., Hertzmark, E., *et al.* (2002) 'Physical activity, body mass index, and ovulatory disorder infertility.' *Epidemiology 13*, 184–190.

Rier, S., Martin, D., Bowman, R., and Becker, J. (1995) 'Immunoresponsiveness in endometriosis: implications of estrogenic toxicants.' *Environmental Health Perspectives 103*, 7, 151–156.

Ritz, B., Wilhelm, M., Hoggatt, K., and Ghosh, J. (2007) 'Ambient air pollution and preterm birth in the environment and pregnancy outcomes study at the University of California, Los Angeles.' *American Journal of Epidemiology 166*, 1045–1052.

Rogan, W., and Chen, A. (2005) 'Health risks and benefits of bis (4-chlorophenyl)-1,1,1-trichloroethane (DDT).' *Lancet 366*, 9487, 763–773.

Rossi Berry, K., Horstein, M., Cramer, D., Ehrlich, S., and Missmer, S. (2011) 'Effect of alcohol consumption on in vitro fertilization.' *Obstetrics and Gynaecology 117*, 136–142.

Safe, S. (2005) 'Clinical correlates of environmental endocrine disruptors.' *Trends in Endocrinology & Metabolism 16*, 4, 139–144.

Sanders, K., and Bruce, N. (1999) 'Psycho-social stress and treatment outcome following assisted reproductive technology.' *Human Reproduction 14*, 1656–1662.

Schneiderman, N., Ironson, G., and Siegel, S. (2005) 'Stress and health: psychological, behavioral, and biological determinants.' *Annual Review of Clinical Psychology 1*, 607–628.

Seaborg, E. (2007) 'Growing evidence links too little sleep to obesity and diabetes.' *Endocrine News*, 14–15.

Sepaniak, S., Forges, T., Gerard, H., Foliguet, B., Bene, M., and Monnier-Barbarino, P. (2006) 'The influence of cigarette smoking on human sperm quality and DNA fragmentation.' *Toxicology 223*, 54–60.

Shanthanagouda, A., and Patil, J. (2013) 'Comparative biochemistry and physiology Part C. *Toxicology & Pharmacology 157*, 2, 162–171.

Sharara, F., Beatse, S., Leonard, M., Navot, D., and Scott, S. (1994) 'Cigarette smoking accelerates the development of diminished ovarian reserve as evidenced by the clomiphene citrate challenge test.' *Fertility and Sterility 62*, 257–262.

Sharma, R., Biedenharn, K., Fedor, J., and Agarwal, A. (2013) 'Lifestyle factors and reproductive health: taking control of your fertility.' *Reproductive Biology and Endocrinology 11*, 66.

Shiverick, K. (2011) 'Cigarette Smoking and Reproductive and Developmental Toxicity.' In R.C. Gupta (ed.) *Reproductive and Developmental Toxicology.* Burlington, MA: Elsevier.

Skakkebaek, N., Meyts, R., and Main, K. (2001) 'Testicular dysgenesis syndrome: an increasingly common developmental disorder with environmental aspects.' *Human Reproduction 16,* 5, 972–978.

Smedley, J., Dick, F., and Sadhra, S. (2007) *Oxford Handbook of Occupational Health.* New York: Oxford University Press.

Soares, S., Simon, C., Remohi, J., and Pellicer, A. (2007) 'Cigarette smoking affects uterine receptiveness.' *Human Reproduction 22,* 543–547.

Steeghers Theunissen, R. (2003) 'Nutrient-gene interactions in early pregnancy: a vascular hypothesis.' *European Journal of Obstetrics and Gynaecology and Reproductive Biology 106,* 2, 115.

Talbot, P., and Riveles, K. (2005) 'Smoking and reproduction: the oviduct as a target of cigarette smoke.' *Reproductive Biology and Endocrinology 3,* 52.

Templeton, A., Morris, J., and Parslow, W. (1996) 'Factors that affect outcome of in-vitro fertilisation treatment.' *Lancet 348,* 9039, 1402.

Terzioglu, F. (2001) 'Investigation into effectiveness of counseling on assisted reproductive techniques in Turkey.' *J. Psychosom. Obstet. Gynaecol. 22,* 133–141.

US Environmental Protection Agency (1993) *Respiratory Effects of Passive Smoking: Lung Cancer and Other Disorders: The Report of the US Environmental Protection Agency.* Monograph 4. NIH Publication No. 93-3605. Washington, DC: US Department of Health and Human Services.

Vaamonde, D., Da Silva-Grigoletto, M., Garcia-Manso, J., Vaamonde-Lemos, R., Swanson, R., and Oehninger, S. (2009) 'Response of semen parameters to three training modalities.' *Fertility and Sterility 92,* 1941–1946.

Valko, M., Morris, H., and Cronin, M. (2005) 'Metals, toxicity and oxidative stress.' *Current Medicinal Chemistry 12,* 1161–1208.

van Waeleghem, K., de Clercq, N., Vermeulen, L., Schoonjans, F., and Comhaire, F. (1996) 'Deterioration of sperm quality in young healthy Belgian men.' *Human Reproduction 11,* 2, 325–329.

Voorhis, B., Dawson, J., Stovall, D., Sparks, A., and Syrop, C. (1996) 'The effects of smoking on ovarian function and fertility during assisted reproduction cycles.' *Obstetrics and Gynaecology 5,* 785–791.

Warhurst, A. (1995) *An Environmental Assessment of Alkylphenol Ethoxylates and Alkylphenols.* Edinburgh and London: Friends of the Earth.

Warren, M., and Perlroth, N. (2001) 'The effects of intense exercise on the female reproductive system.' *Journal of Endocrinology 170,* 3–11.

Waylen, A., Metwally, M., and Jones, G. (2009) 'Effects of cigarette smoking upon clinical outcomes of assisted reproduction: a meta-analysis.' *Human Reproduction Update 15,* 1, 31–44.

Wilmore, J., and Knuttgen, H. (2003) 'Aerobic exercise and endurance improving fitness for health benefits.' *The Physician and Sports Medicine 31,* 5, 45.

Wise, L., Rothman, K., Mikkelsen, E., Sørensen, H., Riis, A., and Hatch, E. (2012) 'A prospective cohort study of physical activity and time to pregnancy.' *Fertility and Sterility 97,* 5, 1136–1142.

# Chapter 12

# Supporting Assisted Reproduction in Women Over 40 Years of Age

*Natasha Claire Dunn, Senior Clinical Embryologist working in London, BSc (Animal Science), Graduate Diploma in Reproductive Sciences and Advanced Diploma of Nutritional Medicine*

## 1. Key issues affecting women over 40

As more women are seeking assisted reproductive techniques (ART) in their later reproductive years (specifically over 40 years of age), many find they are facing a series of issues associated with age and its effects on reproduction. These include the following:

- Poor response to stimulation drugs during ART – meaning that treatment cycles may get cancelled. Doctors may then need to increase doses of ART drugs and add in other drugs such as steroids, which can become very costly.

- When response is poor, cycles may be cancelled due to no follicles or low follicle numbers, or downgraded to IUI (intrauterine insemination).

- Egg quality issues, for example poorer quality oocytes associated with age and increased doses of ART stimulation drugs.

- Higher risk of aneuploidy (chromosomal abnormality) and pregnancy loss/spontaneous abortion.

- Increased immune activity (see Chapter 5 for further information on this).

## 2. Embryo quality

Women are born with approximately two million oocytes. By the time of menarche this number is reduced to approximately 300,000 (Marcus and Brinsden 1996) and continues to fall until menopause. There is also an increase in the rate of follicular decline, which increases from the age of 37.5 years until menopause. This results in a decline in the overall ovarian reserve, an increase in oocyte aneuploidy (chromosome abnormality) and a significantly higher rate of spontaneous abortion. Advancing age is also associated with decreased embryo viability (Marcus and Brinsden 1996).

Embryo quality is influenced by oocyte maturation. This is determined by the nuclear and the mitochondrial genome and the microenvironment provided by the ovary itself (Rienzi, Vajta and Ubaldi 2011). We can confidently conclude that the confounding factor introduced by advancing age is the quality of the oocyte, rather than the endometrium, as a number of studies have shown high pregnancy rates in older women with donated oocytes from younger women (Ziebe *et al.* 2001). It is, however, of course possible for a woman aged over 40 to have a healthy baby naturally and via ART, although there are increased risks in this age category. The remainder of this chapter will outline some of the factors that can influence oocyte maturation, and may prove useful for women in this age group aiming to improve their chances of success.

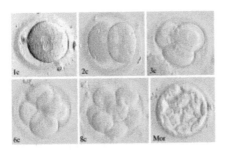

Figure 12.1 Normal human embryos

*A view of normal human embryos taken from under a phase contrast microscopy. The embryos show equal blastomeres and minimal fragmentation, although embryo 3c, which is a 3-cell embryo, shows slightly more fragmentation than the others (Sathananthan 2006)*

## 2.1 Embryo quality: age and spontaneous abortion (pregnancy loss)

Ziebe *et al.* (2001) found that there was no real difference in the fragmentation rate for women under the age of 40, but once they reached 40 and over, the embryo fragmentation rate rapidly increased (embryo fragmentation occurs when portions of the embryo's cells break off and are now separate from the nucleated section of the cell). Ziebe *et al.* (2001) also found that the decline in quality and increased fragmentation in relation to age also corresponds to a significant decrease in the implantation rate for women over 40. This was evident by a correlation between increased miscarriage rates and a decrease in ongoing pregnancy rates, with the mean miscarriage rate higher among pregnant women aged 43±4.8 years (Ziebe *et al.* 2001). Furthermore, they found that embryos at the cleavage stage that were transferred in women aged over 40, and that were at the same cell stage and morphological quality as those of younger women, showed a significant decrease in the implantation rate. This means that even though the embryo grade looked, to the naked eye, morphologically as viable as a younger woman's, there was a decrease in embryo quality with advanced physiological and biological ovarian age.

Scientists have documented in blastocysts (day 5/6 embryos) (Ahlström *et al.* 2011) that as a woman gets older there is a decrease in blastocyst morphology and quality with increasing maternal age. Ahlström *et al.* (2011) concluded that as women age, the expansion of the blastocoel decreases significantly, as does the quality of the trophectoderm cells (cavity inside the blastocyst), and there is a significant decrease in the quality of the trophectoderm cells (which go on to form the placenta) and inner cell mass (ICM – the stem cells that form the foetus). This also lowers the chance of a take-home pregnancy in the over-40s age range. With a lower percentage of embryos reaching blastocyst stage, and with a decrease in blastocoel expansion, the blastocysts also produced a lower quality trophectoderm and ICM.

Irrespective of female age, a greater chance of pregnancy was achieved from blastocysts with grading of 4BA or 3BA, according to a study conducted by Ahlström *et al.* (2011). Most IVF clinics will recommend a day three transfer for women over 40 years old, whereby embryos are transferred before the blastocyst stage. This is due to the decrease in the embryo numbers and their quality. However, it does appear that some clinics may allow a woman aged over 40 to try for a blastocyst transfer if there are four or more good quality embryos.

## 2.2 Paternal age

Rives *et al.* (2014), found that paternal age had an effect on chromosome meiotic segregation in men aged 39 years and over, with an increase in disomic 21 spermatozoa. Duel *et al.* (2012) conducted a large study with azoospermic (low levels to no sperm in ejaculate) and non-azoospermic males, to test if there was a correlation between sperm concentration and chromosomal abnormalities. They found that azoospermic men that had increased gonadotrophin levels were at greater risk of chromosomal abnormalities compared with men that had azoospermia as a result of positive anthological history, such as vasectomy, varicocele, chemotherapy or cryptorchidism. However, the test was too small to conclude whether or not men with high gonadotrophins had the highest prevalence of chromosomal abnormalities compared with those men with normal levels (Duel *et al.* 2012).

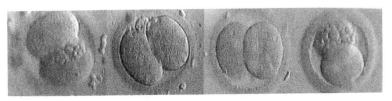

Figure 12.2 Normal 2-cell human embryos showing fragmentation

*Normal 2-cell human embryos viewed under a phase contrast microscopy,*
*showing fragments over the blastomeres (Sathananthan 2006)*

## 2.3 Oocyte quality and ageing

As women age, their oocytes begin to decrease in quality and quantity. Women aged 37 years and over face a higher risk of genetic aneuploidy such as Down's syndrome and spontaneous miscarriage (Fleming and Cook 2008).

In younger women, the organelles in the oocyte are generally more normally organised at the developing meiotic phases. Women aged 37 years and over have been found to experience more spontaneous miscarriages that are genetically abnormal in the majority of cases (Ford 2013). According to a range of literature and studies, this is due to a deterioration in the meiotic process of the oocyte that occurs with age, with women over 37 showing decreased expression in mitochondrial mRNA and proteins in the oocyte, and an increase in vacuoles (Ford 2013). Instances of Down's syndrome have been found to increase with the age of both male and female partners; the syndrome is caused by trisomy 21, thought to result from non-disjunction of the oocytes during meiosis (Yoon *et al.* 1996). The extra chromosome that causes Down's syndrome is approximately 80 per cent from maternal origin and 20 per cent paternal origin, with DNA non-disjunctions being 90–95 per cent maternal and 5–10 per cent paternal (Yoon *et al.* 1996). At the maternal age of 20 years, the risk of Down's syndrome is 1/1667, increasing to 1/30 at the maternal age of 45 years (Heffner 2004). Allen *et al.* (2009) found in their large population-based study that there was a correlation between advanced maternal age and chromosome 21 non-disjunction on oocytes. They found that the errors were greater for those in women ≥40 years of age at the time of their infant's birth.

## 2.4 CoQ10 and oocyte and embryo quality

The quality of the oocyte is the most important factor for achieving a pregnancy. As women age, their oocytes accumulate free radical damage (Turi et al. 2012). Reactive oxygen species (ROS) are a common occurrence in sperm and increase as men age, with 90 per cent of ROS being produced by the mitochondria (Bentov and Casper 2013), but evidence suggests they are also a factor in terms of oocyte quality. Turi et al. (2012) reported that women with unexplained infertility who also produced poor quality embryos had a decrease of glutathione peroxidase in their follicular fluid. The main role of glutathione peroxidase is to protect cells against oxidative damage, along with vitamins C and E and uric acid (the latter can act as an anti-oxidant). Turi et al. (2012) also demonstrated the presence of CoQ10 in women's follicular fluid, where it acts to scavenge free radicals and stimulate oxidative growth.

Turi et al. (2012) reported CoQ10 levels to be higher in the follicular fluid of those with more mature oocytes and a higher grading of embryos. A decline in the concentration of CoQ10 in our tissues and cells is part of human ageing (Bentov and Casper 2013). CoQ10 plays a large metabolic role in our mitochondrial cells and is crucial in energy metabolism. It is thought to have a protective role as an anti-oxidant for sperm and oocytes, and it also stimulates cell growth in both the oocyte and sperm cell, thereby preventing the oxidative damage (Turi et al. 2012).

Bentov and Casper (2013) showed in 52-week-old mouse models that were treated with CoQ10 a significant increase in oocyte numbers at ovulation after they were stimulated, and a lower mitochondrial potential and larger litter size compared with their control mice. Although this is an animal study, it indicates the potential for CoQ10 to have some impact positively on mitochondrial energy function and production in maternal-aged women; however, more research is needed. The impact could potentially be achieved by dietary supplements of CoQ10 or adding CoQ10 to culture media for ATP production (Bentov and Casper 2013). This would be for determination via future studies.

Stojkovic *et al.* (1999) trialled CoQ10 as a supplementation in bovine embryo culture media, and found that it had a positive effect on early cleavage, blastocyst formation, hatching and ATP content of the embryos. Cell proliferation was increased as a result of increasing ATP production from the supplementation of CoQ10, which accelerated the formation of blastocoel cavity and hatching (Stojkovic *et al.* 1999). There is more research needed into CoQ10 and its effects as a supplement in fertility and human reproduction, as it is a very new area.

## 2.5 Essential fats and embryo quality

Omega-3 (n-3), omega-6 (n-6) and omega-9 (n-9) are polyunsaturated fatty acids (PUFAs) essential in the human diet. They include the long chain n-3 PUFAs, eicosapentaenoic acid (EPA) and docosahexanoic acid (DHA). These are found in high levels in oily fish (Wakefield *et al.* 2008). Nehra *et al.* (2012) compared three diets: (i) mimic a diet rich in cold water fish high in omega-3; (ii) mimic a standard western diet of omega-6 (using linoleic acid (LA), with alpha-linoleic acid (ALA) fat provided as soybean oil (SOY diet); (iii) hydrogenated coconut oil (HCO). This was a randomised trial on mice of reproductive age, which produced outcomes that mirror the human model with the three diets (Nehra *et al.* 2012), namely the correlation between decreased mitochondrial quality and spindle segregation, and increasing maternal age leading to a higher rate of aneuploidy and Down's syndrome. Nehra *et al.* (2012) also looked at mature (MII) oocytes amongst the three groups for mitochondrial distribution, revealing extensive mitochondrial aggregation in MIIs. The study also found that four out of five (80%) MII oocytes contained regular spindle morphology from those on a DHA diet, or SOY diet, compared with those on a standard laboratory diet, which showed normal meiotic spindles (refer to Table 12.1).

## Table 12.1 Oocyte morphology on each diet

| MII oocyte morphology corresponding to diet | Standard laboratory diet | SOY diet | DHA diet |
|---|---|---|---|
| MII oocytes with mitochondrial aggregation normal | 0.006% | 0% | 33% |
| Normal meiotic spindles | 80% | 0% | 66% |

(Nehra *et al.* 2012)

Wakefield *et al.* (2008) found that although PUFAs such as n-3s can enhance the downward trend of maternal ageing on oocytes, it has a negative effect on good quality zygotes and lowers the number of embryos cleaving at the 2-cell stage. If this was found to be the case, it was due to the increased level of ROS from the PUFAs, which impair the embryo's development, meaning they would need to be supplemented with anti-oxidants (Wakefield *et al.* 2008). Interestingly, Nehra *et al.* (2012) report litter sizes to be smaller and offspring survival high among those on the omega-3 rich diet, while those on the omega-6 diet had a very low reproductive outcome. By changing diets before maternal ageing begins, and consuming more natural omega-3s and less omega-6 fats, we may be able to improve oocyte quality for the future and decrease aneuploidy rates, with implications for chromosomal disorders such as Down's syndrome as maternal reproduction advances (Nehra *et al.* 2012). Additional randomised controlled studies are needed, as to date only very small study groups and animal models have been used when looking at diet, and oocyte and embryo quality.

## 3. Poor response to IVF stimulation

According to Ferraretti *et al.* (2011) a poor responder is defined as an individual with a poor response to ovarian stimulation, indicated by a reduction in follicular response – with the end result being a reduced number of retrieved oocytes. Typically, a poor ovulation responder (POR) will fall into the category of a peak oestrodial ($E_2$) level of <300pg/ml to 500pg/ml, this metric being crucial for defining POR patients (Ferraretti *et al.* 2011). According to Klinkert *et al.* (2005), advanced female age and elevated basal follicle-stimulating hormone (FSH) levels (>12 or >15mIU/ml) taken on cycle days two or three (Badawy *et al.* 2011) are known to be a risk for developing POR during an IVF cycle. With increased age there is a decline in oocyte quality and quantity, an increase in oocyte aneuploidy and a higher rate of spontaneous abortion (Marcus and Brinsden 1996), which can correspond with a decline in anti-Müllerian hormone (AMH) and increase in FSH taken on days 2–3 of the cycle (Badawy *et al.* 2011) (refer to Table 12.2). Women aged 40 years and over who are categorised as poor responders are faced with two questions: should they attempt IVF and, if so, what stimulation protocol should they use to optimise their chances (Resolve: The National Infertility Association 2014).

## Table 12.2 Summary of age-specific AMH and FSH baselines (Centre for Human Reproduction 2014)

| Age | FSH | AMH |
|---|---|---|
| 38–40 | <8.4mIU/ml | =1.1ng/ml |
| 44+ | <8.5mIU/ml | =0.5ng/ml |

The simplest approach towards POR patients that many clinics took was to increase the dose of gonadotrophins for ovarian stimulation. However, Marcus and Brinsden (1996) found that doubling the dose of gonadotrophins from 225IU to 450IU a day had no effect on ovarian response for these POR patients. For the past 10 years, a standard ovarian stimulation protocol used for PORs has been a GnRH agonist 'long' protocol whereby the agonist is administered for 10 days or longer, followed by the gonadotrophin stimulation. This is now considered a poor choice for a POR patient, as it is thought to remove endogenous gonadotrophins from the system and 'suppress' the ovary stimulation response (Resolve: The National Infertility Association 2014).

The GnRH agonist has led to the suggested use of the flare-up protocol for POR patients as an advised treatment during IVF (Klinkert *et al.* 2005). Using the flare-up protocol, the patient starts the agonist on their menstrual cycle concurrent with the use of gonadotrophins. The downfall with the flare-up is the fact that the standard dose of agonist results in elevated levels of androgens, LH and progesterone in the follicular phase (Resolve: The National Infertility Association 2014). This affects oocyte quality, which is already diminishing in patients over 40, and the quality of the endometrial receptivity (Resolve: The National Infertility Association 2014). Reducing the dose of the agonist and pre-treating patients with an oral contraceptive pill has been found to be one way of helping to eliminate the negative effects of the flare-up protocol (Resolve: The National Infertility Association 2014).

A newer approach for POR patients is the use of a Ganirelix Acetate Injection®, Cetrotide®, which is a GnRH antagonist protocol. This involves gonadotrophin or FSH starting on day two or three of the menstrual cycle, with no oral contraceptive or agonist pre-treatment (Resolve: The National Infertility Association 2014). High doses of FSH are used, and once the scan shows a lead follicle of around 13 to 14mm in diameter, an antagonist is given and gonadotrophins continued. The antagonist stops the LH surge and the high dose of FSH potentially maximises oocyte numbers (Resolve: The National Infertility Association 2014). There are no randomised studies as yet that prove the benefits of the antagonist protocol.

Table 12.3 Summary of stimulation protocol advantages and disadvantages (Resolve: The National Infertility Association 2014)

| Poor response to IVF stimulation protocols | Age | Advantages | Downfalls |
|---|---|---|---|
| Gonadotrophins | 40–44 | None | Removes endogenous gonadotrophins and 'suppresses' ovary stimulation response |
| Flare-up with agonist and gonadotrophins | 40–44 | Reducing dose of agonist can eliminate the negative effects of the flare-up resulting in a better recruitment of oocytes and significant improvements in pregnancy rates | Results in elevated levels of androgens, LH and progesterone |
| GnRH antagonist | 40–44 | No pill or agonist used | High doses of FSH |

## 4. Possible immune activity

Generally the role of the immune system is to fight off infection, such as bacteria and viruses. The foetus is classified with a different genetic pattern from the mother, as it contains genetic material from the father. Thus, the immune system can see the foetus as a foreign body. In a normal pregnancy, the body suppresses the normal immune response and the foetus is not rejected (Human Fertilisation & Embryology Authority 2010).

Natural killer (NK) cells are a type of white blood cell and component of the innate immune system (Ntrivalas *et al.* 2001). NK cells can be found in the blood and also in the uterine lining during early pregnancy – these are known as uterine NK cells. It is now thought that NK cells have some involvement in recurrent spontaneous abortions (RSA). Chapters 8 and 9 provide a more detailed overview of these immunological factors, but they are considered here as there is some evidence that immunological factors affect this age group. NK cells originate from the bone marrow, and make their way to the endometrium or decidua via the interaction between integrin $\beta_2\alpha_4$ and the adhesion of molecule-1 through the blood. Studies have also found the phenotype of uterine NK cells ($CD25^{bright}$ $CD16^-$) is different from that of the NK cells found in peripheral blood ($CD56^{dim}$ $CD16^+$), meaning that testing NK cells in the blood may not be a clear indicator (Rai *et al.* 2005). Rai *et al.* (2005) also documented a reduced rate of implantation associated with an increased absolute count of activated NK cells ($CD56^{dim}$ $CD16^+$ $CD69^+$), and $CD56^+/$ $CD69^+$ cells have been found to be more common in the decidua of patients who have had an RSA, compared with those from a normal pregnancy (Ntrivalas *et al.* 2001). With RSA, patients have been found to show around 12.3 per cent total $CD56^+$ compared with only 6.59 per cent in patients with a normal pregnancy (Ntrivalas *et al.* 2001). Furthermore, RSA patients have been found to show 13.1 per cent in total for $CD56^{dim}$, and 7.29 per cent in patients with a normal pregnancy (Ntrivalas *et al.* 2001).

Some ART clinics offer blood tests to identify levels of NK cells, although these will only test the NK cells present in the blood and not the NK cells in the uterine cells. Treatments that are offered are high-dose steroids, intravenous immunoglobulin (IVIg), and tumour necrosis factor-a (TNF) blocking agents (Human Fertilisation & Embryology Authority 2010). Use of these treatments comes with potential risks, which patients must understand before beginning. Some of these risk factors include headaches, muscle pain, fever and chills, lower back pain, blood clots and kidney failure. Examples of the more extreme risks include the introduction of infections such as hepatitis and HIV, or the onset of lymphatic cancer or tuberculosis (Human Fertilisation & Embryology Authority 2010).

Not only do these treatments carry side-effects, but also they are not licensed in reproductive medicine, nor is there any widely stated conclusive evidence that they work. As such, patient consents must be signed, dated and witnessed (Human Fertilisation & Embryology Authority 2010). Some people use the treatments in conjunction with other drugs, alternative natural therapies and anti-inflammatory foods. Dietary approaches and the evidence around supplementation are reviewed in detail in Chapter 10, but a brief overview is presented below.

## 5. Healthy eating to support the immune system

Foods that are high in sugar and saturated fats (fried and fatty foods) can cause overactivity of the immune system, while omega-6 and animal fats can lead to inflammation, fatigue and damaged blood vessels (Pizzorono, Murray and Joiner-Bey 2002). Anti-inflammatory properties can be gained from a diet of foods that are high in vitamin C and fibre, for example fresh beetroot, as well as oily fish high in omega-3 such as salmon, mackerel, tuna and sardines (Hart 2014). An increase in wholegrains is recommended while avoiding refined grains, such as white breads, cereal, rice and pastas, which can cause inflammation responses to worsen (Hart 2014). Wholegrains have less sugar, and are found to have more fibre.

Eating dark leafy greens is also important, as these contain vitamin E, which protects the body from inflammation-causing cytokines (Byrd-Bredbenner et al. 2009). Highest concentrations of vitamin E can be found in spinach, kale and broccoli; these vegetables also contain good levels of calcium and iron (Hart 2014).

Almonds and walnuts are another good source of vitamin E, fibre, calcium and alpha linoleic acid (ALA) (Hart 2014). Yellow and red capsicum, and chili, are all high in anti-oxidants and have anti-inflammatory properties (Hart 2014). Turmeric and ginger have been shown in studies to have an anti-inflammatory effect (Surh 2002). Turmeric helps to turn off NF-kappa B, which is a protein in the body that regulates the immune system and triggers the inflammation process (Surh 2002). All berries are high in anti-oxidants and have anti-inflammation properties, while tart cherries are said to have the highest anti-inflammatory content of any food (Hart 2014).

## 6. Importance of AMH in planning treatment of over-40s

Anti-Müllerian hormone (AMH) is expressed in both the male and female reproductive organs. One characteristic of AMH is its expression in the ovarian granulosa cells from as early as 36 weeks from gestation, through to menopause. When AMH levels decrease, this indicates a woman reaching exhaustion of her follicular reserve (La Marca and Volpe 2006). AMH is produced by the granulosa cells, from pre-antral and antral follicles inhibiting the early stages of follicular development. AMH is not expressed in atretic follicles and theca cells (La Marca et al. 2010). Oestradiol and AMH work together to cause a down regulation effect of AMH and AMH type II receptor on the ovaries, suggesting an FSH-induced steroidogenesis (La Marca et al. 2010).

As a woman ages, generally there will be an increase in FSH and a decrease in inhibin B and antral follicle count (AFC), the levels of which are recorded using blood tests and scans. This was previously the most reliable marker for investigating a women's ovarian reserve before the introduction to AMH (La Marca et al. 2010). In recent years there have been more studies involving AMH, and it has been proven to be a good predictor of a woman's ovarian reserve, especially for those women undergoing ART. It has been found that AMH is a better marker to reflect continuous decline of the oocyte/follicle ratio in comparison with age decline (La Marca and Volpe 2006).

Women suffering from polycystic ovary syndrome (PCOS) have been found to have an increased level of AMH compared with healthy women of the same age. This is thought to be due to an excessive increase of granulosa cell AMH secretion, and increased accumulation of antral follicles (La Marca *et al.* 2010). Interestingly, higher levels of AMH occur in PCOS patients. The levels are similar to those measured in obese and insulin-sensitive patients, a group in which common traits are observed – those being higher in insulin-resistance and weight gain (La Marca *et al.* 2010). The non-PCOS obese patients showed a reduced level of inhibin B, as well as reduced levels of AMH, revealing obesity to be a lone factor associated with reduction in ovarian reserve (La Marca *et al.* 2010).

AMH levels are also thought to decline during an IVF cycle with the administration of FSH. This is due to the maturation of multiple follicles, as serum AMH corresponds with AFC, inhibin B and FSH in relation to age (La Marca and Volpe 2006).

Other factors that have been found to affect the levels of AMH in women are smoking, alcohol, race or ethnicity, and the use of gonadotrophins, although in a study by La Marca *et al.* (2010) it was determined that, prior to the administration of gonadotrophin, AMH was a good predictor for identifying women who do not respond, or respond poorly, to this IVF drug. On the other end of the scale, it is also thought to be a predictor for detecting ovarian hyperstimulation syndrome (OHSS), as the hyper-ovarian response to the FSH is a result of high AMH (La Marca *et al.* 2010).

It is significant to note that a correlation was found between AMH in follicular fluid and embryo implantation, clinical pregnancy and embryo morphology/quality. With an increase in AMH these variables also increase, while there was no conclusive correlation found between these variables and serum AMH (La Marca *et al.* 2010). It has been concluded that, when compared with other ovarian tests, the testing of AMH levels is the best marker for reflecting a woman's decline in reproductive function (La Marca and Volpe 2006).

## 7. Strategies for improving ovarian reserve

Some clinics have also found that the use of dehydroepiandrosterone supplementation (DHEA), which is an endogenous steroid from the adrenal and theca cells that also declines with age (around age 30), may help increase the precursor hormones in the ovarian reserve (Yilmaz *et al.* 2013). Yilmaz *et al.* (2013) found that by giving women DHEA supplementation, spontaneous pregnancy was increased before ART, while the chance of pregnancy of those undergoing ART also increased.

Gleicher and Barad (2011) found that not only was there an increase in oocytes per cycle when women were supplemented with DHEA, but there was also an increase in oocyte and embryo quality and therefore pregnancy success, with a decline in the rates of miscarriage. In one case, a 43-year-old US woman used DHEA and other remedies to overcome POR, and in her first IVF cycle she only produced one oocyte. After using supplements of DHEA she produced three oocytes in her second cycle and by her ninth cycle she was producing 17 oocytes and made 16 embryos (Gleicher and Barad 2011).

DHEA is an androgen, which, if used continuously at high doses during an IVF cycle, can lead to unwanted side-effects. Barad and Gleicher (2006) gave women a 25mg dose of DHEA three times per day for 16 weeks prior to their IVF treatment. The patients who received DHEA showed increases in oocyte yield, fertilisation rate and embryo quality, but also experienced side-effects such as increased sebum, acne, a feeling of being unwell, and increased libido. None of the women reported increased hirsutism (Barad and Gleicher 2006).

A patient using more than 75mg of DHEA per day over a long period of time may experience side-effects including acne, deepening of the voice, and facial hair. However, it has been clinically demonstrated that even long term therapy of DHEA of similar dosage is safe, although this drug is still under controlled randomised investigation studies (Barad and Gleicher 2006).

## 8. Increased occurrence of aneuploidy in over-40s

As a woman's reproductive age increases, there is a greater tendency towards aneuploidy with oocyte maturation. This is due to the fact that the human oocyte, unlike the sperm cell, lacks checkpoints that recognise chromosomal abnormalities (Fleming and Cooke 2008), Such abnormalities increase with age due to the structural differences in the meiotic spindles. Abnormalities in human embryos cause around 60 per cent of RSA in ART, and these abnormalities contribute not only genetically and chromosomally, but also morphologically and physiologically, which is also largely attributed to maternal age (Fleming and Cooke 2008). It has been found that of all reasons for embryo abnormalities, aneuploidy was the most common, with frequencies ranging from 10.8 per cent to 34.8 per cent (Fleming and Cooke 2008).

Using chromosomes from the oocyte polar bodies of mature patients, a study utilising fluorescence in situ hybridisation (FISH) analysis found that aneuploidies were the most common occurrence, ranging from 43 per cent to 52 per cent and deriving from meiosis I and II errors (Fleming and Cooke 2008). It is common for abnormalities to occur in cleavage stage embryos, and it is more common to see this trend in maternal-aged women as the chromosomal abnormality at the cleavage stage is around 90 per cent, with the most common irregularity being aneuploidy (Fleming and Cooke 2008).

Studies have shown that blastocyst stage embryos exhibit mosaicism, polyploidy and aneuploidy, with a higher rate of mosaicism, and chromosomal abnormalities that have also been shown to have a common correlation with IVF patients presenting with low AMH (Fleming and Cooke 2008). Studies have also shown that RSA and trisomic offspring in women with low AMH can be reduced when using pre-genetic screening (PGS and PGD) in aneuploidy screening, and it has been found that it is possible to reliably screen more than eight or nine chromosomes. This can improve IVF implantation rates for women ≥37 years (Fleming and Cooke 2008).

A combination of maternal and paternal patients aged 35 years and above significantly increases the chances of conceiving a child with Down's syndrome and moderately increases these chances further when either maternal or paternal patients are of advanced age (Fisch et al. 2003). In a 15-year study, Fisch et al. (2003) found that there was no paternal influence on the offspring being born with Down's syndrome until the paternal age was 35 years or older, and the results were most pronounced at maternal age 40 and above.

## 9. Other ART options for over-40s: egg donation

Many couples find they need to use egg donation as a final resort, after discussion with IVF specialists, each other and counsellors to make sure this is the correct decision. There are a number of ways to go about finding an egg donor. In some cases the couple may be lucky enough to know a family friend or have a family member (altruistic donor) willing to undergo the surgical egg extraction procedure in order to donate their oocytes to the receiving couple. Those not so lucky may have to purchase oocytes from another country, egg share with another woman, advertise, or in some countries wait for an anonymous donor on a registry list. See Table 12.4, and also Chapter 2 where egg donation is considered briefly.

Table 12.4 Four categories that egg donation can fall into (Ahuja et al. 1997)

| Categories for egg donation | Category I | Category II | Category III | Category VI |
|---|---|---|---|---|
| Altruistic-anonymous donors | Women who volunteer to undergo egg donation to women unknown to them | | | |
| Altruistic-anonymous donors | | Women who accept money for their services | | |
| Known-anonymous donors | | | Donor is matched and the recipient and donor remain anonymous to each other | |
| Infertile-anonymous donors (egg share) | | | | Where the patient (donor) offers to donate some of their oocytes in return for a subsidised IVF cycle |

Egg sharing is a popular option in the UK, as the patient and donor are both needing drugs for their cycle and the egg collection procedure, which is invasive. This option also provides another with donor oocytes, leaving no third party taking risks. Egg sharing is not available in all countries; while in some countries, such as Denmark and Israel, it is the only option for egg donation (Ahuja *et al.* 1997).

Ahuja *et al.* (1997) found that donors generally come from well-educated middle class families who are able to address issues with the clinics themselves and understand both the procedures and what was expected of them. Offers of cash support are rejected, family support is ensured and a secure commitment to the recipient couple is made, with 63 per cent responding that if required they would donate again (Ahuja *et al.* 1997). The study by Ahuja *et al.* (1997) also found that counselling plays a very important role in the egg donation process, with 25 per cent of donors developing stress from a seeming lack of care and concern during the treatment by staff at the clinic attended.

A more positive correlation to those that underwent egg sharing was found, as people who egg-shared were more likely to do this again. Ahuja *et al.* (1997) further found that anonymous donors experienced disappointment at not knowing if the recipient became pregnant, describing the feeling as like 'giving a gift that was never acknowledged'.

The physical treatment of drugs and invasive procedures were considered the worst part of donating (Ahuja *et al.* 1997).

As part of the HFEA requirements in the UK, all parties must be sufficiently briefed before egg donation takes place. Egg donors in the UK are only anonymous if they are shared egg donors or known egg donors. As part of the donor process, correct consents are filled out and signed and bloods and screenings thoroughly checked (Ahuja *et al.* 1997). In the USA it is most common to find an anonymous donor, while in some cases it will be a known donor, usually a family member or friend. In the UK, a full medical evaluation of the donor will take place including blood types, testing for STDs, and genetic tests and counselling (Fleming and Cooke 2008).

## 10. Review of success rates

The decline of female fertility begins at around 25 years of age, and accelerates in a woman's mid-30s until menopause is reached (Mills *et al.* 2011). An increasing number of couples and single women are seeking ART to support them in creating a family later in their lives (Mills *et al.* 2011). The following is an overview of current statistics on success rates and factors that can affect outcomes in this age group.

In the UK, the Human Fertilisation & Embryology Authority (HFEA) is the governing body that regulates IVF clinics and information from laboratories. According to data collated by the HFEA from cycles beginning in 2011 and ending in 2012, the national average of the predicted chance that women aged 40 to 42 will have a pregnancy resulting in a live birth using any form of ART suitable to them is 13.5 per cent. With women aged from 43 to 44 the average is 5.5 per cent, and according to data collated on women over 44 it is 0.9 per cent (Human Fertilisation & Embryology Authority 2014).

In the year ending 2011, the national average for women in the UK aged 40 to 42 who underwent some form of ART and achieved a successful embryo transfer and a live birth was 7.5 per cent. For women aged 43 to 44 it was 3.2 per cent, and for women over 44 it was 0.6 per cent (Human Fertilisation & Embryology Authority 2014). Note that these were a mixture of multiple embryos replaced and different ART procedures used, such as IUI, IVF, DI and ICSI.

### Table 12.5 UK national average live birth success rates (Human Fertilisation & Embryology Authority 2014)

| Assisted reproductive technique (ART) | Age | Cycles ending year | UK national average success rate |
|---|---|---|---|
| DI Stimulated | 40–42 | 2013 | 7.7% |
| DI Unstimulated | 40–42 | 2012 | 6.2% |
| DI Stimulated | 43–44 | 2013 | 2.7% |

| Assisted reproductive technique (ART) | Age | Cycles ending year | UK national average success rate |
|---|---|---|---|
| DI Unstimulated | 43–44 | 2013 | 3.5% |
| Stimulated IUI | 40–42 | 2013 | 5% |
| Unstimulated IUI | 40–42 | 2013 | N/A |
| Stimulated IUI | 43–44 | 2013 | 3.9% |
| Unstimulated IUI | 43–44 | 2013 | 4.1% |
| IVF/ICSI | 40–42 | 2012 | 13.6% |
| IVF/ICSI | 43–44 | 2012 | 4.5% |

It is estimated that the rate of decline in a woman's fecundity is 17 per cent from menarche to the age of 40 and increases to 55 per cent by 45 years of age. Only 44 per cent of pregnancies by women at the age of 40 result in a live birth (Mills *et al.* 2011); however, it is important to note that this figure is potentially misleading because additional factors such as spontaneous abortion – experienced by approximately 20 per cent of women in the over-40s age group – and the increased risk of chromosomal abnormalities affect pregnancies at this age (Mills *et al.* 2011).

## 11. Women aged between 40 and 44: stimulated vs. unstimulated cycles

For women aged 40 to 42 years who used stimulated IUI in 2013 in the UK, the national average of success was 5 per cent, while for women aged 43 to 44 years the success rate was 3.9 per cent. These figures can be seen in Table 12.5 (Human Fertilisation & Embryology Authority 2014c). Note that these were a mixture of multiple embryos replaced. There were no women aged over 44 years using IUI (Human Fertilisation & Embryology Authority 2014c), which was a significant decrease from the previous year's statistics, indicating a decline in pregnancy with age. Is this a product of lifestyle, diet, stress factors, or the pressure placed on woman in current times?

The HFEA report reveals that no women aged 40–42 or 44 used a natural IUI (unstimulated) cycle, but among women aged 43 years the success rate with a live birth was 4.1 per cent (Table 12.5). There were no women over the age of 44 who used this procedure in the UK (Human Fertilisation & Embryology Authority 2014d).

With regard to women aged from 40 to 42 who used unstimulated donor insemination (DI), for cycles ending with a live birth in 2012 the national average was 6.2 per cent. For women aged 43 to 44 years the average was 3.5 per cent for a live birth. There were no women who used this procedure who were over the age of 44. These results are clearly seen in Table 12.5 (Human Fertilisation & Embryology Authority 2014b).

The UK national average for women aged 40 to 42 years who used stimulated DI cycles ending in 2013 with a live birth was 7.7 per cent; for women aged 43 to 44 it was 2.7 per cent for live births. No women over 44 opted to use DI stimulated or unstimulated in 2011, as seen in Table 12.5 (Human Fertilisation & Embryology Authority 2014a,b).

For women who underwent fresh IVF/ICSI cycles starting in 2011 and finishing in 2012, the national average live birth rate according to the HFEA for women aged 40 to 42 was 13.6 per cent; for women aged 43 to 44 it was 4.5 per cent; and for women aged 44 and over it was 1 per cent (Human Fertilisation & Embryology Authority 2014e,f).

According to the HFEA in 2012, the national averages of women in these age groups (40–44) who used their own oocytes in a frozen cycle and produced a live birth were as follows: 15.2 per cent for women aged 40–42; 1 per cent for women aged over 44 (Table 12.5) (Human Fertilisation & Embryology Authority 2014e,f).

In the USA, information from clinics is reported to the Society for Assisted Reproductive Technology (SART). In 2012 SART reported women aged 41–42 undergoing a fresh cycle having 16.2 per cent of transfers resulting in a live birth, with the average number of embryos transferred being 2.9. For women aged over 42, 6.1 per cent resulted in a live birth with the average number of embryos replaced being 2.9 (SART 2014).

The NICE guidelines in the UK state that women aged 40 to 42 years of age who have not conceived naturally after two years of unprotected sex, or 12 cycles of artificial insemination, where six or more of these are IUI, are eligible for one full cycle of IVF or ICSI, provided they have not undergone IVF in the past. There must also be no evidence of low ovarian reserve, and they must be made fully aware of any additional implications of IVF and pregnancy at this age (NICE 2013).

··· BOX 12.1 A DONOR'S REFLECTION ·····························

'I am a 34-year-old woman who has twice been an egg donor to a known recipient in Australia. I first donated my oocytes when I was in my late 20s. I was working in an IVF clinic as an embryologist in Australia where anonymous egg donation is close to non-existent. I saw many couples desperate for a family, and I wanted to do more. I felt I had something that could offer to help these people. I was single, and I had no desire for children at that stage in my life, I was career driven and wanted to travel.

'I added my name to the donor registry list, and became an egg donor just as I had become an organ donor. A clinician who knew a couple that was looking for a donor approached me, thinking that I would be a good match. After some discussion he put us in contact. The couple wanted to know more about my family and personal medical histories. Due to concerns about my epilepsy and other family genetic medical histories, they wanted reassurance of my commitment to proceed with the egg donation, as it was a very stressful time for them.

'I found the couple to be loving and caring, and felt that I could not have wished to donate to more wonderfully grateful recipients. I was more than reassured that this was what I wanted to do. If I could make a difference in two people's lives by as small a gesture as giving a genetic gift, then this was something I wanted to do. I went through many blood tests, genetic tests, tests for sexually transmitted infections, scans and counselling before I was allocated the drugs to stimulate my ovaries. During my first cycle I did not tell my family or many friends, so I found the process very daunting and lonely. I had no one to speak to about my feelings of anxiety and what I was going through. I was in a new relationship and was trying to hide injections from my partner, which proved to be much harder than I expected when I was visiting interstate.

'My first cycle went as well as I could have hoped. I managed to produce all mature oocytes, and enough to grow to blastocyst stage, with one viable embryo that went on to produce a beautiful baby girl. Following the procedures, my body underwent a lot of stress. I bled heavily for four days, my stomach bloated out like a pregnant woman's, and I was in pain. I cannot describe this in any other way; I felt as if my body had aged physically around five years as a result of the drugs, anaesthetics and stress.

'My body never fully bounced back to where it was before my first stimulation cycle, but that couldn't have been further from my mind on the day my recipient couple sent me a picture of their newborn baby girl. Seeing such a proud happy family smiling with a small bundle in their arms was the greatest feeling I have ever experienced in my life. Words cannot describe it and I knew from that moment that it was all worth it.

'A few years later my recipient couple approached me about donating again to give their daughter a sibling. I thought this through with a lot of care, remembering how I had felt after the first cycle, how my body did not react well during the experience, and how I had felt so isolated due to having kept the procedure a secret for personal reasons. It had been hard.

'My brother is my "rock" in life, someone I can always turn to in need. He was always there for me growing up, and I felt that no one should be denied the opportunity to experience a sibling as amazing as my brother, so I agreed to participate in one more cycle irrespective of whether the outcome was positive or negative. I started my drugs again, followed by an egg collection that resulted in one viable blastocyst for transfer, and ultimately a beautiful son for the couple and brother for their daughter was born.

'Unfortunately this time I experienced complications – I hyperstimulated and became very ill for a long while. Again I had not told many people, including my family, about my egg donation and due to a lack of medical empathy and care I soon developed post-traumatic depression, which lasted nearly 12 months. This would have to have been the hardest and loneliest 12 months of my life.

'However, not once do I regret donating. When I see this beautiful family it makes me so happy to have been able to be a part of their lives, and offer them a small genetic gift that has given them so much joy. I also thank them for the kindness they have shown towards me. They are truly the most amazing people I have ever met. The advice that I give to all women now going through treatment is never isolate yourself, always use counsellors, ask as many questions as necessary and above all tell family and friends, as you need a support network. Family and friends will always be there for you – no matter how strong we think we might be, we always need a web of support to hold ourselves together.'

## ··· BOX 12.2 A RECIPIENT'S REFLECTION ·······················

'My husband and I stopped using contraception when I was 34. We were busy with work, holidays and study, but expected that a pregnancy would eventuate sometime in the next year. After a year we tried harder, taking it seriously – counting days, testing for ovulation, and timing sex to maximise chances of pregnancy. After another year we became concerned, and sought help. I had a slightly high FSH and slightly low anti-Müllerian hormone – I was told my ovaries were more like those of a 40-year-old than a 36-year-old. My husband had slightly more than expected abnormal sperm in his semen analysis. IVF with ICSI was recommended. We saw a counsellor, signed consent forms, had a police check, and discussed what to do with leftover frozen embryos.

'We started IVF with hope – this was the year we were going to have a child. I tolerated the drugs well, but found the progesterone made me teary to anything emotional (I would sob at reality television programs: "Look at that woman – she looks so happy after her makeover"). We tolerated injections, vaginal scans, producing sperm samples in locked rooms in hospitals, and anaesthetics for egg collections. Low numbers of eggs were collected at each egg collection, and not all would be able to be fertilised. In some cycles there was not an embryo to transfer as none had made it that far. The difficult part wasn't the injections, the anaesthetics, the blood tests or the scans. It was the not knowing; the feeling that life was on hold. The feeling of standing at an intersection, in front of two possible paths in life – one with no children, and one with children. We didn't know whether to buy a house with enough room for kids, or a smaller place for just the two of us. We didn't know whether to book a holiday in six months' time, or to look at prams. Or whether to take on that promotion at work, or wind back a little.

'Friends and family sympathised and tried to keep our spirits up. Comments like "I knew someone who just got pregnant on a holiday after years of trying" didn't help. Comments like "You are going through a hard time – let me know if you want a chat or a night out" helped.

'Two years and eight stimulated IVF cycles later, we asked – should we keep on trying? Our lovely IVF specialist suggested a second opinion and recommended someone. We tried a different regime, a different IVF laboratory, but still no pregnancy. We sought the opinion of a third specialist, and began looking at other options: adoption, donor egg, or a child-free existence. The hardest part was trying to decide when to stop. We kept thinking, maybe just one more time – the next time might work. Adoption in Australia takes over five years. We were already getting older and wanted to be young enough to run and play with a child. Egg donation in Australia relies on altruistic donation. Unlike in some countries, such as America, it is illegal to pay people for egg donation in Australia – so there are very few people who volunteer to donate eggs, and those that do generally do so for a relative or a close friend. Anonymous donation is very rare, and the IVF clinics had closed their waiting lists as the wait for a donor was in excess of five years.

'We were coming to the conclusion that we would be heading down the path of a life without children. We started to talk about all the places we could travel together, the small apartment we could buy near the city, and all the nieces and nephews we had whose lives we could be a part of. Then our IVF specialist said that he knew someone who might be interested in donating eggs – a scientist working in the IVF laboratory, who saw first-hand the couples having IVF. We considered the possibility. How attached were we to my genes? My chromosomes that gave me my hair colour, my eye colour, my stubbornness, my large bottom, my intelligence, my humour, and my calmness. How much of me was nature and how much was nurture? This woman who was considering donating her eggs was clearly kind, thoughtful and generous – surely these were great qualities. We decided to meet with her and talk about it. Obviously as a scientist she understood the process she would have to go through. We told her our IVF journey. She ran through her family's medical history. We talked about why she wanted to do this amazingly kind gift of egg donation. Then we each took time to think about all the issues. And we all decided we wanted to go ahead.

'The next step was mandatory counselling for all of us through the IVF centre, and then the donor had to go through medical tests. Medication was used to align our cycles and she underwent a stimulation cycle, scans, and an anaesthetic for the egg pick-up. My husband produced sperm in the hospital and an embryo was created. I was grateful – whatever the end result. This amazing woman, a virtual stranger, tried her best to help us. I was also concerned for her. Was it difficult for her? Did she have side-effects of the medications? Did she have people in her life to take care of her during the injections, the scans and the egg pick-up and recovery?

'One beautiful embryo was produced and transferred into me on day five. And it worked. For the first time ever I was pregnant. We shared the news with the donor, who was delighted. We sent her copies of every scan we had, and nine months later our perfect daughter was born.

'While I was pregnant I will admit that I had moments of anxiety – will this child look very different from me? Will I love this child, as a mother should? Will they see me as their mother? From the moment our daughter was born I can whole-heartedly say that she could not be more beautiful, more loved and more loving. And I don't think of her as 'not mine'. Occasionally when people comment that she looks like me (I think she looks like herself most of all, and a bit like her dad), I will remember that she doesn't have any of my genetic material in her. Instead she has the genetic material of a wonderful woman who put herself through tests and medical procedures just to try to help us. And that makes me happy.

'Two years later, we also have a little boy. Our lovely donor agreed to undergo another cycle to give our daughter the opportunity to have a sibling. She has met both our children, and when they are old enough to understand, it is our intention to let our children know that they were conceived with the help of this wonderful woman.'

## Dedication

Natasha Dunn dedicates this chapter to Dr Robert H.L. Dunn, Marianne Dunn, John Basil 'Lofty' Dunn and James M.E. Dunn.

## References

Ahlstrom, A., Westin, C., Reismer, E., Wikland, M.,Hardarson, T. (2011) 'Trophectoderm morphology: an important parameter for predicting live birth after single blastocyst transfer'. *Human Reproduction 26*, 12, 3289–3296

Ahuja, K.K., Mostyn, B.K., and Simons, E.G. (1997) 'Egg sharing and egg donation: attitudes of British egg donors and recipients.' *Human Reproduction 12*, 12, 2845–2852.

Allen, E.G., Freeman, S.B., Druschel, C., O'Leary, L.A., *et al.* (2009) 'Maternal age and risk for trisomy 21 assessed by the origin of chromosome nondisjunctions: a report from the Atlanta and National Down Syndrome Projects.' *Human Genetics 125*, 1, 41–52.

Badawy, A., Wageah, A., El Gharib, M., Osman, E.E. (2011) 'Prediction and diagnosis of poor ovarian response: The dilemma'. *Journal of Reproduction and Infertility 12*,4, 241–248

Barad, D., and Gleicher, N. (2006) 'Effect of dehydroepiandrosterone on oocyte and embryo yields, embryo grade and cell number in IVF.' *Human Reproduction 21*, 11, 2845–2849.

Bentov, Y., and Casper, R.F. (2013) 'The aging oocyte – can mitochondrial function be improved?' *Fertility and Sterility 99*, 1, 18–22.

Byrd-Bredbenner, C., Moe, G., Beshgetoot, D., and Berning, J. (2009) *Wardlaw's Perspectives in Nutrition* (8th edition). New York: McGraw Hill.

Centre for Human Reproduction (2014), www.centerforhumanreprod.com/infertilityedu/causes/highfsh/levels.

Duel, E.C., Groen, H., Van Ravenswaaij-Arts, C.M., Dijkhuizen,T., van Echten-Arends, J., and Land, J.A. (2012) 'The prevalence of chromosomal abnormalities in subgroups of infertile men.' *Human Reproduction 27*, 1, 36–43.

Ferraretti, A.P., Marca, A., La Fauser, B.C., Tarlatzis, J.M., Nargund, G., and Gianaroli, L. (2011) 'ESHRE consensus on the definition of "poor response" to ovarian stimulation for in vitro fertilization: the bologna criteria.' *Human Reproduction 26*, 7, 1616–1624.

Fisch, H., Hyung, G., Golden, R., Hensle, T.W., Olsson, C.A., and Liberson, G.L. (2003) 'The influence of paternal age on Down syndrome.' *Journal of Urology 169*, 6, 2275–2278

Fleming, S. and Cooke, S. (2008) *Textbook of Assisted Reproduction for Scientists in Reproductive Technology: Scientists in Reproductive Technology (SIRT); Fertility Society of Australia.* Australia: VIVID Publishing.

Ford, J.H. (2013) 'Reduced quality and accelerated follicle loss with female reproductive aging – does incline theca dehydroepiandrosterone (DHEA) underlie the problem?' *Journal of Biomedical Science 20*, 93, 1–9.

Gleicher, N., and Barad, D.H. (2011) 'Dehydorpianrosterone (DHEA) supplementation in diminished ovarian reserve (DOR).' *Reproductive Biology and Endocrinology 9*, 67–78.

Hart, J. (2014) *Eat Pretty: Nutrition for Beauty, Inside and Out.* San Francisco, CA: Chronicle Books.

Heffner L.J. (2004) 'Advanced maternal age – how old is too old?' *New England Journal of Medicine 351*,19.

Human Fertilisation & Embryology Authority (2010) *Reproductive Immunology.* Available at www.hfea.gov.uk/fertility-treatment-options-reproductive-immunology. html, accessed on 28 May 2015.

Human Fertilisation & Embryology Authority (2014a) *DI Data: Stimulated Donor Insemination (DI) Cycles in the Year Ending 2nd Quarter 2013.* Available at http:// guide.hfea.gov.uk/guide/HeadlineData.aspx?code=88&s=p&pv=W1B1QJ&d =0&nav=7&rate=d&rate_sub=DI_STIM, accessed on 28 May 2015.

Human Fertilisation & Embryology Authority (2014b) *DI Data: Unstimulated Donor Insemination (DI) Cycles in the Year Ending 2nd Quarter 2013.* Available at http://guide.hfea.gov.uk/guide/ HeadlineData.aspx?code=88&s=p&pv=W1B1QJ&d=0&nav=8&rate=d&rate_ sub=DI_UNSTIM, accessed on 28 May 2015.

Human Fertilisation & Embryology Authority (2014c) Available at http://guide.hfea. gov.uk/guide/HeadlineData.aspx?code=88&&s=p&pv=W1B1QJ&d=0&nav= 9&rate=u&rate_sub=STIMhttp://guide.hfea.gov.uk/guide/HeadlineData. aspx?code=88&&s=p&pv=W1B1QJ&d=0&nav=9&rate=u&rate_sub=STIM.

Human Fertilisation & Embryology Authority (2014d) Available at http:// guide.hfea.gov.uk/guide/HeadlineData.aspx?code=88&s=p&pv=W1B1Q &d=0&nav=10&rate=u&rate_sub=UNSTIM.

Human Fertilisation & Embryology Authority (2014e) *IVF and ICSI Data. Why Are We Showing Different Success Rates?* Available at http://guide.hfea.gov.uk/guide/ HeadlineData.aspx?code=88&&s=p&pv=W1B1QJ&d=0&nav=11&rate=i&rate_ sub=FSO, accessed on 28 May 2015.

Human Fertilisation & Embryology Authority (2014f) *IVF and ICSI Data. Why Are We Showing Different Success Rates?* Available at http://guide.hfea.gov.uk/guide/ HeadlineData.aspx?code=88&s=p&pv=W1B1QJ&d=0&nav=12&rate=i&rate_ sub=FERO, accessed on 28 May 2015.

Klinkert, E.R., Broekmans, F.J., Looman, C.W.N., Hannema, J.D.F., and te Velde, E.R. (2005) 'Expected poor responders on the basis of an antral follicle count do not benefit from higher starting dose of gonadotrophins in IVF treatment: a randomized controlled trial.' *Human Reproduction 20*, 3, 611–615

La Marca, A., and Volpe, A. (2006) 'Anti-Müllerian hormone (AMH) in female reproduction: is measurement of circulating AMH a useful tool?' *Clinical Endocrinology 64*, 603–610.

La Marca, A., Sighinolfi, G., Radi, D., Argento, C., *et al.* (2010) 'Anti-Müllerian hormone (AMH) as a predictive marker in assisted reproductive technology (ART).' *Human Reproduction Update 16*, 2, 113–130.

Marcus, S.F., and Brinsden, P.R. (1996) 'In-vitro fertilization and embryo transfer in women aged 40 years and over.' *Human Reproduction 2*, 6, 459–468.

Mills, M., Rindfuss, R., McDonald, P., and Velde, E. (2011) 'Why do people postpone parenthood? Reasons and social policy incentives'. *Human Reproduction* Update 17, 6, 848–860

Nehra, D., Lee, H.D., Fallon, E.M., Carlson, S.J., *et al*. (2012) 'Prolonging the female reproductive lifespan and improving egg quality with dietary omega-3 fatty acids.' *Aging Cell 11*, 1046–1054.

NICE (National Institute for Health and Care Excellence) (2013) *Updated NICE Guidelines Revise Treatment Recommendations for People with Fertility Problems*. Available at www. nice.org.uk/guidance/cg156/resources/updated-nice-guidelines-revise-treatment-recommendations-for-people-with-fertility-problems, accessed on 28 May 2015.

Ntrivalas, E.I., Kwak-Kim, J.Y.H., Gilman-Sachs, A., Chung-Bang, H., *et al*. (2001) 'Status of peripheral blood natural killer cells in women with recurrent spontaneous abortions an infertility of unknown aetiology.' *Human Reproduction 16*, 5, 855–861.

Pizzorono Jr., E.J., Murray, T.M., and Joiner-Bey, H. (2002). *The Clinician's Handbook of Natural Medicine* (2nd edition). New York: Churchill Livingstone.

Rai, R., Sacks, G., Trew, G. (2005) 'Natural Killer Cells and reproductive failure-theory, practice and prejudice'. *Human Reproduction 20*, 5, 1123–1126.

Resolve: The National Infertility Association (2014) *Poor Responder*. Available at www. resolve.org/diagnosis-management/infertility-diagnosis/poor-responder.html, accessed on 28 May 2015.

Rienzi, L., Vajta, G., and Ubaldi, F. (2011) 'Predictive value of oocyte morphology in human IVF: a systematic review of the literature.' *Human Reproduction 17*, 1, 34–45.

Rives, N., Langlois, G., Bordes, A., Siméon, N., and Macé, B. (2014) 'Cytogenetic analysis of spermatozoa from males aged between 47 and 71 years.' *British Medical Journal of Genetics 39*, 1–5.

SART Cors (2014) *Clinic Summary Report: All SART Member Clinics*. Available at www. sartcorsonline.com/rptCSR_PublicMultYear.aspx?ClinicPKID=0, accessed on 28 May 2015.

Sathananthan, A.H. (2006) *Early Human Development: The Beginning of Life*. CD-ROMs of images of human fertilisation and embryos (preview). Available at www.sathembryoart. com, accessed on 28 May 2015.

Stojkovic, M., Westesen, K., Zakhartchenko, V., Stojkovic, P., Boxhammer, K., and Wolf, E. (1999) 'Coenzyme Q10 in submicron-sized dispersion improves development, hatching, cell proliferation, and adenosine triphosphate content of in vitro-produced bovine embryos.' *Biology of Reproduction 61*, 541–547.

Surh, Y.-J. (2002) 'Anti-tumor promoting potential of selected spice ingredients with antioxidative anti-inflammatory activities: a short review.' *Food and Chemical Toxicology 40*, 8, 1091–1097.

Turi, A., Sterano, R.G., Francesca, B., Principi, F., *et al*. (2012) 'Coenzyme Q10 content in follicular fluid and its relationship with oocyte fertilization and embryo grading.' *Reproductive Medicine 285*, 1173–1176.

Wakefield, S.L., Lane, M., Schilz, S.J., Herbart, M.L., Thompson, J.G., and Mitchell, G. (2008) 'Maternal supply of omega-3 polyunsaturated fatty acids alter mechanisms involved in oocyte and early embryo development in the mouse.' *American Journal of Physiology and Endocrinology and Metabolism 294*, E425–E434.

Yilmaz, N., Uygur, D., Inal, H., Gorkem, U., Cicek, N., and Mollamahmutoglu, L. (2013) 'Dehyroepiandrosterone supplementation improves predictive markers for diminished ovarian reserve: serum AMH, inhibin B and antral follicle count.' *European Journal of Obstetrics & Gynaecology and Reproductive Biology 169*, 257–260.

Yoon, P.W., Freeman, S.B., Sherman, S.L., Taft, L.F., *et al.* (1996) 'Advanced maternal age and the risk of Down syndrome characterized by the meiotic stage of the chromosomal error: a population-based study.' *American Journal of Human Genetics 58*, 625–633.

Ziebe, Z., Loft, A., Petersen, J.H., Andersen, A., *et al.* (2001) 'Embryo quality and developmental potential is compromised by age.' *Acta Obstericia et Gynecologica Scandinavica 80*, 2, 169–174.

## Chapter 13

# Acupuncture in Assisted Reproduction

*Irina Szmelskyj DipAc, MSc, MBAcC, Lead Clinician, True Health Clinics and Founder of The Fertility Foundation, Godmanchester, Huntingdon, UK. Lecturer, MSc Supervisor and Examiner, Northern College of Acupuncture, York, UK; Guest Lecturer, University of Lincoln, Lincoln, UK; New Zealand School of Acupuncture and Traditional Chinese Medicine, Wellington, New Zealand*

## 1. What is acupuncture?

Acupuncture is a therapeutic modality where very thin needles are inserted into specific points in the body, referred to as 'acupuncture points'. It has been practised for over 2500 years.

Acupuncture is based on the Traditional Chinese Medicine (TCM) model. According to TCM a special energy called *Qi* (pronounced 'chee') flows through the human body. The role of Qi is to keep a person healthy, nourished, warm and protected from external invasions (Larre and Rochat de la Vallee 1999).

In disease, the flow of Qi is affected and this can lead to various Qi imbalances, such as deficiency, blockage, too much or not enough Qi, and/or Qi that is too hot or cold. Inserting very thin sterile acupuncture needles into specific acupuncture points can help to rebalance the energy, and this initiates natural healing. Acupuncture points are usually chosen according to TCM diagnosis, although in some cases acupuncture points can be chosen based on their anatomical location.

When treating patients, acupuncturists may use other supplementary techniques. The most commonly used techniques in reproductive medicine are listed in Box 13.1.

### BOX 13.1 THE MOST COMMONLY USED ACUPUNCTURE TECHNIQUES IN REPRODUCTIVE ··· MEDICINE (BRITISH ACUPUNCTURE COUNCIL 2014) ···

▶ *Moxibustion.* Acupuncture points are warmed with heat generated by burning a herb called mugwort or by putting a heat lamp over acupuncture points. The use of heat is believed to be beneficial in cases where Qi is too cold or stagnant.

▶ *Electro-acupuncture.* A very gentle electrical current is transferred through the needles into the body. This helps to improve the blood flow and relax the muscle tissue.

▶ *Auricular acupuncture.* Needles are inserted into acupuncture points located on the ear. These points can be used to supplement body acupuncture or can be used on their own as a separate style of acupuncture.

Many acupuncturists are also trained to offer dietary advice based on TCM principles, thereby encouraging patients to eat energetically appropriate foods for their constitution.

Over the years, several other styles of acupuncture have evolved. For example, Korean acupuncture tends to use points on the hands. In Japanese acupuncture, thinner needles are used, and they are inserted more shallowly. Dry needling 'acupuncture' and trigger point acupuncture are two styles of acupuncture that are often practised by conventionally trained medical practitioners (for example osteopaths, doctors, physiotherapists). The needles are inserted into areas on the body that are associated with certain nerve pathways or associated dermatomes.

# 2. Mechanisms of acupuncture, with particular emphasis on reproduction

## 2.1 Acupuncture improves uterine blood flow

Good uterine blood flow at all stages of the reproductive cycle is considered to lead to better reproductive outcomes. Research studies show that implantation rates are improved if there is good uterine blood flow on the last day of gonadotrophin stimulation (Ozturk *et al.* 2004), on the day of final oocyte maturation trigger injection (Ivanovski *et al.* 2012) and on the day of embryo transfer (Chien *et al.* 2004).

A growing body of evidence shows that acupuncture may help to improve uterine blood flow. In a small prospective study carried out by Stener-Victorin *et al.* (1996), eight sessions of electro-acupuncture resulted in a significant reduction of the mean pulsatility index of the uterine arteries (Stener-Victorin *et al.* 1996). Ho *et al.* (2009) in their randomised controlled trial found that four sessions of electro-acupuncture significantly reduced the pulsatility index of the uterine arteries. In another controlled study by Yu *et al.* (2010), acupuncture treatment significantly reduced pulsatility index and resistance index in the uterine arteries of women suffering from dysmenorrhoea.

## 2.2 Acupuncture improves ovarian blood flow

Having a good blood supply to the ovaries and follicles is also important. It improves:

- follicular recruitment (Bassil *et al.* 1997)
- follicular development (Balakier and Stronell 1994)
- oocyte recovery rates (Nargund *et al.* 1996; Ozturk *et al.* 2004)
- grades of embryos (Nargund *et al.* 1996; Ozturk *et al.* 2004)
- pregnancy rates (Borini *et al.* 2001; Coulam, Goodman and Rinehart 1999; Ozturk *et al.* 2004).

A limited body of evidence based on animal studies suggests that acupuncture treatment may help to improve ovarian blood flow. In two studies done on rats, low-frequency electro-acupuncture treatment significantly increased ovarian blood flow. The increase in the ovarian blood flow was abolished once ovarian sympathetic nerves were severed, suggesting that acupuncture works via ovarian sympathetic nerves (Stener-Victorin, Kobayashi and Kurosawa 2003; Stener-Victorin *et al.* 2004).

## 2.3 Acupuncture improves the endometrial lining

A thin endometrial lining can negatively impact outcomes of assisted reproductive techniques (ART). A 2014 systematic review and meta-analysis found that there was a trend towards lower ongoing pregnancy and live birth rates in women who had an endometrial lining ≤7mm in thickness (Kasius *et al.* 2014).

In a 2013 randomised controlled trial, patients who received acupuncture treatment had statistically significantly thicker endometrial lining compared with control and sham acupuncture groups (10.3mm vs. 8.7mm vs. 6.5mm respectively) (Isoyama Manca di Villahermosa *et al.* 2013).

## 2.4 Acupuncture may possibly reduce uterine motility

Difficulties during the embryo transfer procedure can lead to significantly lower pregnancy rates. This is thought to be due to initiation of uterine contractions (motility), which can be triggered by a simple contact with the fundus part of the uterus or through cervical manipulation (Mains and Van Voorhis 2010).

Animal studies suggest that acupuncture treatment can reduce uterine motility (Kim *et al.* 2003; Kim, Shin and Na 2000), but a study on patients undergoing IVF did not observe any reductions in their uterine motility (Paulus *et al.* 2003). The acupuncture points used in this study were different from the ones used in the rat studies, and this may have possibly affected the outcome. More research is needed on human participants before any conclusions can be made about acupuncture effect on uterine motility.

## 2.5 Acupuncture possibly improves IVF embryo implantation rates

Over 40 clinical trials have assessed what effect acupuncture treatment has on IVF outcomes. In the majority of these studies, the focus on the use of acupuncture was on embryo transfer day. The acupuncture points commonly used in these studies (such as LI4, SP6, ST36, ST29, LIV3, SP8) are hypothesised to improve embryo implantation rates.

At least ten systematic reviews have been published assessing the efficacy of acupuncture treatment upon improving IVF outcomes (Shen *et al.* 2015; Cheong *et al.* 2013; Manheimer *et al.* 2013; Zheng *et al.* 2012; Qu, Zhou and Ren 2012; Rubio *et al.* 2009; El-Toukhy *et al.* 2008; Manheimer *et al.* 2008; Cheong *et al.* 2010). The results are mixed, in this author's opinion primarily due to studies utilising underpowered acupuncture treatment. For example, the number of treatment sessions administered in the majority of these studies is too low to produce meaningful, measurable results.

Other factors that affect the findings in these research studies include (Szmelskyj and Aquilina 2014):

- too small sample sizes in the studies and therefore studies being underpowered to detect changes
- choice of control intervention, with sham acupuncture not being totally inert
- treatment protocols often not being individualised
- poor timing of acupuncture intervention in relation to key stages of reproductive treatments.

## 3. Acupuncture reduces stress

Some research suggests that stress can significantly reduce the probability of natural conception (Louis *et al.* 2011) and conception through IVF (Matthiesen *et al.* 2011). High levels of the stress hormone cortisol can also increase the risk of miscarriages (Nepomnaschy *et al.* 2006).

Several studies have assessed the effect of acupuncture on mental/emotional wellbeing of women undergoing IVF treatment and found significant improvements in mental/emotional health outcomes (Balk *et al.* 2010; Isoyama *et al.* 2012; Kovárová, Smith and Turnbull 2010; Smith *et al.* 2011).

In their review paper, Grant and Cochrane (2014) conclude that acupuncture treatment of IVF patients can help to reduce anxiety and stress levels and improve socio-psychological coping.

## 4. Acupuncture in the management of common complex conditions

### 4.1 Acupuncture and polycystic ovary syndrome (PCOS)

WHO classifies ovulatory disorders into three categories (Broekmans 2010):

- Grade I: Hypogonadotrophic hypogonadal anovulation

- Grade II: Normogonadotrophic normo-oestrogenic anovulation

- Grade III: Hypergonadotrophic hypo-oestrogenic anovulation.

Around 85 per cent of patients with anovulation fall into the normogonadotrophic normo-oestrogenic anovulation category, and the majority of these patients suffer from PCOS (Broekmans 2010). PCOS can lead to oligovulation or anovulation. Many women who have PCOS may also suffer from hyperglycaemia and hyperandrogenism.

Conventional medical management of these patients includes lifestyle changes such as weight loss (Broekmans 2010; Thessaloniki ESHRE/ASRM-Sponsored PCOS Consensus Workshop Group 2008) and adoption of a low glycaemic index diet (Moran *et al.* 2013), ovulation induction (Thessaloniki ESHRE/ASRM-Sponsored PCOS Consensus Workshop Group 2008) and ovarian surgery (Thessaloniki ESHRE/ASRM-Sponsored PCOS Consensus Workshop Group 2008). In cases where these treatments fail, ART such as IVF may be necessary.

A diagnosis of PCOS can complicate IVF treatments. For example, research shows that women with PCOS require longer gonadotrophin stimulation (Heijnen *et al.* 2006), most likely due to having excessive body excessive weight. Also, women with PCOS and/or polycystic ovaries (PCO) are at higher risk of developing ovarian hyperstimulation syndrome (OHSS) (Swanton *et al.* 2010).

In natural conception cases in women with PCOS, acupuncture can help to re-establish ovulatory menstrual cycles and regulate irregular cycles. In a small longitudinal prospective study, women with PCOS were treated with electro-acupuncture. Regular ovulatory cycles were re-established in one-third of the cases (Stener-Victorin *et al.* 2000). In a recent controlled trial, 84 women with PCOS were randomised into one of the three groups: low frequency electro-acupuncture, physical exercise or no intervention. Menstrual regularity and hyperandrogenism improved in the low frequency electro-acupuncture and physical exercise groups, but electro-acupuncture was superior to physical exercise (Jedel *et al.* 2011).

In women with PCOS undergoing IVF, acupuncture may help to improve response to gonadotrophin stimulation, improve embryo quality and reduce the risks of OHSS. In a randomised controlled trial, women with PCOS undergoing IVF treatment who received electro-acupuncture had significantly higher fertilisation and cleavage rates and better quality embryos compared with a standard care group (Cui *et al.* 2011). In another randomised controlled trial, PCOS patients who received electro-acupuncture had a statistically significant higher number of embryos compared with women who received standard care (Rashidi *et al.* 2013).

## BOX 13.2 ILLUSTRATIVE CASE STUDY:
··· ACUPUNCTURE AND PCOS ······································

Anna presented for acupuncture treatment to help to prepare her for IVF treatment. Anna was 33 years of age and was diagnosed with PCOS. She presented after failed conception following six rounds of ovulation induction with clomiphene citrate and metformin. Prior to that Anna and her husband had tried to conceive naturally for two years.

Anna's BMI was 32, but she was otherwise in good health. She reported being very stressed due to subfertility and work pressures. Her TCM primary diagnosis was Excess Fire. It was agreed that Anna would receive two to three months of weekly acupuncture treatments in preparation for IVF. She was also encouraged to increase exercise levels and follow a low glycaemic index diet.

Unexpectedly, Anna conceived naturally after just three acupuncture treatments. She continued to have weekly acupuncture treatments during the first trimester. A scan at 12 weeks showed one healthy foetus.

## 4.2 Acupuncture and endometriosis

Endometriosis is a condition whereby endometrial tissue is found outside the uterus, including in the bladder, the bowel or on the ovaries. Thirty to 50 per cent of women who have endometriosis can find it difficult to conceive (Missmer *et al.* 2004; The Practice Committee of the American Society for Reproductive Medicine 2012).

Endometriosis has been shown to affect natural conception and IVF treatment outcomes in several ways (The Practice Committee of the American Society for Reproductive Medicine 2012):

- Pelvic cavity anatomy may be distorted due to adhesions and scarring from endometriosis.
- Inflammation.
- The menstrual cycle may be abnormal, in particular long follicular phase and short luteal phase.
- Impaired embryo implantation.
- Poor quality eggs and embryos.

Conventional medical management of endometriosis includes expectant management, surgery and suppression of ovulation with pharmacological drugs (Macer and Taylor 2012). Ovulation suppression is not a viable option in patients who are trying to conceive naturally, but three to six months of ovulation suppression treatment prior to starting IVF may improve IVF outcomes (Sallam *et al.* 2006).

In this author's experience, women with endometriosis do not favour conventional treatment options. Surgery carries the risk of infection and adhesions, and ovulation suppression drugs' side-effects (in particular menopausal type hot flushes, vaginal dryness and depression) are not well tolerated (Dunselman *et al.* 2014).

Limited evidence suggests that acupuncture may offer a viable alternative treatment option for endometriosis and natural conception cases and may also help to improve IVF outcomes in patients with endometriosis. Other strategies for natural management of endometriosis are covered in Chapter 5.

As far as this author is aware, no research has been published that has specifically evaluated the effects of acupuncture on endometriosis-related subfertility. However, several studies have assessed the effects of acupuncture on endometriosis-related pain. For example, in a small randomised controlled trial, patients who received sixteen treatments of Japanese-style acupuncture had significantly lower pain scores compared with patients who received sham acupuncture (Wayne *et al.* 2008). In another randomised controlled study, electro-acupuncture treatment was found to significantly reduce endometriosis-related pain levels (Jin, Sun and Jin 2009). Other studies of various methodologies seem to provide additional evidence that acupuncture improves endometriosis-related pain (Kiran *et al.* 2013; Liu *et al.* 2014; Ma *et al.* 2013; Xiong *et al.* 2012).

It can, therefore, be hypothesised that if acupuncture can decrease endometriosis-related pain, it is possible that other endometriosis-related health outcomes may improve with acupuncture treatment.

## BOX 13.3 ILLUSTRATIVE CASE STUDY: ··· ACUPUNCTURE AND ENDOMETRIOSIS ·····················

Lisa presented for acupuncture treatment to help her conceive. She was 29 years of age and in good health. However, she suffered from cyclical abdominal and shoulder pain, which she suspected was a symptom of endometriosis. Her doctor refused to investigate the pain, dismissing it as muscle spasm. The pain improved after a two-month course of acupuncture. However, Lisa did not conceive.

In the meantime, her husband's semen analysis showed sub-optimal semen parameters. Lisa decided to privately fund an MRI scan, which revealed that she had endometrial patches in her pelvis.

Lisa and her husband proceeded with IVF treatment. Lisa received acupuncture treatment during the first round of IVF. She had only one good quality embryo, which was transferred on day five. The treatment cycle resulted in a healthy pregnancy.

··············································································

# 5. Practical considerations

## 5.1 Choosing an acupuncturist

Reproductive acupuncture is a specialist subject that is usually not covered in enough detail as part of the undergraduate acupuncture training programme. Therefore, patients seeking acupuncture treatment to help them conceive should look for acupuncturists with a specialist interest and postgraduate training in reproductive acupuncture. To find a registered acupuncturist, in the UK go to the British Acupuncture Council (BAcC) website at www.acupuncture.org.uk and in the USA visit the National Certification Commission for Acupuncture and Oriental Medicine (NCCAOM) website at www.nccaom.org. Patients are then recommended to check what training their acupuncturist has in reproductive medicine.

## 5.2 Treatment timing

Ideally, patients should begin their acupuncture treatment at least two to three months before they begin their IVF medication. It takes approximately a year for ovarian follicles to develop from their dormant phase (Gougeon 1986), while during the last four to five months of their development (Gougeon 1996) follicles are particularly affected by the environment in which they are developing. These last few months provide an ideal window when acupuncture can positively influence follicular development and therefore the quality of the eggs that these follicles release.

Sperm also takes around three months to be produced (Amann 2008). Therefore, in couples with male factor subfertility the cumulative effects of acupuncture will be maximised after three months.

## 5.3 Dose effect

Research suggests that the effectiveness of acupuncture is dependent on the dose of acupuncture administered. The dose of acupuncture can be measured as the number of treatment sessions per course of treatment, the number of acupuncture points used during each session and the strength of stimulation of each point.

An example of dose-related acupuncture treatment effects on conception is provided by Cridennda and her colleagues. In their

2005 retrospective clinical study they found that IVF patients who conceived following acupuncture treatment received on average 8.4 electro-acupuncture sessions, whereas patients who did not conceive only received 5.1 electro-acupuncture sessions (Cridennda, Magarelli and Cohen 2005).

## 6. Concluding remarks

A growing body of evidence suggests that acupuncture can influence ART outcomes in a number of ways. This includes promoting a better utero-ovarian blood flow, development of a better quality endometrial lining, possible reduction in uterine motility, as well as reduction in stress levels. The effectiveness of acupuncture treatment depends on factors such as the experience and level of training of the acupuncturist administering the treatment and the duration and intensity of acupuncture provided.

## References

Amann, R.P. (2008) 'The cycle of the seminiferous epithelium in humans: a need to revisit?' *Journal of Andrology 29*, 5, 469–487.

Balakier, H., and Stronell, R.D. (1994) 'Color Doppler assessment of folliculogenesis in in vitro fertilization patients.' *Fertility and Sterility 62*, 6, 1211–1216.

Balk, J., Catov, J., Horn, B., Gecsi, K., and Wakim, A. (2010) 'The relationship between perceived stress, acupuncture, and pregnancy rates among IVF patients: a pilot study.' *Complementary Therapies in Clinical Practice 16*, 3, 154–157.

Bassil, S., Wyns, C., Toussaint-Demylle, D., Nisolle, M., Gordts, S., and Donnez, J. (1997) 'The relationship between ovarian vascularity and the duration of stimulation in in-vitro fertilization.' *Human Reproduction (Oxford, England) 12*, 6, 1240–1245.

Borini, A., Maccolini, A., Tallarini, A., Bonu, M.A., Sciajno, R., and Flamigni, C. (2001) 'Perifollicular vascularity and its relationship with oocyte maturity and IVF outcome.' *Annals of the New York Academy of Sciences 943*, 64–67.

British Acupuncture Council (2014) *Styles of Acupuncture.* Available at www.acupuncture. org.uk/public-content/public-styles/styles-of-acupuncture.html, accessed on 10 June 2015.

Broekmans, F. (2010) 'The Initial Fertility Assessment: A Medical Check-up of the Couple Experiencing Difficulties Conceiving.' In N. de Haan, M. Spelt and R. Gobel (eds), *Reproductive Medicine: A Textbook for Paramedics.* Amsterdam: Elsevier Gezondheidszorg.

Cheong, Y., Nardo, L.G., Rutherford, T., and Ledger, W. (2010) 'Acupuncture and herbal medicine in in vitro fertilisation: a review of the evidence for clinical practice.' *Human Fertility 13*, 1, 3–12.

Cheong, Y.C., Dix, S., Hung Yu Ng, E., Ledger, W.L., and Farquhar, C. (2013) 'Acupuncture and assisted reproductive technology.' *Cochrane Database of Systematic Reviews 7*, CD006920.

Chien, L.W., Lee, W.S., Au, H.K., and Tzeng, C.R. (2004) 'Assessment of changes in utero-ovarian arterial impedance during the peri-implantation period by Doppler sonography in women undergoing assisted reproduction.' *Ultrasound in Obstetrics & Gynaecology: The Official Journal of the International Society of Ultrasound in Obstetrics and Gynaecology 23*, 5, 496–500.

Coulam, C.B., Goodman, C., and Rinehart, J.S. (1999) 'Colour Doppler indices of follicular blood flow as predictors of pregnancy after in-vitro fertilization and embryo transfer.' *Human Reproduction (Oxford, England) 14*, 8, 1979–1982.

Cridennda, D., Magarelli, P., and Cohen, M. (2005) 'Acupuncture and in vitro fertilization: does the number of treatments impact reproductive outcomes?' *Society for Acupuncture Research 301*, 85–88.

Cui, W., Li, J., Sun, W., and Wen, J. (2011) 'Effect of electroacupuncture on oocyte quality and pregnancy for patients with PCOS undergoing in vitro fertilization and embryo transfervitro fertilization and embryo transfer.' *Zhongguo Zhen Jiu 31*, 8, 687–691.

Dunselman, G.A., Vermeulen, N., Becker, C., Calhaz-Jorge, C., *et al.* (2014) 'ESHRE guideline: Management of women with endometriosis.' *Human Reproduction (Oxford, England) 29*, 3, 400–412.

El-Toukhy, T., Sunkara, S.K., Khairy, M., Dyer, R., Khalaf, Y., and Coomarasamy, A. (2008) 'A systematic review and meta-analysis of acupuncture in in vitro fertilisation.' *International Journal of Obstetrics and Gynaecology 115*, 10, 1203–1213.

Gougeon, A. (1986) 'Dynamics of follicular growth in the human: a model from preliminary results.' *Human Reproduction (Oxford, England) 1*, 2, 81–87.

Gougeon, A. (1996) 'Regulation of ovarian follicular development in primates: facts and hypotheses.' *Endocrine Reviews 17*, 2, 121–155.

Grant, L-E., Cochrane, S. (2014) 'Acupuncture for the mental and emotional health of women undergoing IVF treatment: A comprehensive review'. *Australian Journal of Acupuncture & Chinese Medicine, 9*, 1, 5–12.

Heijnen, E.M., Eijkemans, M.J., Hughes, E.G., Laven, J.S., Macklon, N.S., and Fauser, B.C. (2006) 'A meta-analysis of outcomes of conventional IVF in women with polycystic ovary syndrome.' *Human Reproduction Update 12*, 1, 13–21.

Ho, M., Huang, L.C., Chang, Y.Y., Chen, H.Y., *et al.* (2009) 'Electroacupuncture reduces uterine artery blood flow impedance in infertile women.' *Taiwanese Journal of Obstetrics and Gynaecology 48*, 2, 148–151.

Isoyama Manca di Villahermosa, D., Dos Santos, L.G., Nogueira, M.B., Vilarino, F.L., and Barbosa, C.P. (2013) 'Influence of acupuncture on the outcomes of in vitro fertilisation when embryo implantation has failed: a prospective randomised controlled clinical trial.' *Acupuncture in Medicine 31*, 3, 157–161.

Isoyama, D., Cordts, E.B., de Souza van Niewegen, A.M., de Almeida Pereira de Carvalho, W., Matsumura, S.T., and Barbosa, C.P. (2012) 'Effect of acupuncture on symptoms of anxiety in women undergoing in vitro fertilisation: a prospective randomised controlled study.' *Acupuncture in Medicine 30*, 2, 85–88.

Ivanovski, M., Damcevski, N., Radevska, B., and Doicev, G. (2012) 'Assessment of uterine artery and arcuate artery blood flow by transvaginal color Doppler ultrasound on the day of human chorionic gonadotropin administration as predictors of pregnancy in an in vitro fertilization program.' *Akusherstvo I Ginekologia (Sofia) 51*, 2, 55–60.

Jedel, E., Labrie, F., Odén, A., Holm, G., *et al.* (2011) 'Impact of electro-acupuncture and physical exercise on hyperandrogenism and oligo/amenorrhea in women with polycystic ovary syndrome: a randomized controlled trial.' *American Journal of Physiology, Endocrinology and Metabolism 300*, 1, E37–E45.

Jin, Y.B., Sun, Z.L., and Jin, H.F. (2009) '[Randomized controlled study on ear-electroacupuncture treatment of endometriosis-induced dysmenorrhea in patients].' *Zhen Ci Yan Jiu 34*, 3, 188–192.

Kasius, A., Smit, J.G., Torrance, H.L., Eijkemans, M.J., *et al.* (2014) 'Endometrial thickness and pregnancy rates after IVF: a systematic review and meta-analysis.' *Human Reproduction Update 20*, 4, 530–541.

Kim, J.S., Na, C.S., Hwang, W.J., Lee, B.C., Shin, K.H., and Pak, S.C. (2003) 'Immunohistochemical localization of cyclooxygenase-2 in pregnant rat uterus by sp-6 acupuncture.' *American Journal of Chinese Medicine 31*, 3, 481–488.

Kim, J.-S., Shin, K.H., and Na, C.S. (2000) 'Effect of acupuncture treatment on uterine motility and cyclooxygenase-2 expression in pregnant rats.' *Gynaecologic and Obstetric Investigation 50*, 4, 225–230.

Kiran, G., Gumusalan, Y., Ekerbicer, H.C., Kiran, H., Coskun, A., and Arikan, D.C. (2013) 'A randomized pilot study of acupuncture treatment for primary dysmenorrhea.' *European Journal of Obstetrics, Gynaecology, and Reproductive Biology 169*, 2, 292–295.

Kovárová, P., Smith, C.A., and Turnbull, D.A. (2010) 'An exploratory study of the effect of acupuncture on self-efficacy for women seeking fertility support.' *Explore (NY) 6*, 5, 330–334.

Larre, C., and Rochat de la Vallee, E. (1999) *Essence Spirit Blood and Qi.* Kings Lynn, Norfolk: Monkey Press.

Liu, C.Z., Xie, J.P., Wang, L.P., Liu, Y.Q., *et al.* (2014) 'A randomized controlled trial of single point acupuncture in primary dysmenorrhea.' *Pain Medicine (Malden, Mass.) 15*, 6, 910–920.

Louis, G.M., Lum, K.J., Sundaram, R., Chen, Z., *et al.* (2011) 'Stress reduces conception probabilities across the fertile window: evidence in support of relaxation.' *Fertility and Sterility 95*, 7, 2184–2189.

Ma, Y.X., Ye, X.N., Liu, C.Z., Cai, P.Y., *et al.* (2013) 'A clinical trial of acupuncture about time-varying treatment and points selection in primary dysmenorrhea.' *Journal of Ethnopharmacology 148*, 2, 498–504.

Macer, M.L., and Taylor, H.S. (2012) 'Endometriosis and infertility: a review of the pathogenesis and treatment of endometriosis-associated infertility.' *Obstetrics and Gynaecology Clinics of North America 39*, 4, 535–549.

Mains, L., and Van Voorhis, B.J. (2010) 'Optimizing the technique of embryo transfer.' *Fertility and Sterility 94*, 3, 785–790.

Manheimer, E., van der Windt, D., Cheng, K., Stafford, K., *et al.* (2013) 'The effects of acupuncture on rates of clinical pregnancy among women undergoing in vitro fertilization: a systematic review and meta-analysis.' *Human Reproduction Update 19*, 6, 696–713.

Manheimer, E., Zhang, G., Udoff, L., Haramati, A., *et al.* (2008) 'Effects of acupuncture on rates of pregnancy and live birth among women undergoing in vitro fertilisation: systematic review and meta-analysis.' *British Medical Journal 336*, 7643, 545–549.

Matthiesen, S.M., Frederiksen, Y., Ingerslev, H.J., and Zachariae, R. (2011) 'Stress, distress and outcome of assisted reproductive technology (ART): a meta-analysis.' *Human Reproduction (Oxford, England) 26*, 10, 2763–2776.

Missmer, S.A., Hankinson, S.E., Spiegelman, D., Barbieri, R.L., Marshall, L.M., and Hunter, D.J. (2004) 'Incidence of laparoscopically confirmed endometriosis by demographic, anthropometric, and lifestyle factors.' *American Journal of Epidemiology 160*, 8, 784–796.

Moran, L.J., Ko, H., Misso, M., Marsh, K., *et al.* (2013) 'Dietary composition in the treatment of polycystic ovary syndrome: a systematic review to inform evidence-based guidelines.' *Human Reproduction Update 19*, 5, 432.

Nargund, G., Bourne, T., Doyle, P., Parsons, J., *et al.* (1996) 'Associations between ultrasound indices of follicular blood flow, oocyte recovery and preimplantation embryo quality.' *Human Reproduction (Oxford, England) 11*, 1, 109–113.

Nepomnaschy, P.A., Welch, K.B., McConnell, D.S., Low, B.S., Strassmann, B.I., and England, B.G. (2006) 'Cortisol levels and very early pregnancy loss in humans.' *Proceedings of the National Academy of Sciences of the United States of America 103*, 10, 3938–3942.

Ozturk, O., Bhattacharya, S., Saridogan, E., Jauniaux, E., and Templeton, A. (2004) 'Role of utero-ovarian vascular impedance: predictor of ongoing pregnancy in an IVF embryo transfer programme.' *Reproductive Biomedicine Online 9*, 3, 299–305.

Paulus, W.E., Zhang, M., Strehler, E., and Sterzik, K. (2003) 'Motility of the endometrium after acupuncture treatment.' *Fertility and Sterility 80*, 3, 131.

Qu, F., Zhou, J., and Ren, R.X. (2012) 'Effects of acupuncture on the outcomes of in vitro fertilization: a systematic review and meta-analysis.' *Journal of Alternative and Complementary Medicine 18*, 5, 429–439.

Rashidi, H., Tehrani, S., Hamedani, A., and Pirzadeh, L. (2013) 'Effects of acupuncture on the outcome of in vitro fertilisation and intracytoplasmic sperm injection in women with polycystic ovarian syndrome.' *Acupuncture in Medicine 31*, 2, 151–156.

Rubio, C., Giménez, C., Fernández, E., Vendrell, X., *et al.* (2009) 'Acupuncture and in vitro fertilization: Updated meta-analysis.' *Human Reproduction 24*, 8, 2045–2047.

Sallam, H.N., Garcia-Velasco, J.A., Dias, S., and Arici, A. (2006) 'Long-term pituitary down-regulation before in vitro fertilization (IVF) for women with endometriosis.' *Cochrane Database of Systematic Reviews 1*, CD004635.

Shen, C., Wu, M., Shu, D., Zhao, X., and Gao, Y. (2015) 'The role of acupuncture in in vitro fertilization: a systematic review and meta-analysis.' *Gynaecologic and Obstetric Investigation 79*, 1–12.

Smith, C.A., Ussher, J.M., Perz, J., Carmady, B., and Lacey, S.D. (2011) 'The effect of acupuncture on psychosocial outcomes for women experiencing infertility: a pilot randomized controlled trial.' *Journal of Alternative and Complementary Medicine (New York, N.Y.) 17*, 10, 923–930.

Stener-Victorin, E., Kobayashi, R., and Kurosawa, M. (2003) 'Ovarian blood flow responses to electro-acupuncture stimulation at different frequencies and intensities in anaesthetized rats.' *Autonomic Neuroscience: Basic and Clinical 108*, 1–2, 50–56.

Stener-Victorin, E., Kobayashi, R., Watanabe, O., Lundeberg, T., and Kurosawa, M. (2004) 'Effect of electro-acupuncture stimulation of different frequencies and intensities on ovarian blood flow in anaesthetized rats with steroid-induced polycystic ovaries.' *Reproductive Biology and Endocrinology 26*, 2, 16.

Stener-Victorin, E., Waldenström, U., Andersson, S.A., and Wikland, M. (1996) 'Reduction of blood flow impedance in the uterine arteries of infertile women with electro-acupuncture.' *Human Reproduction (Oxford, England) 11*, 6, 1314–1317.

Stener-Victorin, E., Waldenström, U., Tägnfors, U., Lundeberg, T., Lindstedt, G., and Janson, P.O. (2000) 'Effects of electro-acupuncture on anovulation in women with polycystic ovary syndrome.' *Acta Obstetricia et Gynecologica Scandinavica 79*, 3, 180–188.

Swanton, A., Storey, L., McVeigh, E., and Child, T. (2010) 'IVF outcome in women with PCOS, PCO and normal ovarian morphology.' *European Journal of Obstetrics, Gynaecology, and Reproductive Biology 149*, 1, 68–71.

Szmelskyj, I., and Aquilina, L. (2014) 'Acupuncture During ART.' In A. Szmelskyj (ed.), *Acupuncture for IVF and Assisted Reproduction. An Integrated Approach to Treatment and Management* (1st edition). London: Churchill Livingstone.

The Practice Committee of the American Society for Reproductive Medicine (2012) 'Endometriosis and infertility: a committee opinion.' *Fertility and Sterility 98*, 3, 591–598.

Thessaloniki ESHRE/ASRM-Sponsored PCOS Consensus Workshop Group (2008) 'Consensus on infertility treatment related to polycystic ovary syndrome.' *Fertility and Sterility 89*, 3, 505–522.

Wayne, P.M., Kerr, C.E., Schnyer, R.N., Legedza, A.T., *et al.* (2008) 'Japanese-style acupuncture for endometriosis-related pelvic pain in adolescents and young women: results of a randomized sham-controlled trial.' *Journal of Pediatric & Adolescent Gynaecology 21*, 5, 247–257.

Xiong, J., Liu, F., Zhang, M.M., Wang, W., and Huang, G.Y. (2012) 'De-qi, not psychological factors, determines the therapeutic efficacy of acupuncture treatment for primary dysmenorrhea.' *Chinese Journal of Integrative Medicine 18*, 1, 7–15.

Yu, Y.P., Ma, L.X., Ma, Y.X., Ma, Y.X., *et al.* (2010) 'Immediate effect of acupuncture at sanyinjiao (SP6) and xuanzhong (GB39) on uterine arterial blood flow in primary dysmenorrhea.' *Journal of Alternative and Complementary Medicine (New York, N.Y.) 16*, 10, 1073–1078.

Zheng, C.H., Huang, G.Y., Zhang, M.M., and Wang, W. (2012) 'Effects of acupuncture on pregnancy rates in women undergoing in vitro fertilization: a systematic review and meta-analysis.' *Fertility and Sterility 97*, 3, 599–611.

## Chapter 14

# Reflexology to Assist With Fertility

*Deborah Cook, Senior Lecturer,*
*University of Worcester, Reflexologist,*
*MAHE, BSc (Hons), RGN, RNT, MAR*

## 1. Introduction

This chapter gives a brief introduction to reflexology, its origins and an explanation of how this therapy is believed to help with some clients who may encounter difficulties with conception. By using the available research it explores how this type of complementary therapy can be used with clients presenting with fertility issues. However, it must be remembered that a reflexologist cannot diagnose medical conditions but can help with the overall wellbeing of the person undergoing treatment.

The exact origins of reflexology are unclear. However, in common with other complementary therapies, reflexology is underpinned with the belief that a person needs to achieve a 'balance' of the physical, psychological and spiritual to maintain wellbeing. It is believed that Chinese society has been using a type of reflexology, in the form of meridian therapy, for over 5000 years. In Egypt, a wall painting was discovered in the tomb of Ankhmahor in Saqqara, the 'Tomb of the Physician', probably dating from 2330 BC; this individual was the highest ranking official after the Pharaoh. There are several wall paintings, some indicating recognisable modern surgical procedures; however, one shows a person being touched on the foot and another on their hand, and it is accompanied with hieroglyphics reading 'Do not let it be painful' by one of the patients and 'I do as you please' as a reply from the practitioner. The hand and feet treatment, and underpinning philosophy, are the basis for modern reflexology.

Reflexology in one format or another has also been found in both the Inca and North American Indian cultures. However, it was not until the early 14th century that this type of therapy was documented in Europe.

## 2. Reflexology today

The western approach to reflexology is based on zone therapy, where it is considered that energy runs through the body longitudinally in ten zones, from the head to the feet, dividing the body into ten sections. The understanding is that the energy passes through the body in each zone ending on the feet and hands, leaving a map of the body.

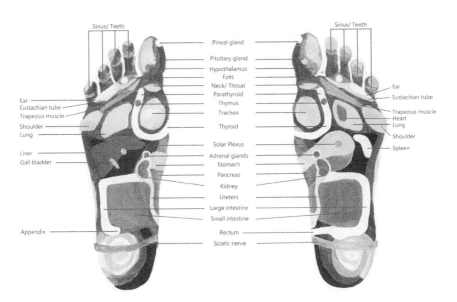

Figure 14.1 Zonal map (reproduced with kind permission from the Association of Reflexologists)

Should there be any problems in the body, mind and/or spirit, the energy does not have a clear flow and this imbalance can be found in the final map. The reflexologist locates these areas of imbalance on the foot or hand and massages them, which allows the energy to flow freely again, to regain balance. The areas of imbalance can be a little uncomfortable to the patient, or feel 'different' to the therapist. These areas of sensitivity are held until the uncomfortable feeling is diminished, and the points are probably worked two or three times during a complete treatment, usually with the sensitivity reducing. As well as feeling uncomfortable points on the feet, the client may also experience other sensations in their body or become emotional.

The published maps, which were produced mostly as a teaching aid, are all similar. However, there may be some variation when locating specific points on the feet, which should be expected as no two humans are exactly the same. The exact mechanism of how the energy moves through the body or where the energy comes from is still unclear.

A typical treatment lasts about an hour, with the client seated in a reclining chair or on a treatment couch, with their feet accessible to the therapist. Opening massage manoeuvres are used to allow the client to become accustomed to having their feet touched, and this gives the therapist time to examine and feel the feet. The therapist then undertakes a specific reflexology treatment to ensure that all of the reflex points are examined and massaged. The treatment is usually completed with a final massage and relaxation techniques. Although the therapist conducts an assessment and tailors the sessions to the individual needs of the client, it is usual to have a course of weekly treatments for six weeks, then to assess the effects of the therapy and to devise a suitable ongoing treatment plan.

## 3. Evidence to support reflexology

As with most complementary therapies, the scientific evidence to support reflexology treatment is scant, with small sample sizes and generally a qualitative methodology, which is not considered to be as robust as quantitative approaches. Ernst, Posadzki and Leekaur (2011) conducted a systematic review of randomised controlled trials concerning reflexology, finding only 23 studies within their inclusion criteria, and they concluded that these studies did not indicate convincingly that reflexology was effective for any medical condition. Many of the studies explored offered a foot massage compared with a reflexology treatment, and then found no significant change in outcomes for either group (Ernst *et al.* 2011). A reflexologist may argue that even a non-specific foot massage would stimulate some the reflex points, and therefore a 'significant' lack of difference in results would be expected. Many of the qualitative studies relate personal experiences and effects of treatments, and perhaps there is currently not enough understanding of human physiology to explore how these treatments act within the body.

In recent studies in Indian (Kaur, Kaur and Bhardwaj 2012) and Turkish (Korhan, Khorshid and Uyar 2014) intensive care units, reflexology was found to lower blood pressure and pulse rate in sedated patients, and this reduced the level of sedative drugs needed. The sample sizes and type of patients in these studies may be limited, but the fact that reflexology causes physiological changes to occur in unconscious patients warrants further exploration as to the mechanism of the response, and perhaps this is where the current understanding of human physiology is not sufficient. There have also been other studies that have clearly demonstrated measurable physiological changes in specific areas of their body whilst a client is undergoing reflexology in that specific region (Sudmeier *et al.*1999; Mur *et al.* 2001; Jones *et al.* 2012; Miura *et al.* 2013).

Although the studies are few, together they negate the notion that only relaxation occurs with reflexology and perhaps this is not because of a placebo effect of treatments. Even with this poor scientific underpinning of complementary and alternative therapies (CAMs), Thompson (2005) notes that patients may seek this form of care because of their increased interest in their personal wellbeing and the low technology of the treatments, which encourages a more 'self-care' model of health, which may be very important with the technical approaches of assisted reproductive techniques (ART). Reflexology is a touch therapy, and therapeutic touch in any form may also be seen as a positive adjunct to ART (Kissinger and Kaczmarek 2006).

## 4. Reflexology and fertility

In the realm of infertility, reflexology has been used as a supportive complementary therapy, for patients with a definitive diagnosis such as polycystic ovary syndrome (PCOS) or with idiopathic infertility issues, and to support clients undertaking a range of fertility treatments. A Google search of 'reflexology infertility' gives over 400,000 hits, which range from patient testimonials to therapists offering treatments and expertise with patients with fertility issues. Despite the majority of sites offering no scientific support for this complementary therapy, there is a wealth of positive reports where reflexology has been utilised and a pregnancy followed.

However, a report in 2009 found that patients who chose to use CAMs with ART actually had a reduced level of ongoing pregnancy/live birth rate, compared with those who did not use CAMs (Boivin and Schmidt 2009). This paper, based in Denmark, noted that of the group that opted to use CAMs, 54.3 per cent had reflexology, but they also noted that this group had a greater number of cycles of ART and there is no explanation as to why this was the case – perhaps their cause of infertility was more complex. The study did not explore the levels of anxiety or any psychological scores of the all-female participants included in the study, which may be a significant factor in lack of pregnancy/live birth.

There are many reflexologists who have treated clients with infertility issues, all of whom have developed their skills from their basic training, and many go on to specialise in this area; there are some forms of reflexology that have been particularly developed for clients with these needs. Ann Gillanders (2006) guides reflexologists on working with women through the lifespan, and includes advice when treating during pre-conception and pregnancy. Susanne Enzer (2004) has developed techniques that aim to balance the endocrine system, which is a key element in fertility issues. Jan Williamson (2010) teaches precision reflexology, where the therapist uses intuition and practical experience to link key areas, increasing the levels of relaxation and the restoration of whole body balance. These are a few of many therapists who have chosen to specialise in this particular area of a person's wellbeing.

The author qualified as a reflexologist in 2002 and since then has worked with a great range of self-referred clients, ranging from patients with long-term conditions such as multiple sclerosis to acute presentations such as constipation or back pain. After a year-long basic training, the author undertook extra training in vertical reflexology techniques (VRT) (Booth 2000), which are not specifically related to fertility issues but have been found to be useful in these cases. By background the author is an emergency nurse, who is now employed as university senior lecturer teaching healthcare-related topics. As a therapist it was challenging to reconcile the lack of scientific evidence to support reflexology, after coming from a profession that is constantly changing in the light of new research. However, the subjective evidence demonstrated that reflexology offered clients a different approach to maintaining their wellbeing. The following are some of the case histories of patients treated by the author. After an initial assessment, the treatments addressed individual concerns, but concentrated on the key areas of pituitary gland, pelvis and relaxation points, using both a basic reflexology pattern and some of the vertical techniques.

## 5. Case studies

··· BOX 14.1 CASE STUDY 1 ·················································

A 34-year-old nanny, general good physical health, 4–5 years previously had occasional depression; more recently felt low, but not clinical depression. Was prone to be anxious and stressed, used relaxation tapes sporadically. Menstrual cycle was a regular 26–28 days. Had been trying to conceive for two years; a hysterosalpingogram showed no obvious problems. There were existing spine issues that were treated and maintained by an osteopath. No prescribed medication on initial assessment, but taking folic acid and zinc.

*Treatments:* Seven treatments over nine weeks for the client and one treatment for her husband, at the end of the course of treatments. The spine reflexes were always sensitive, so these were worked well in addition to the other areas. The solar plexus and diaphragm were worked at the beginning, middle and end of sessions to increase the levels of relaxation; some time was taken to develop deep breathing techniques. At the start of the sessions the patient was unable to take a slow deep breath in and out, but as time progressed this improved enormously. During the course of treatments the areas of sensitivity and imbalance were reduced, but the spine reflexes, particularly around the lumbar region, remained sensitive.

*Outcomes:* From this initial course of treatments there was a successful pregnancy. This lady returned three years later for similar treatments over a ten-month period, but at this time was also undergoing ART. During this second course of sessions, the timings were adjusted to fit with the ART processes and there was one early miscarriage and then a successful pregnancy.

··· BOX 14.2 CASE STUDY 2 ················································

A 37-year-old air stewardess. Good general physical health, very busy life and often out of the country. Smoked 5–10 cigarettes per day and diet was good when at home and able to cook. Diagnosed with mild endometriosis six months prior to first treatment, periods painful, but tended to be every 30 days. Had been trying to conceive for 3½ years. There was some question as to whether an appendicectomy at age 11 had damaged the right fallopian tube, but there was no empirical evidence. The patient was taking folic acid, and took zinc sporadically.

*Treatments:* Six sessions over ten weeks, then intermittently over the following six months, it being difficult to fit treatments with her work patterns. The pituitary gland reflex was present in every treatment and only reduced slightly in its sensitivity through the course.

*Outcomes:* No conception during these initial sessions. This lady returned three years later, still leading a very busy life, had undergone ART but resulted in a miscarriage, and now was going to have ART a final time, so felt that reflexology would optimise the changes of conception. Unfortunately, this round of ART was also unsuccessful.

## ··· BOX 14.3 CASE STUDY 3 ·················································

A 24-year-old nurse. Good general health, busy and stressful professional life. Well-balanced diet, took regular exercise, non-smoker. Stopped oral contraceptive after taking for five years; there was no menstrual period for the following year, and then a menstrual cycle of five weeks became the norm, and it had been noted that during this time there was no ovulation. Had been trying to conceive for three years, and had been given a course of Clomid, which led to conception but early miscarriage. Ovarian drilling was performed one month prior to the reflexology, and at the time of sessions no prescribed medications were being taken, but the patient was taking folic acid and began to take zinc supplements at week four. The initial progesterone levels were very low.

*Treatments:* Seven sessions over nine weeks, then monthly treatments. The first session the feet were very quiet with very little response; however, the sensitivity was increased as treatments progressed, and then became quieter again. There was a significant increase in progesterone levels – 28ng/ml after treatment 3, then 59ng/ml after treatment 5.

*Outcomes:* After seven sessions there was a successful pregnancy. The client had monthly treatments throughout the pregnancy. Two years later the client had a second child with no interventions.

## ··· BOX 14.4 CASE STUDY 4 ·················································

A 30-year-old office manager. Was taking oral contraceptive for over six years, then stopped; no period for 6–8 months, ultrasound scan revealed polycystic ovaries. At the time of the first session had already undertaken two courses of ART, needing Clomid and gonadotrophin – resulted in one conception, but early miscarriage. Was prescribed metformin for insulin intolerance, folic acid and over-the-counter remedy for seasonal hay fever. Tried to maintain a healthy diet, but sometimes IBS symptoms. Non-smoker, drank about 1–1½ bottles of wine per week, which she was aiming to reduce. Was due to complete another round of ART.

*Treatments:* Six weekly sessions, then fortnightly over the next six months. Treatments were adjusted to fit with the ART process. A second course of six treatments, then monthly treatments. The feet became sweaty on the first few treatments but this settled down.

*Outcomes:* After the first course of treatments one pregnancy – second semester miscarriage. After the second course of treatments and another round of ART, successful pregnancy – twins. Patient had reflexology during both pregnancies and after the birth of the twins.

These four clients had different presentations but had commonalities: all were stressed or anxious to a lesser or greater degree about the ART and/or the lack of pregnancy, they were all open to the idea that reflexology would help in some way, and used this type of treatment as an adjunct to other more conventional approaches. In all cases the patients felt relaxed after a treatment, and many chatted about their concerns during their sessions. Stress can manifest itself in many ways and this may be detrimental to the physical function, as well as to the emotional aspects of the patient wellbeing, which may affect fertility (Sanders and Bruce 1997; Peterson *et al.* 2006; Kondoh *et al.* 2009).

The four clients experienced a whole range of emotions during their courses of treatments: anxiety, sadness, elation, guilt. Despite the weakness in the evidence to support reflexology, the opportunity for the client to express concerns to an objective listener and to take time to reflect cannot be underestimated in these cases. Some reflexologists concentrate their treatments to balance the emotional aspects of wellbeing, which may be useful in fertility cases (Talkington 2013).

History-taking and initial assessment is vital for treatment planning. In relation to cases with fertility issues, more specific advice is given by the Association of Reflexologists (Smith and Earlam 2012) as to where to direct the assessment, but this does not extend to how to explore a client's sexual health history. Taking a sexual health history is often poorly completed by health professionals (Peate 1997; Skelton and Matthews 2001; Peate 2010), so perhaps this is an area in which therapists may need education and guidance. There is no stipulation that CAM therapists have a healthcare background:

they undergo training in their particular therapy, where history-taking is taught to be holistic and often includes a greater assessment of lifestyle factors that may not be present using a medical model. Coming from an emergency nursing background, at the time of these cases the understanding of ART was limited for the author, and this was addressed with research and networking with other therapists. However, it was an advantage to have a good understanding of anatomy and physiology in these cases.

The cases here were treated about ten years before this publication; and with those clients undergoing ART procedures, at the time of increased ovulation there were no reflexology sessions. It was believed that reflexology could reduce the effectiveness of the hormones being used to increase egg production, as the key aim of the reflexology was to encourage a balanced body. However, current thought is that the level of medication used would not be adversely affected by the treatments (Smith and Earlam 2012). In all cases the pituitary gland reflex was present and was paid particular attention, as this gland is considered to be a control centre for hormonal balance. Paying particular attention to the endocrine system during a treatment session correlates with the Enzer reflexology approach (Enzer 2004).

In all of the cases the progression of the menstrual cycles was apparent in the treatments. The uterus reflex was often present just before the period began, and in some cases ovulation was felt in the ovary reflex, though this did not occur always and this may be related to the existing fertility issues. If and when the patient was pregnant, a small red mark was seen on the lumbar region of the spinal reflex; in fact with case 3, the red mark was there one week before pregnancy was confirmed by the medical team. In some cases reflexology treatments were continued through pregnancy, with a small egg-shaped swelling developing in the lumbar curve of the spinal reflex as the baby developed. During these treatments the clients felt relaxed, and reported that ailments such as constipation and lumbar back pain, associated with their pregnancy, were improved after the sessions. After the birth of the babies, the author was kindly allowed to give them a gentle treatment, which everyone enjoyed.

The Association of Reflexologists in the UK offers guidance to its practitioners when treating clients with fertility issues. They recommend that both partners have treatments prior to conception (Smith 2013), which is very difficult to achieve; the clients mentioned above, like many others, had been trying to conceive for several years before opting to have reflexology. Infertility is not usually investigated until two years have been spent attempting conception (NICE 2013), so perhaps pre-conception reflexology may be an unrealistic expectation. In only one of the mentioned cases did the husband receive a reflexology treatment, and this took two or three attempts to make an appointment, and there was only one treatment. It was not ideal in this situation to have a stand-alone treatment but it did give the husband an opportunity to experience reflexology and to discuss his thoughts.

## 6. Concluding remarks

The Tsambika Monastery is perched at the top of a 300m hill in Rhodes, and legend has it that the final 350 steps are walked barefoot by any woman with fertility issues, to the small Byzantine church dedicated to 'Our Lady', to pray to the Virgin, and then she will be blessed with children. This may seem bizarre, but it seems to be quite successful on the island – perhaps the small stones on the path stimulate the reflexes on the soles of the feet.

This ancient form of complementary therapy has little scientific evidence to explain how it works; however, using a holistic approach to the care of patients with fertility issues reflexology seems to be a useful part of a multidisciplinary approach. The notion that the body is in some way imbalanced in these cases correlates well to the philosophy of gaining and maintaining balance that underpins modern reflexology. Reflexologists can use their basic training or extend their practice in this specialist area, but the treatments need to concentrate on the endocrine system, the pelvic area and relaxation techniques. It is vital that the therapist conducts a holistic assessment, ensuring that it includes sexual health and conception history, and tries to treat both partners on a regular basis.

# References

Boivin, J., and Schmidt, L. (2009) 'Use of complementary and alternative medicines associated with a 30% lower ongoing pregnancy/live birth rate during 12 months of fertility treatment.' *Human Reproduction 24*, 7, 1626–1631.

Booth, L. (2000) *Vertical Reflexology: A Revolutionary Five-minute Technique to Transform Your Health.* London: Piatkus.

Enzer, S. (2004) *Maternity Reflexology Manual.* Soul to Sole Reflexology.

Ernst, E., Posadzki, P., and Leekaur, M.S. (2011) 'Reflexology: an update of a systematic review of randomised clinical trials.' *Maturitas 68*, 116–120.

Gillanders, A. (2006) *Reflexology for Women: Simple Step-by-Step Treatments for Women of All Ages.* London: Octopus.

Jones, J., Thomson, P., Lauder, W., Howie, K., and Leslie, S.J. (2012) 'Reflexology has an acute (immediate) haemodynamic effect in healthy volunteers: a double-blind randomised controlled trial.' *Complementary Therapies in Clinical Practice 18*, 4, 204–211.

Kaur, J., Kaur, S., and Bhardwaj, N. (2012) 'Effect of "foot massage and reflexology" on physiological parameters of critically ill patients.' *Nursing and Midwifery Research Journal 8*, 3, 223–233.

Kissinger, J., and Kaczmarek, L. (2006) 'Healing touch and fertility: a case report.' *The Journal of Perinatal Education 15*, 2, 13–20.

Kondoh, E., Okamoto, T., Higuch, T., Tatsumi, K., *et al.* (2009) 'Stress affects uterine receptivity through an ovarian-independent pathway.' *Human Reproduction 24*, 4, 945–953.

Korhan, E.A., Khorshid, L., and Uyar, M. (2014) 'Reflexology: its effects on physiological anxiety signs and sedation needs.' *Holistic Nursing Practice 28*, 1, 6–23.

Miura, N., Akitsuki, Y., Sekiguchi, A., and Kawashima, R. (2013) 'Activity in the primary somatosensory cortex induced by reflexological stimulation is unaffected by pseudo-information: a functional magnetic resonance imaging study.' *BMC Complementary and Alternative Medicine 13*, 114 –126.

Mur, E., Schmidseder. J., Egger, I., Bodner, G., *et al.* (2001) 'Influence of reflex zone therapy of the feet on intestinal blood flow measured by color Doppler sonography.' *Forsch Komplementarmed Klass Naturheilkd 8*, 2, 86–89.

National Institute for Health and Care Excellence (NICE) (2013) *NICE Guidelines CG 156.* Available at www.nice.org.uk/guidance/CG156/chapter/introduction, accessed on 11 June 2015.

Peate, I. (1997) 'Taking a sexual health history: the role of the practice nurse.' *British Journal of Nursing 6*, 17, 978–983.

Peate, I. (2010) 'Privacy please… Taking a sexual health history.' *British Journal of Health Care Assistants 4*, 2, 71–74.

Peterson, B.D., Newton C.R., Rosen K.H., and Skaggs, G.E. (2006) 'Gender differences in how men and women who are referred for IVF cope with infertility stress.' *Human Reproduction 21*, 9, 2443–2449.

Sanders, K.A., and Bruce, N.W. (1997) 'A prospective study of psychosocial stress and fertility in women.' *Human Reproduction 12*, 10, 2324–2329.

Skelton, J.R., and Matthews, P.M. (2001) 'Teaching sexual history taking to health care professionals in primary care.' *Medical Education 35*, 603–608.

Smith, T. (2013) 'Fertility or conception?' *Reflexions*, June, 13–15.

Smith, T., and Earlam S. (2012) *The Conception Journey: A Guide for Reflexologists.* Taunton, Somerset: Association of Reflexologists.

Sudmeier, I., Bodner, G., Egger, I., Mur, E., Ulmer, H., and Herold, M. (1999) 'Changes of renal blood flow during organ-associated foot reflexology measured by color Doppler sonography.' *Forsch Komplementarmed 6*, 3, 129–134.

Talkington, J. (2013) 'Fertility and emotional reflexology.' *Reflexions*, June, 21–22.

Thompson, A. (2005) *A Healthy Partnership: Integrating Complementary Healthcare Into Primary Care.* London: The Prince of Wales's Foundation for Integrated Health.

Williamson, J. (2010) *The Complete Guide to Precision Reflexology* (2nd edition). London: Quay Books.

## Further information

Association of Reflexologists: www.aor.org.uk. Information about reflexology; reflexologist locator.

Krogsgard, D., and Lund Frandsen, P. (2006) *Round About: Infertility.* Available at www.touchpoint.dk/wss/touchpointuk.asp?page=8171, accessed on 11 June 2015.

Smith, T., and Earlam S. (2012) *The Conception Journey: A Guide for Reflexologists.* Taunton, Somerset: Association of Reflexologists.

# Chapter 15

# Yoga to Support Fertility

*Lisa Attfield BTEC, HND, BWY Dip*

## 1. Introduction to yoga

Yoga is both a physical and a spiritual practice. There are many types of yoga but the most popular style practised in the UK is Hatha Yoga, which is differentiated into many forms including Iyengar, Bikram, Ashtanga and Vinyasa. These consist of elements of yoga postures (*asana*), breath awareness (*pranayama*) and relaxation and meditation. The meaning of the word yoga is 'to join', derived from the Sanskrit verb *yuj ~ to join*. It is believed that yoga practice helps people make connections between the mind, body and soul and that this helps to provide overall harmony and balance.

Yoga is one of the orthodox systems of Indian philosophy, systematised by Patanjali in his classical work the *Yoga Sutras*, written in Sanskrit dating from 200 BC. Important authoritative texts include the *Bhagavad Gita*, where Sri Krishna explains to Arjuna the meaning of yoga philosophy. Other texts include the *Upanishads* and *Hatha Yoga Pradipika* (*Light on Hatha Yoga*) complied by Yogi Swatmarama. The *Hatha Yoga Pradipika* explains that Hatha Yoga is not only for health and fitness but for awakening the vital energies: *pranas*, *chakras* and *kundalini shakti*.

Yogic practice has direct physical benefits, regardless of any spiritual aims. Physical and mental therapy are both important achievements of yoga as it works on the holistic principles of harmony and unification.

## 1.1 Asana

'Prior to everything, *asana* is spoken of as the first part of Hatha Yoga. Having done *asana*, one attains steadiness of the body and mind, freedom from disease and lightness of the limbs' (Muktibodhananda 2002).

*Asana* is a state of being in which one can remain mentally and physically calm, steady, quiet and comfortable. The mind and body are not separate entities, as the practice of *asana* integrates and harmonises the connection of body and mind. Both the body and the mind can harbour tension so the aim of *asana* is to release mental tension by dealing with it on a physical level acting somato-psychically, through the body to the mind. Muscular knots can occur anywhere in the body and through yoga *asana*, combined with other yoga practices *pranayama* and meditation, it is believed the tightness can be effectively eliminated, tackling it on both a physical and a mental level.

## 1.2 Prana

*Prana*, the vital energy, corresponds to *chi* in Chinese medicine and it is believed to pervade the whole body following flow patterns called *nadis* (Muktibodhananda 2002). It is thought that *nadis* are responsible for maintaining all individual cellular activity, and if the *prana* is blocked then toxins can accumulate in the body. The belief is that when *prana* begins to flow the toxins are removed from the system, ensuring health of the body as a whole.

## 1.3 Kundalini and chakras

The purpose of yoga is to awaken the *kundalini shakti*, defined as the evolutionary energy of a human being. By practising *asana* the *chakras* are stimulated, distributing the generated *kundalini* energy around the body. Once balance is created between interacting processes and activities of mental and *pranic* forces then the central pathway in the spine awakens the *sushumna nadi*, through which *kundalini shakti* rises to the highest *chakra sahasrara*, thought to be the highest centre of human consciousness.

There are seven major *chakras* located along the pathway of the *sushumna*, originating in the perineum then flowing through the spinal cord to the top of the head. The *chakras* are connected to the network of *nadis* and they correspond with nerves on a more subtle level. In yogic terms *chakras* are vortices of *pranic* energy at specific areas of the body, which control the circulation of *prana*.

On a physical level, *chakras* are associated with the major endocrine glands and nerve plexuses in the body. Specific *asanas* have a particularly beneficial effect on one or more of these glands or plexuses. Yoga *asana* also promotes the general health of specific areas of the body. Each type of *chakra* energy vibrates at a different rate and is associated with specific psychosomatic functions and correlates with the nerve plexuses of the physical body. The second *chakra*, *Svadhisthana*, is located in the area of the sacrum and relates to male and female reproductive organs and hormones. The *chakra* is depicted with a symbol of fertility in the formation of an aquatic creature resembling a crocodile (Feuerstein 2001).

## 2. Yoga's links to anatomy and physiology

B.K.S. Iyengar, 'the man who helped bring yoga to the West' (British Wheel of Yoga 2014), published the best-seller *Light of Yoga* in 1966. This book is still in print and the Open University's Suzanne Newcombe (British Wheel of Yoga 2014) explains that it contains a 'systemic and rigorous attention to detail of yoga postures (*asana*)'. Iyengar details the techniques and effects of over 200 Hatha Yoga postures and provides a section on curative *asana* for various diseases based on over 25 years of experience with his pupils (Iyengar 1991).

In Dr H.D. Coulter's book *Anatomy of Hatha Yoga* (2001) he explains Hatha Yoga in demystified, scientific terms. The book has become a modern authoritative source that correlates the study of Hatha Yoga with anatomy and physiology. The text outlines specific yoga postures and explains the effects these have on the body from an anatomical and physiological view. Dr Coulter explains the connections to the nervous system throughout the body. He examines the effect of the breath on the functions of the somatic and autonomic nervous system. The somatic nervous system controls the skeletal muscle action, whilst the autonomic nervous system looks at the internal function of the body – glands, body pressure, digestive system and so on. Breathing techniques play a part in relaxation on the autonomic nervous system (Coulter 2001). Fight or flight responses, known as acute stress, refers to the physiological reaction of a threat of danger triggering the sympathetic nervous system to release hormones stimulating the adrenal glands, preparing the body for emergencies.

Trying to conceive naturally, especially at a more 'advanced' age, can prove to be stressful and patients may experience a rollercoaster of different emotions. Yoga can help a person to relax, and so works to help alleviate stress. This can help to provide inner strength and confidence to continue a journey to parenthood, either with or without assisted reproductive techniques (ART) such as IVF. The author of this chapter has developed a series of *asanas* and produced a DVD, called *Fertility Yoga*. This is designed to reduce stress, and focuses on therapeutic yoga postures to benefit reproductive health. It concentrates on specific yoga postures to encourage blood flow to the reproductive area and relaxation techniques that de-stress the mind and body.

··· BOX 15.1 FERTILITY YOGA ·············································

The author's system of Fertility Yoga is designed to:

▶ increase energy and blood flow to the pelvic area

▶ stimulate the reproductive system

▶ balance hormones

▶ reduce stress and calm negative thinking

▶ enhance connections between mind and body.

Scientists have been studying the positive impact of yoga as a therapy on various health conditions; for example: 'Practicing yoga can improve better cardiovascular health, stronger nervous and immune system and has a positive effect on the reproductive system' (Trimarchi n.d.). It is important to mention that yoga used as a therapy for infertility cannot treat medical infertility problems such as blocked tubes, but can help infertility issues caused by stress and the stress associated with conditions such as cysts and endometriosis. Chronic psychological stress can alter the body's ability to regulate hormones, which in turn may cause problems with ovulation, sperm quality, egg fertilisation and other complications that may affect the reproductive system. See Chapters 4, 5 and 6 for further details about this.

## 3. Yoga and female infertility

*Asanas* working the area of the pelvis create energy and blood circulation for the reproductive system and may help strengthen the abdominal region and protect the back. There are some postures involving inversion, where the legs are elevated or the body is lowered; these are thought to be beneficial, as inverted yoga postures stimulate the pituitary gland and in turn the reproductive system, and forward bend *asanas* have a positive effect in supplying pure blood to the pelvic organs (Iyengar 2005). Iyengar (2005) also explains that *asanas* prove to be beneficial to helping with infertility, menstrual disorders and miscarriage as they strengthen the pelvic muscles, improve blood circulation in the pelvic region, strengthen the reproductive area and exercise the spine (the channel for the *chakras*).

··· BOX 15.2 OTHER BENEFITS OF YOGA ························

Yoga may aid the healing process by playing an active role in the journey towards 'positive mind state healing' (Woodyard 2001):

▶ The practice of yoga generates balance energy which is vital to the function of the immune system.

▶ Yoga is recognised as a form of mind–body medicine that integrates an individual's physical, mental and spiritual components to improve aspects of health, particularly stress-related illness.

▶ Yoga increases blood flow and levels of haemoglobin and red blood cells which allows for oxygen to reach the body cells, enhancing their function.

··· BOX 15.3 CASE STUDY ·················································

A 31-year-old female living in the UK in generally good physical health. She had a very stressful job with long hours and travel. She had a slight scoliosis of the spine affecting general back health; this was aggravated by stress and time spent sitting at a desk using a computer. She was managing this with ongoing physiotherapy and acupuncture. Her menstrual cycle was a regular 28–30 days. She had been trying to conceive for six years and had been through a gynaecology referral, but there had been no investigations. She had six-monthly reviews where the specialist confirmed that lifestyle factors were the main issues (principally stress and diet).

Along with changes to her diet and a reduction in alcohol the client managed stress and increased physical activity with yoga to improve spine mobility and strength. She also used deep breathing techniques. After two further years of good health, regular yoga practice and changes in lifestyle, the NHS finally undertook investigations and confirmed that IVF was the only option due to blocked fallopian tubes.

She left her job and used yoga and relaxation to manage the stress and anxiety associated with the IVF processes. The first cycle of IVF was a success but unfortunately ended in a miscarriage at 11 weeks. The second IVF produced a chemical pregnancy resulting in hCG blood testing over a period of time, which the client found very stressful. Next a frozen transfer was undertaken; this was successful but initial bleeding meant that she had to take progesterone injections until 12 weeks pregnant. The client practised yoga during pregnancy and used postnatal yoga to aid a return to good physical shape. She embarked on another frozen embryo transfer three years later aged 38, but sadly this was unsuccessful. A fifth IVF cycle produced a successful twin pregnancy. Modified yoga and deep relaxation were used during the multiple pregnancy.

····························································································

## 4. Male reproductive health and yoga

It is claimed that regular yoga practice in men may also be beneficial 'to enhance male reproductive health to produce the probability of successful conception' (Sengupta, Chaudhuri and Bhattacharya 2013). As well as the positive effects yoga has on stress reduction and wellbeing, the authors report that 'regular yoga practice can improve the quality of sperm if one has an issue with sperm count or motility' (Sengupta *et al.* 2013). If men practice yoga *asanas* it is thought they work to activate the second *chakra* in the pelvic area and that this can release energy blockages relating to sensual or sexual issues. This is thought to be important as 'the links between infertility and stress are complex and not fully understood, but cortisol, the so-called stress hormone, can interfere with normal reproductive functions' (Sengupta *et al.* 2013). It has also been claimed that reducing stress through yoga can boost fertility: 'In 2000 Domar found 55 per cent of infertility patients had a baby within one year of practicing yoga and meditation along with other relaxation techniques' (Sengupta *et al.* 2013).

## References

British Wheel of Yoga (2014) *B.K.S. Iyengar: The Man Who Helped Bring Yoga to the West.* Available at www.bwy.org.uk/bks-iyengar-the-man-who-helped-bring-yoga-to-the-west, accessed on 12 June 2015.

Coulter, H.D. (2001) *Anatomy of Hatha Yoga.* Honesdale, PA: Body and Breath.

Feuerstein, G. (2001) *The Yoga Tradition.* Prescott, AZ: Hohm Press.

Iyengar, B. (1991) *Light of Yoga.* London: Thorsons/HarperCollins.

Iyengar, G. (2005) *Yoga: A Gem for Women.* Kootenay, Canada: Timeless Books.

Muktibodhananda, S. (2002) *Hatha Yoga Pradipika.* Munger, Bihar: Yoga Publications Trust.

Sengupta, P., Chaudhuri, P., and Bhattacharya, K. (2013) 'Male reproductive health and yoga.' *International Journal of Yoga 6,* 2, 87–95.

Trimarchi, M. (n.d.) *How Can Yoga Increase Fertility?* Available at http://health.howstuffworks.com/pregnancy-and-parenting/pregnancy/fertility/yoga-increase-fertility1.htm, accessed on 12 June 2015.

Woodyard, C. (2001) 'Exploring the therapeutic effects of yoga and its ability to increase quality of life.' *International Journal of Yoga 4,* 2, 49–54.

# Subject Index

# Author Index

CPI Antony Rowe
Eastbourne, UK
June 20, 2023